Cancer Prevention

A Guide

Dr. M. Vijayakumar

Dr. Nanda Rajaneesh

Dr. Rohan Thomas Mathew

STARDOM BOOKS

www.StardomBooks.com

STARDOM BOOKS

112 Bordeaux Ct.

Coppel, TX 75019, USA

FIRST EDITION DECEMBER 2023

STARDOM BOOKS, LLC.

112 Bordeaux Ct. Coppel, TX 75019, USA

www.stardombooks.com

Stardom Books, United States

Stardom Alliance, India

CANCER PREVENTION-A GUIDE

Dr. Nanda Rajaneesh

p. 424
cm. 15.24 X 22.86

Category: HEALTH & FITNESS/ Diseases & Conditions/ Cancer MEDICAL / Oncology / General

ISBN: 978-1-957456-33-1

DEDICATION

This book is dedicated to The Society for Prevention of Cancer.

CONTENTS

PREFACE   xi
SOCIETY FOR PREVENTION OF CANCER   xiii
FOREWORD   xv-xviii
CONTRIBUTORS   xix-xxiii

1   LIFESTYLE FACTORS CAUSING CANCER   1

2   VIRAL CARCINOGENESIS   13

3   STRESS, IMMUNITY AND CANCER   51

4   ROLE OF NUTRITION IN PREVENTION OF CANCER   67

5   ROLE OF YOGA IN PREVENTING CANCER   75

6   HOLISTIC THERAPIES TO PREVENT A CANCER RELAPSE   81

7   MUSIC THERAPY TO PREVENT THE RECURRENCE OF CANCER   95

8   PRECANCEROUS CONDITIONS: A RADIOLOGIST'S PERSPECTIVE   105

9   EARLY DETECTION OF PRECANCEROUS CONDITIONS- A PATHOLOGIST'S PERSPECTIVE   119

10	ROLE OF PUBLIC AWARENESS AND HYGIENE IN CANCER PREVENTION	143
11	HABITS AND CANCER	153
12	FAMILY HISTORY OF CANCER. IS IT SIGNIFICANT?	163
13	INFLUENCE OF CIRCADIAN RHYTHM AND SLEEP ON CANCER	171
14	GERIATRIC ONCOLOGY. CAN WE PREVENT CANCER AMONG ELDERLY?	177
15	BARIATRIC SURGERY. ITS IMPACT ON REDUCING CANCER RISK	187
16	AUTOIMMUNITY AND CANCER	195
17	SCOPE OF RESEARCH AND CHALLENGES IN PREVENTION OF CANCERS	213
18	BREAST CANCER PREVENTION	227
19	INFERTILITY AND IVF TREATMENT AND RISK OF BREAST CANCER	241

20	COLORECTAL CANCER PREVENTION	247
21	PREVENTION OF MULTIPLE MYELOMA AND LYMPHOMA	259
22	PREMALIGNANT LESIONS OF THE ORAL CAVITY	267
23	PREVENTION OF GASTRIC CANCER	277
24	PANCREATIC CANCER: IS IT PREVENTABLE?	285
25	OVARIAN CANCER PREVENTION AND ROLE OF HORMONES	297
26	PREVENTION OF CERVICAL CANCER: AN OVERVIEW	309
27	PREVENTION OF LUNG CANCER AND IMPACT OF AWARENESS	315
28	PREVENTION OF UROLOGICAL CANCERS AND EARLY DETECTION OF PRECANCEROUS CONDITIONS	321

PREFACE

The incidence of cancer is increasing at an alarming rate. The surge in cancer cases is an ever-growing concern, casting a shadow of urgency over our world. As humanity triumphs over infectious ailments, non-communicable diseases assume an increasingly dominant role in our health landscape. A significant portion of these conditions can be attributed to lifestyle choices, rendering prevention a formidable strategy. While researchers explore groundbreaking therapies and pharmaceutical interventions capable of transforming cancer into a chronic ailment, the timeless wisdom encapsulated in the maxim "Prevention is better than cure" remains resoundingly pertinent. With this book, we have assembled a consortium of esteemed experts from diverse backgrounds, weaving together their wisdom and insights to forge a tapestry of holistic approaches to safeguard against the clutches of cancer. Cancer, both the disease itself and its arduous treatment, frequently exacts a heavy toll on patients, causing profound suffering while simultaneously burdening their families with immense distress. Regrettably, it stands among the leading causes of mortality worldwide. Although there have been notable advancements in novel therapeutic approaches and pharmacological interventions, their widespread accessibility remains hindered by exorbitant costs. In light of this, the imperative lies in prioritizing cancer prevention strategies and implementing screening programs for early detection, as they emerge as the most pragmatic and economical means of curbing the morbidity and mortality associated with this affliction. Paradoxically, despite their tremendous potential to mitigate the impact of cancer, the vital domains of prevention and early diagnosis are often relegated to the periphery of public health concerns, overshadowed by other competing priorities. In pursuit of its noble objective, the Society for Prevention of Cancer (SPOC) was established in January 2021. Its purpose is to elevate consciousness regarding cancer prevention and foster an understanding of how lifestyle modifications rooted in scientific insights can deter cancer occurrence and recurrence. With utmost humility, we present this book, a profound exposition that encompasses the breadth and depth of cancer prevention, aiming to galvanize a collective movement. It is our sincere aspiration that medical practitioners, public health specialists, aspiring healthcare professionals, and scholars in allied scientific disciplines will unite with us, forging ahead together in this noble endeavor. We thank all our authors for their time and effort in contributing towards this book.

Dr. M. Vijayakumar
Dr. Nanda Rajaneesh
Dr. Rohan Thomas Mathew

The Editorial Team

SOCIETY FOR PREVENTION OF CANCER

Until now, extensive scientific research has been done on various diseases and ways to treat them. Due to the covid outbreak, the focus is shifting towards immunity building and disease prevention. The need for cancer prevention has also been highlighted in the recent discovery of a Japanese scientist, Professor Yoshinori Ohsumi, on the way cells consume themselves, a process that plays a key role in cancer and other diseases.

Throughout history, our ancient Vedas and revered Ayurvedic teachings have consistently emphasised the critical importance of prevention. At the heart of this philosophy is the resonating motto "Let the well be well and help the sick," which captures the essence of proactive care. The Atharva Veda, brimming with profound meditative and medical wisdom, is regarded as an invaluable treasure by ancient Indian physicians. The importance of prevention is further emphasised in various sections of the renowned Charaka Samhita, immortalising its enduring relevance.

In the contemporary world, the significance of prevention through dietary and lifestyle modifications has resurfaced and regained prominence. Within the realm of medical terminology, this aligns with the concept of 'Public Health,' which endeavors to avert issues before they manifest in the population, epitomizing the timeless adage: "Prevention is better than cure."

In pursuit of its noble objective, the Society for Prevention of Cancer (SPOC) was established in January 2021. Its purpose is to elevate consciousness regarding cancer prevention and foster an understanding of how lifestyle modifications rooted in scientific insights can deter cancer occurrence and recurrence. With utmost humility, we present this book, a profound exposition that encompasses the breadth and depth of cancer prevention, aiming to galvanize a collective movement. It is our sincere aspiration that medical practitioners, public health specialists, aspiring healthcare professionals, and scholars in allied scientific disciplines will unite with us, forging ahead together in this noble endeavor.

This book represents the Society's latest endeavor to impart comprehensive knowledge to students and the general public regarding cancer prevention and its prevention of recurrence. It serves as a valuable resource, equipping readers with the necessary information to proactively safeguard against cancer and its reoccurrence.

Dr. Nanda Rajaneesh

Chairman, Society for Prevention of Cancer

FOREWORD

It is an honor and privilege to be asked to write the foreword for this well-timed book on "Cancer Prevention." I have had the good fortune to interact with some of the authors. I am aware of their immense dedication and eminence in the field. They all have decades of experience and are very humane in treating patients, rising above all considerations. It is laudable that these eminent cancer doctors have taken the time to write this altruistic book on the prevention and early detection of cancer. As a non-medical professional, it is fascinating to see how the authors have holistically gone about addressing the root causes of cancer in patients and the prevention of the many cancers that can afflict humanity. The authors provide a roadmap to take charge of one's life in the journey of preventing cancer.

The Mayo Clinic has aptly defined cancer as, "Any one of a large number of diseases characterized by the development of abnormal cells that divide uncontrollably and have the ability to infiltrate and destroy normal body tissue. Cancer often has the ability to spread throughout your body. Cancer is the second-leading cause of death in the world. But survival rates are improving for many types of cancers, thanks to improvements in cancer screening, treatment and prevention."

"Cancer Prevention" is thus a very timely book. This book is written by eminent Indian doctors specializing in cancer treatment and cure. Currently, cancer as a disease is making headlines, and many cancer treatment facilities are being opened in India. In fact, the 3rd of February is observed as World Cancer Day.

The authors have combined their vast expertise to bring out this book on Cancer Prevention. They cover the gamut of subjects in three broad categories: causes and risk factors of cancer, early detection, the prevention of various cancers. The book has an earlier section on holistic methods individuals can implement to avert cancer. The section that describes the effect of stress, anxiety, the role of nutrition, yoga and holistic therapies would be an eye-opener, and very beneficial for the common people.

The reader will benefit from studying the life cycle factors that cause cancer and minimize and hopefully avoid it. A very pertinent chapter on family history covers the genetic factors that indicate potential cancer development in patients. And this is followed by the chapter on early detection methods of pre-cancerous and cancer symptoms. It is prompt detection and treatment that saves lives.

Another interesting section is on non-medical measures to curtail the chance of getting cancer. The chapters on reducing stress and anxiety, nutrition, and yoga will be beneficial to lessen other ailments like heart disease. The final chapter on holistic therapies should appeal to a broad section of readers.

In conclusion, this book is a timely addition targeted at the common people to raise awareness of the causes of cancer and the prevention of various cancers. It is valuable for its description of the active steps individuals can take on their own and under general physician's guidance to reduce the chances of contracting cancer. It is not often that so many specialists devote their valuable time to bringing forth such knowledge for the benefit of the common people. Verily as it is said "Forewarned is forearmed!" This book is a valuable resource and excellent asset which will go a long way in helping reduce the number of cancer patients and improving the quality of life for them and their families.

Venkata M Durvasula,

Northern California

FOREWORD

Modern living has brought several comforts. Medical science also has increased healthy longevity. However, there are attendant adverse effects too, the lifestyle diseases. These are often referred to as noncommunicable diseases (NCDs), but paradoxically they are spreading very fast. Some call this a silent epidemic. These form a mixed group of diseases affecting different organ systems. The origins of the factors leading to these conditions could be seen as exogenous, (e.g., toxins, infections), autogenous (e.g., stressed lifestyle) or endogenous (e.g., genetic). However, there is a complex interplay of these factors that result in the outcome, such as developing the NCD or being protected from it. Oncogenes form an example of the interplay between environmental insult by viral infections affecting the existing genes in our body. At the same time, control of our lifestyle could mitigate the risk of cancer, despite being inherited with a gene and/or being exposed to a risky environmental lifestyle.

Cancer has emerged as the second largest among the NCDs after the cardiovascular disorders. Cancer also brings in many other concerns. From stigma to financial crisis, the implications from cancer vary widely. There is an urgent need to prevent the occurrence of this condition and lower the incidence. There is also a need to mitigate the secondary effects such as stigma from the cancer.

In this direction, the authors led by a team led by Dr. Nanda Rajaneesh, Dr Vijayakumar and Dr Rohan have done a commendable academic exercise. In this book they have compiled the risk factors and the need to prevent cancers in different systems. The description of the risk factors that will lead to understanding the methods by which we can prevent cancer is elaborated in these multiple chapters.

The public health approach should address preventing the risk factors, preventing the emergence of the cancer in the general population as well as in those who are at risk. Prevention also is equally relevant even after the detection of cancer. Detecting early with right intervention has a good chance complete remission. Likewise, evidence-based approaches to the treatment of cancer could prevent multiple disabilities, including the psychological damage.

The authors of these chapters have several things in common while addressing the issue of prevention. Lifestyle changes can mitigate the development of the risk factor. Proper hygiene, avoiding intoxicants, ensuring exercise, and controlling body weight, leading a life that is a void of exposure to external carcinogens or some examples that the authors have in common. Most of these preventive lifestyle practices to lower the risk of developing the risk factors are simple and easy. Actively engaging in other healthier lifestyles is equally important. These include reducing stress and the practice of yoga.

The authors have demonstrated in their literature review that yoga forms a healthy lifestyle practice. For example, a comprehensive yoga practice includes not just performing some of the exercises as yoga asanas, but also facilitate practice of healthy diet and meditation leading to stress reduction.

The book can be considered as a comprehensive reference text for use in the public health management. Educating the public as part of community health services, hence takes the main stage. The public education using the information documented in this book is hence very valuable. For that matter, the referred lifestyle practices if made inclusive, could help not just preventing cancer, but also reduce risk and morbidity for a range of NCDs.

The exhaustiveness with which the authors have collected information is hence commendable. The book serves as a reference text not just for oncologists but also for everyone who is working in public health services. Practitioners of the traditional systems of health care, including Ayurveda and Yoga, will also benefit from understanding various causative factors in cancer. Such an understanding will help them formulate better interventions in subjects at risk for cancer and for those who have developed the disease that has been detected early in its course. The authors also demonstrate the potential for such interventions in reducing consequences of cancer.

The book is a useful addition to our reference library. In particular, those who were working with cancer subjects will benefit greatly. If simplified, with respect to the length and the technical content, the book could in a different format, can also help a wide range of community health workers. The latter will be the potential human resource to be able to educate masses, and hence produce better results.

Detecting cancer has a dramatic experience for the subject. Preparedness of an individual to manage the consequences can help improving the morale and motivation to participate in early interventions that can have better outcome, including prevention of complications.

Therefore, cancer mitigation is possible but needs empowerment to the masses of all approaches and awareness of preventive lifestyle.

Dr. B.N. Gangadhar

Professor Emeritus, Department of Integrative Medicine.

Former Senior Professor of Psychiatry & Director

National Institute of Mental Health and Neurosciences

Bengaluru, 560029.

CONTRIBUTORS

1. Mr. *Aryaan Iqbal Shoaib*
Bachelor of Science,
Virginia Commonwealth University,
VA, USA.

2. Dr. *Ashwini Kumar Kudari*
M.Ch (Surgical Gastroenterology),
Senior Consultant,
Narayana Health,
Bangalore.

3. Dr. *BG Dharmanand*
MD, DM Consultant Rheumatologist,
Manipal Hospital, Millers Road, Bangalore.

4. Mr. *Bharath A Kashyap*
Sophomore, Virginia Polytechnic Institute and State University,
VA, USA

5. Dr. *Govindarajan M J*
MBBS, MD
Consultant Radiologist -Oncoimaging,
Apollo Hospitals,
Bangalore.

6. Dr. *Kalaivani V*
MS FRCS FIAGES PGDHHM
Professor of Surgery,
Sapthagiri Institute of Medical Sciences and Research Centre,
Past President SSBASICC,
EC Member, KSC ASI.

7. Dr. *K.Govind Babu*
MD (Medicine) ,DM(Medical Oncology),
Consultant - HCG hospitals and St.Johns Medical College Hospital,
Bangalore.

8. Dr. K Lakshman
FRCS (Eng) FRCS (Edin)
Consultant Surgeon,
Shanti Hospital and Research Centre, Bangalore.

9. Dr. Malathi M
Professor,
Dept. of Oncopathology,
Zulekha Yenepoya Institute of Oncology,
Yenepoya Medical College,
Mangalore- Karnataka

10. Dr. Meena Kumari B.T
M.B.B.S, PGDGM
Geriatrician,
Entrepreneur Director
Ramaiah Capital

11. Dr. Monika Pansari
MBBS, MS, DNB (Surgical Oncology)
FIAGES, Fellowship in Breast & GYN Oncology (USA),
HOD & Senior Consultant Surgical Oncologist,
(Breast & GYN Oncology),
BGS Gleneagles Global Hospital, Bangalore.

12. Dr. Mythri Shankar
MD (USA), IBLM, AFMCP
Nuclear Medicine - Lead Consultant, Aster Hospitals - Bangalore.
Co-Founder: The Green Foundation India.
Author: EASE (Amazon Bestseller)
TEDx Speaker.

13. Dr. Nagesh N S
Director and Professor Surgical Gastroenterology,
Institute of Gastroenterology and organ transplant,
Bangalore.

14. Dr. Poonam Maurya
MBBS DNB,
Consultant Medical Oncology,
Apollo Hospitals and KIMS, Bangalore

15. Dr. Pradeep Chowbey
MS, MNAMS, FRCS(London), FIMSA,
FAIS, FICS, FACS, FIAGES, FALS, FAMS.
Chairman - Max Institute of Laparoscopic, Endoscopic & Bariatric Surgery,
Chairman - Surgery & Allied Surgical Specialities,
Max Super Speciality Hospital,
New Delhi-110017 (India).

16. Dr. Raghunath S.K
MS, DNB (Urology)
Fellowship in Uro-oncology (RGCI, Delhi)
Fellowship in Laparoscopic and Robotic Urology (Taiwan),
Fellowship in Molecular Oncology of Prostate cancer,
CPDR, Washington DC, USA.
Uro-oncologist and Robotic surgeon,
Director and Head - Dept of Urological Oncology and Robotic Surgery.
Director- Robotic surgery program, HCG
HCG Cancer Hospital,
TEDx Speaker
Secretary- Society of Genitourinary Oncologists (SOGO) India.
Bengaluru.

17. Dr. Rajeev Vijayakumar
DNB Medical Oncology MRCP,
ESMO-certified Medical Oncologist
Consultant, BGS Gleneagles Global Hospital.

18. Ms. Ruchika Dawar
MSc. (Yoga),
SVYASA University.

19. Dr. Rudrapatna Jayshree Subramanyam
M.Sc. (Medical Microbiology); PhD (Medical Microbiology)
Former Professor and Head,
Department of Microbiology,
Kidwai Memorial Institute of Oncology,
Bangalore.

20. Dr. Samara Mahindra
Integrative Oncology Specialist,
Founder and Direct of CARER –
Personalised Cancer Care & India's first Integrative Oncology Company
New Delhi

21. Dr. Samhitha Venkatesh
Resident, General Surgery,
Malteser Waldkrankenhaus St. Marien,
Erlangen, Germany.

22. Dr. Sampath Chandra Prasad Rao
MS, DNB, FACS, FEB-ORLHNS, FEAONO
Consultant Skull Base,
Otolaryngology-Head and Neck Oncosurgeon,
Manipal Hospital, Head & Neck Sciences,
Bangalore.

23. Dr. Sandhya Ravi
M.S, Consultant General Surgeon,
Managing Director, Prameya Health, Bangalore.

24. Dr. Sharan B Singh M
Professor And HOD Physiology,
Principal,
Svims-Sri Padmavathi Medical College For Women,
Tirupati-517507.

25. Ms. Sharanya Shastry
Sports and Clinical Nutritionist-Dietitian,
Masters in Sports Sciences from ISST PUNE,
Masters in Therapeutic Dietetics and Applied Nutrition MAHE, Manipal Udupi,
Certified Bariatric Nutritionist (SVT, Mumbai) and Certified Diabetes Educator,
Life Member of IDA (Indian Dietetic Association),
SAI Delhi, India.

26. Ms. Sujatha Visweswara
CEO & Co-founder DiGiNxtHlt Solutions, Bangalore.
MTech in Computer Science and Automation and MBA from IIM Bangalore.

27.   Dr. Sumita Shankar
M.Ch. (Plastic Surgery),
Director Research and Development, DrYSR University of Health Sciences, VJW.
Carl-Zeiss fellow in Hand and Microsurgery,
Cranio Facial Fellow (Taiwan), Cosmetic Surgery fellow (USA, Barcelona),
Surgical Leader at Harvard Graduate.

28.   Dr. Veena Viswanath
Sr Registrar,
Manipal Hospital, Millers Road, Bangalore.

29.   Prof. (Dr.) Vishwanath Sathyanarayanan
MBBS MD DM Fellowship,
MD Anderson Cancer Centre,
Senior Consultant Medical Oncology,
Apollo Hospitals, Bangalore.

1

LIFESTYLE FACTORS CAUSING CANCER
Dr. M Vijayakumar, Dr. Rohan Thomas Mathew

Introduction

Lifestyle factors are modifiable habits and ways of life that can significantly influence overall health and well-being. A healthy lifestyle will reduce the incidence of Cancers, cardiovascular diseases, and other lifestyle-associated diseases. Broadly the causes of Cancer can be divided into genetic predisposition versus environmental exposure. Only 5 – 10 % of Cancer have a clear genetic basis. Although the underlying cause of most Cancers is multidimensional, exposure to exogenous factors contributes to disease development and progression.

More than 80% of Cancer occur due to environmental factors such as infectious agents (viruses and bacteria), tobacco, diet, air pollution and occupational exposures. A carcinogen is a substance, organism, or agent capable of causing Cancer. Carcinogens may occur naturally in the environment (such as ultraviolet rays in sunlight) or may be generated by humans (such as automobile exhaust fumes and cigarette smoke). The aim should be to alter our lifestyles to reduce exposure to these agents.

We must be aware of the various lifestyle factors that can cause carcinogenesis. Broadly carcinogens are divided into biological, chemical, and physical agents. Biological agents include infective, bacterial, viral, and fungal agents. Chemical carcinogens are organic and inorganic compounds such as Polycyclic Aromatic Hydrocarbons (PAH), alkylating agents, and aromatic amines that can cause Cancer. Physical agents are ionizing and non-ionizing radiation, heat, etc.

Chemical carcinogens

The International Agency for Research on Cancer (IARC) maintains a list of known carcinogens and updates it regularly as new evidence emerges. For IARC to designate an agent as carcinogenic, it should be "capable of increasing the incidence of malignant neoplasms, reducing their latency or increasing their severity or multiplicity, induction of benign neoplasm." The risk factors include the dose, route, and length of exposure, metabolism, and genetic factors. The first reported association between an environmental agent and Cancer was by Dr. Percival Pott in 1775. He observed an increased incidence of scrotal Cancer in patients who worked as chimney sweepers as children. These young workers were chronically exposed to high levels of soot and tar and developed Cancer later.

Presently over 400 known agents are blamed for developing Cancer. Chemical carcinogens are a large group of structurally diverse organic and inorganic compounds which can affect a wide range of species and tissue. Most of these are organic compounds divided into genotoxic and non-genotoxic. Genotoxic compounds can damage genetic material such as DNA. It occurs via the generation of DNA adducts which results in oxidative damage of DNA or by inducing DNA single or double-strand breaks. If they are not repaired, it will lead to the formation of mutations during replication. Examples of genotoxic chemicals are Polycyclic Aromatic Hydrocarbons (PAH), alkylating agents, aromatic amines, and amides. Some agents act as direct genotoxins, which can cause Cancer at the exposure site. Generally, genotoxic chemicals require metabolic activation from a procarcinogen to an ultimate carcinogen that damages the DNA. Carcinogenesis commonly occurs in the organ mediating biotransformation.

Nongenotoxic carcinogens do not directly impact the DNA, but they affect gene expression, disrupt normal cellular homeostasis, interact with cellular receptors, and increase cellular proliferation or decrease apoptosis. These chemicals usually promote tumor growth and progression: repeated exposures are necessary to elicit an effect. Agents that can cause the formation of reactive oxygen and nitrogen species can induce Cancer via both genotoxic and nongenotoxic mechanisms. Other mechanisms include chemicals producing abundant cytotoxicity with resultant compensatory hyperplasia. Many nongenotoxic carcinogens cause receptor-mediated actions as well. The complete mechanism of action of chemical carcinogens and the various pathways is beyond the scope of this chapter.

The most typical area where a person can get exposed to chemical carcinogens is occupation related. Many of the known major human chemical carcinogens were discovered from epidemiologic studies of populations exposed to large doses for a long time.

Common chemical carcinogens

Aflatoxins
Aristolochic Acids
Arsenic
Asbestos
Benzene
Benzidine
Beryllium
1,3-Butadiene
Cadmium
Coal Tar and Coal-Tar Pitch
Coke-Oven Emissions
Crystalline Silica (respirable size)
Erionite

Ethylene Oxide
Formaldehyde
Hexavalent Chromium Compounds
Indoor Emissions from the Household Combustion of Coal

Tobacco

Tobacco is the most common and significant lifestyle factor which causes Cancer. According to the Global Adult Tobacco Survey – 2 (GATS) India 2017, 28.6% of all adults, 42.4 % of all men, and 14.2 % of all women use some form of tobacco. In the United States of America, approximately 16% of men and 13% of women use only cigarettes, according to a report from 2015. Smokeless tobacco is much more common in India, with 21.4% of adults using it regularly. Smokeless tobacco is used by 29.6% of men and 12.8% of women. Tobacco smoking is prevalent among 19.0% of men, 2.0% of women, and 10.7% of all adults. Khaini and beedi are the most common forms of tobacco used: approximately 11% use khaini, and 8% use beedi. Although compared to GATS–1, there is a six-percentage point reduction in the number of current tobacco users, tobacco usage is still a significant public health problem that needs to be addressed. Data from the USA and other Western countries show that good policies with effective implementation can reduce the number of tobacco users.

Tobacco is often termed the total carcinogen as it has numerous agents which can cause initiation, promotion, and progression of Cancer. According to IARC, there are 72 measurable carcinogens in cigarette smoke and smokeless tobacco. The most dangerous are PAHs, N-nitrosamines, benzene, 1,3-butadiene, aromatic amines, and cadmium due to their increased concentration and higher carcinogenicity. The primary driver of smoking is nicotine, the principal addictive substance and reinforcer of continued smoking. Carbonyl compounds, such as formaldehyde and acetaldehyde, are also present in cigarette smoke from the combustion of sugars and cellulose. Toxic metals, including beryllium, cadmium, lead, and polonium-210, are also in measurable quantities. The commonest nitrosamines present in tobacco are 4-(methylnitrosamino)-1-(3-pyridyl)-1-butanone (NNK), which is derived from nitrosation of nicotine, and N'- nitrosonornicotine (NNN), which is derived from nitrosation of nornicotine. N-nitrosamines are well-established carcinogens, and both compounds are tobacco-specific. NNN and NNK primarily form during the curing process for tobacco. NNK is known to be a potent lung carcinogen and shows tumor induction activity in the nasal cavity, the pancreas, and the liver.

In contrast, NNN has been shown to induce tumors along the respiratory tract and esophagus in various animal models. Smokeless tobacco products, although not burned, nonetheless contain substantial levels of carcinogens, most prominently N-nitrosamines. Smokeless products also can contain PAH and carbonyl compounds, likely derived from fire-curing the constituent tobacco. Like cigarettes, smokeless products would also contain toxic metals. Electronic nicotine delivery systems and heat-not-burn products also generally have lower concentrations of these concerning compounds, although the evidence is limited.

Tobacco associated cancers (TAC)

1.	Oral Cavity	2.	Liver
3.	Larynx & Pharynx	4.	Pancreas
5.	Lung	6.	Kidney
7.	Esophagus	8.	Bladder
9.	Stomach	10.	Cervix
11.	Colon & Rectum	12.	Leukemia

Physical Carcinogens UV rays

Solar ultraviolet radiation is the major physical carcinogen in our environment and the primary cause of human skin Cancer. Depending on the wavelength, UV light is categorized into UVA (320 to 400 nm), UVB (290 to 320 nm), and UVC (240 to 290 nm) radiation. The ozone layer absorbs most of the UVC light emitted from the sun in the atmosphere, and thus, living organisms are mostly exposed to UVA and UVB irradiation. UVC light is more damaging to DNA than UVA and UVB because the absorption maximum of DNA is around 260 nm. UV light is a potent carcinogen because it can initiate carcinogenesis by inducing DNA lesions and suppressing the immune system, resulting in a higher risk. The destruction of the ozone layer has resulted in increased intensity of UV-B radiation, resulting in a higher risk for human skin Cancer. The phenotypic characteristics of light skin complexion, ease of sunburning, and light hair color enhance the risk of skin Cancer.

Ionizing Radiation

Ionizing radiation has the energy to ionize molecules by displacing electrons from atoms. The discovery of ionizing radiation in the early 20th century led to various health problems among researchers. Toxicity, radiation burns, and Cancer were observed among those who handled radioactive materials regularly. The death of Marie Curie from Cancer has been attributed to high radiation exposure.

Radiation-induced damage to cellular target molecules, such as DNA, proteins, and lipids, can be direct or indirect. The immediate action of radiation is due to the deposition of energy directly to the target molecule, resulting in damage. The indirect action is due to the radiolysis of water molecules. After initial absorption of radiation energy, it becomes excited and generates different radiolysis products, such as the reactive hydroxyl radical, which can damage DNA and proteins. As the hydroxyl radical is very reactive, it does not diffuse more than a few nanometers after it is formed before it reacts with other molecules. Thus, only radicals formed near the target molecule will contribute to the damage of that target. However, due to the chemical recombination of radiolysis products, hydrogen peroxide is created, which can produce hydroxyl radicals later, away from the initial site of energy deposition.

Ionizing radiation can be electromagnetic such as x-rays or gamma rays, or consist of particles, such as electrons, protons, neutrons, alpha particles, or carbon ions. Natural radiation sources comprise about 80% of human exposure, and medical sources account for the remaining 20%.

Radon is the most common natural source of radiation exposure. It is encountered in hard rock mining for iron, tin, fluorspar, and Uranium. Radon is a radioactive gas formed as a decay product of radium in the decay chain of Uranium. The decay of Radon produces alpha particles. Although seen in mining shafts, the gas can accumulate in poorly ventilated basements in houses built on Uranium-containing rock. People with high radon exposure have an elevated risk of lung Cancer. Radon gas is USA's second most common cause of lung Cancer.

Another source of human exposure to ionizing radiation is medical X-ray devices. There is a growing concern about using whole-body CT scans for diagnostic purposes. For a typical CT scan, a patient will receive about 100 times more radiation than from a routine mammogram. It is recommended that whole-body CT scans for children should be avoided due to the elevated risk of developing radiation-induced Cancer for this age group.

Radiation therapy is another area of concern, more so in young patients. This is because children who receive radiation therapy are more prone to developing secondary tumors induced by radiation therapy. They also have a good chance of achieving a complete cure from primary Cancer and would have a long life-expectancy. Childhood Cancers have underlying genetic defects, making them more susceptible to genetic damage induced by radiation, leading to secondary Cancer. The standard secondary Cancers have been found in bone marrow, thyroid, breast, and lungs.

Although there are safe limits to which a person may get exposed without adverse events, the official view is that 'no dose is safe.

Interested readers can refer to standard oncology textbooks for the detailed mechanism of how ionizing radiation interacts with the cell and DNA, causing damages which can lead to the formation of malignancy.

Radiofrequency radiation (RFR) and Microwave radiation (MR)

FR is electromagnetic radiation in the frequency range of 3 kHz to 300 MHz, whereas MR is in the frequency range between 300 MHz and 300 GHz. RFR and MR do not have sufficient energy to cause ionization in target tissues; instead, the radiation energy is converted into heat as the radiation energy is absorbed. Sources of RFR and MR include mobile phones, radio transmitters of wireless communication, radars, medical devices, and kitchen appliances.

In 2011 the IARC, a component of the WHO, appointed an Expert Working Group to review all available evidence on the use of cell phones. The group classified cell phone use as "possibly carcinogenic to humans" based on limited human studies, little evidence of radiofrequency radiation and Cancer in rodents, and consistent evidence from mechanistic studies.

THE ELECTROMAGNETIC SPECTRUM

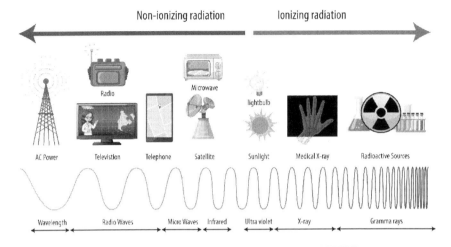

Figure 1: Electromagnetic Spectrum

In 2011 the IARC, a component of the WHO, appointed an Expert Working Group to review all available evidence on the use of cell phones. The group classified cell phone use as "possibly carcinogenic to humans" based on limited human studies, little evidence of radiofrequency radiation and Cancer in rodents, and consistent evidence from mechanistic studies.

However, the group note that the evidence is complex and does not show a direct link between mobile phone use and increased risk of Cancer. Other organizations, such as the FDA, CDC, and FCC, note that no scientific evidence links mobile phone usage and Cancer incidence. Extensive studies such as the Interphone, Danish, and Million Women studies found no association. It has been postulated that the increased use of mobile phones is causing increased brain tumors. But such studies have not checked the effect of mobile phones on Cancer in children or other health risks. Increased use of mobile phones is linked to neurological deficits and reduced attention span affecting memory and learning. It is also known to cause distracted driving leading to accidents.

Use of Microwave Ovens

The microwave oven converts electrical energy to low-frequency electromagnetic frequency waves, which are used to vibrate the water molecules in the food to heat them. The microwaves are generated inside the oven using a magnetron, and the metal walls bounce these waves around. No evidence exists that using microwave ovens to heat food can cause Cancer.

Dietary factors and Cooking Styles

The most critical impact of diet and lifestyle on Cancer risk is body weight. Obesity and inactivity are major contributors to Cancer risk. Obesity and the role of bariatric surgery in reducing the risk are discussed in another chapter.

Alcohol consumption is an established dietary risk factor for developing Cancer. It is classified as a carcinogen by the IARC. Consumption of alcohol increases the risk of numerous Cancers, including those of the liver, esophagus, pharynx, oral cavity, larynx, breast, and colorectum, in a dose-dependent fashion. Enough evidence is present to link excessive alcohol consumption with an increased risk of primary liver Cancer. At least 75% of Cancers of the esophagus, pharynx, oral cavity, and larynx are attributable to alcohol and tobacco, with a marked increase in risk among drinkers who smoke, suggesting a supplementary effect.

The mechanisms for this include direct damage to the cells, modulation of DNA methylation, which affects susceptibility to DNA mutations; and an increase in acetaldehyde, the primary metabolite of alcohol, which enhances the proliferation of epithelial cells, forms DNA adducts, and is a recognized carcinogen.

In 2015 the IARC declared red meat and processed meat 'possibly carcinogenic' based on epidemiological studies. There are various definitions for red meat; however, meat from mammals is considered red meat. Increased red meat consumption is primarily associated with an increased risk for colorectal Cancers. There are also increased risks for pancreatic, prostate and, stomach Cancers. Mechanisms through which red meat may increase Cancer risk include anabolic hormones routinely used in meat production, heterocyclic amines, polycyclic aromatic hydrocarbons formed during cooking at high temperatures; the high amounts of heme iron in red meat; and nitrates and related compounds in smoked, salted, and some processed meats which can convert to carcinogenic nitrosamines in the colon.

Certain items such as smoked food, food cooked with an open flame, soot on cooked food, and spiced and pickled food are also considered high risk for carcinogenesis. Heterocyclic amines (HCAs) and polycyclic aromatic hydrocarbons (PAHs) are chemicals formed when muscle meat is cooked using high-temperature methods, such as pan frying or grilling directly over an open flame. HCAs and PAHs are found to be mutagenic in some studies. PAHs are also formed when fat and juices from meat are grilled directly over a heated surface or open fire drip onto the surface or fire, causing flames and smoke. The smoke contains PAHs that then adhere to the surface of the meat. PAHs can also be formed during the smoking of meats. Whatever the type of meat, however, meats cooked at high temperatures, significantly above 300°F (as in grilling or pan frying) or cooked for a long time tend to form more HCAs. Cooking methods that expose meat to smoke also contribute to PAH formation.

To reduce the risks, avoid direct exposure of meat to an open flame or a hot metal surface and avoid prolonged cooking times (especially at high temperatures). This can reduce HCA and PAH formation. The meat should be continuously turned over on a high heat source. This can substantially reduce HCA formation compared to leaving the meat on the heat source without flipping it often. Before consumption removing charred portions of meat and refraining from using gravy made from meat drippings can also reduce HCA and PAH exposure.

Recommendations by the American Cancer Society in 2012 regarding lifestyle factors and Cancer prevention

1. Engage in regular physical activity. Physical activity is a primary method of weight control, and it also reduces the risk of several Cancers, especially colon Cancer, through independent mechanisms. Moderate to vigorous exercise for at least 30 minutes on most days is a minimum, and more will provide additional benefits.

2. Avoid being overweight and weight gain in adulthood. A positive energy

balance that results in excess body fat is one of the most important contributors to Cancer risk.

3. Limit alcohol consumption. Alcohol consumption contributes to the risk of many Cancers and increases the risk of accidents and addiction.

4. Consume lots of fruits and vegetables. Frequent consumption of fruits and vegetables during adult life is not likely to majorly affect Cancer incidence but reduces the risk of cardiovascular disease.

5. Consume whole grains and avoid refined carbohydrates and sugars. Regularly consuming whole-grain products instead of fine flour and low consumption of refined sugars lower the risk of cardiovascular disease and diabetes. The effect on Cancer risk is less clear.

6. Replace red meat and dairy products with fish, nuts, and legumes. Red meat increases the risk of colorectal Cancer, diabetes, and coronary heart disease and should be largely avoided. Frequent dairy consumption may increase the risk of prostate Cancer. Fish, nuts, and legumes are excellent sources of valuable mono- and polyunsaturated fats and vegetable proteins and may contribute to lower rates of cardiovascular disease and diabetes.

7. Consider taking a vitamin D supplement. Most of the population, especially those living at higher latitudes, have suboptimal vitamin D levels. Many adults may benefit from taking 1,000 IU of vitamin D3 daily during months of low sunlight intensity. Vitamin D supplementation will, at a minimum, reduce bone fracture rates, probably colorectal Cancer incidence, and possibly other Cancers.

Dos and Don'ts

1. Continuous vigilance is required to identify, reduce, or eliminate workplace chemical carcinogen exposure.

2. Avoid tobacco at all costs.

3. Avoid prolonged exposure to sunlight and use appropriate sunscreens if going out in the sun for a long time.

4. Reduce exposure to ionizing radiation as much as possible. "No dose is safe."

Reduce the use of mobile phones as much as possible. Use hands-free technology whenever possible while talking on the phone to create a distance between the phone and the user.

5. Reduce alcohol consumption.

6. Reduce red meat and processed meat.

7. Avoid direct exposure of meat to an open flame or a hot metal surface and avoid prolonged cooking times.

8. Before consumption, remove charred portions of meat and avoid gravy made from meat drippings over the flame.

2

VIRAL ONCOGENESIS

Dr. Rudrapatna Jayshree Subramanyam

Introduction

Some viral infections are linked with the causation of Cancer; however, as a rule, Cancer is not the mainstream sequel of viral infections. A transformed cell is an impasse for the virus. The first clue of viral association with tumors was obtained in 1910 in experiments on chicken with Rous Sarcoma Virus (RSV), for which Peyton Rous was awarded the Nobel Prize in Physiology and Medicine in 1966. This topic remained of peripheral importance for a long time since viruses were not considered of any consequence for human Cancers. Electron microscopic detection of Epstein Barr Viral (EBV) particles in cultures of Burkitt Lymphoma (BL) cells marked the beginning of an indication of viral etiology of human Cancers.[5] Around the same time came the recognition of cellular "oncogenes" and the discovery of the role of retroviruses in transferring these genetic elements from cell to cell. The latter finding fetched Harold E Varmus and Michael J Bishop the Nobel Prize in Physiology and Medicine in 1989.[6] Oncogenes are mutated forms of genes involved in cell growth and differentiation and are prefixed with either a '*c*' or '*v*' to indicate their cellular or viral origin, respectively. Viral oncogenes have been recognized for nearly all oncogenic viruses and are often homologs of cellular oncogenes. The ones discovered so far are listed in **Table 1.** The field has vastly expanded since this significant breakthrough and was accompanied by an explosion in molecular biological techniques. Subsequently, Harald Zur Hausen was credited with the Nobel Prize in Medicine and Physiology in 2008 for uncovering the causative connection between Human Papilloma Virus (HPV) and cervical Cancer (CxCa). KSHV and MCpyV were identified through subtractive analysis of transcriptomic data of the respective tumor tissues in 1994 and 2008, respectively.[7] Today, about a sixth of all Cancers are ascribed to infectious etiologies, most are due to viruses and bacteria (>99%).[8] This, however, may be an underestimate considering that:

(a) Cancer registries are still not present in all developing countries, and

(b) There is less appreciation of some newly recognized viral etiologies of Cancer, e.g., MCPyV and novel association of known oncogenic viruses with other Cancers, e.g., EBV, whose association is higher with Gastric Carcinoma than Lymphoma.[7]

These oncogenic viruses have been labeled "Group I Human Carcinogens" by the International Agency for Research on Cancer (IARC) [9-12] (Table 2).

Although these viruses belong to diverse types like DNA, RNA, and retroviruses, they appear to use similar mechanisms to dysregulate cell growth and metabolism, producing Cancer's core hallmark capabilities. Hence, understanding molecular aspects of viral oncogenesis imparts a clear concept of oncogenesis. Additionally, preventing and treating Cancer caused by oncogenic viruses is an achievable target worth pursuing with all vigor. In this chapter, viral oncogenesis of seven viruses will be discussed, viz. high risk (hr)-HPV, Hepatitis B Virus (HBV), Hepatitis C Virus (HCV), Human Herpes Virus 4 (HHV- 4)/(EBV), HHV-8 or KSHV, HTLV-1 and, MCPyV.

Viral Life Cycle – Lytic and Persistent infections

Acute viral infections produce infectious particles at the end of a lytic cycle. Following recovery from the acute phase of infection, some oncogenic viruses persist latently in nearly all infected individuals (EBV, MCPyV). In contrast, others remain so only in a small minority of infected people (<10% for HPV), thereby establishing chronic infections (HPV, HBV, HCV, HTLV1 and KSHV). In oncogenic DNA viruses, the viral genome is maintained latently as multicopy, covalently closed circular forms within the host cell nuclei, called **Episomes or Plasmids**. Episomes are part of the viral life cycle and are linked to carcinogenesis. The episomal form in HBV is called ccc DNA. These forms reside as nuclear minichromosomes bound to both viral and host proteins - episome maintenance proteins (EMP) which monitor gene expression, epigenetic programming, repression of genes of the viral lytic cycle, binding/tethering of episomes to host metaphase chromosomes, playing a crucial role in synchronizing its replication with host cell division and ensuring distribution of viral genome into daughter cells during mitosis. Examples of EMPs for EBV, KSHV, and HPV are EBNA1, LANA, and E2, respectively.[13]

Integration: HBV's double-stranded linear (DSL) DNA forms are normally exocytosed from the infected cell. These forms could gain entry into the nucleus of a new cell as a new infection or can re-enter an infected cell nucleus by intracellular trafficking. Here DSL DNA can be incorporated into the host genome using nonspecific cellular machinery that handles ds DNA breaks. This process often results in insertions and deletions in the sequences of the integrant.[14-15] HPV integration is non-random at fragile sites.[16] HPV-driven tumors have all three forms of the virus, viz. episomes, integrants and, a combination of both. Viral integration is found in >80% of squamous cell CxCa. Cervical tumors with more episomal forms do better than those with higher viral integrants.[17] Linear forms of MCPyV DNA integrate at one or two sites of the host genome, albeit not at any 'hot spots'.[14] EBV is primarily known to remain latent as episomes within the nucleus. Expression of specific EBV latency genes (Latency I, II, or III) is characteristic of different EBV-associated diseases.[19] Reverse transcribed HTLV1 genomic RNA – the cDNA integrates randomly into the host DNA: TAX,and HBZ are two viral proteins incriminated in the pathogenesis of ATL.[20]

"Every killer leaves behind a trail." Locard's principle in forensic medicine is well known, which holds that "The perpetrator of a crime will bring something into the crime scene and leave with something from it.".".This analogy is very apt for viral-induced human Cancers, and the concept is easily understood with DNA viruses like HPV, EBV, HBV, MCPyV, and KSHV, wherein transformed cells display incriminating evidence of the presence of copies of viral genomes as nuclear episomes and part or whole of viral genomes integrated into the genomes of tumor cells. Contrarily, the footing of HCV-based Cancers is indirect and dependent on the virus' unique ability to induce prolonged standing inflammation due to chronic infection.[21]

Tissue Microenvironment in viral infections

Upon encountering host cells, viruses face a myriad of antiviral substances triggered by molecular signaling following the interaction of surface membrane, cytosolic and endosomal pathogen recognition receptors (PRRs) viz. Toll-Like receptors (TLRs), RIG Like Receptors (RLRs) etc., with specific Pathogen Associated Molecular Patterns (PAMPs) viz. viral capsid proteins (surface TLRs 2 and 4), viral RNA (endosomal TLRs 3, 7, and 8; cytosolic RLR) and viral DNA (TLR9). Molecules released by the cascade of signaling events within the cell are inflammatory cytokines, chemokines, and antiviral effectors viz. interferons - type I (IFNα, IFNβ) and II (IFNγ) etc. This effector antiviral response of the host can control most acute viral infections. If a virus is not eliminated, a bilateral dialogue ensues between the host and the virus, which eventually determines the fate of the virus.

Further, it is intriguing that only a fraction of chronic viral infections ultimately progresses to malignancies. Hence the virus requires the assistance of a wide range of cofactors to convert a chronic disease to Cancer. Extracellular vesicles (EV) or exosomes generated by cells infected with oncogenic viruses are a bag containing viral nucleic acids, oncoproteins, mRNA, miRNA, metabolites, etc. These not only transmit the infection to neighboring cells but are also a means of instructing and conditioning the tissue microenvironment to survive persistently infected cells.[22]

Oncogenesis is a dynamic process that has been best explained as the three 'E's' of Cancer immunoediting, viz. the first phase of *Elimination* wherein transformed cells that may have arisen in the background of chronic viral infection are destroyed; the second phase of *Equilibrium* when the transformed cells continue to survive in apparent "harmony" with the antitumor immune responses; and the third phase of *Escape* – wherein cells with a unique phenotype get selected out as the tumor evolves.[23] All three phases are exemplified by the interplay of pro and anti-tumorigenic factors in the tissue microenvironment, the ultimate consequence of which depends upon which of these two factors prevails. The tumor microenvironment (TME) essentially comprises varied and interactive populations of cells and factors encompassing the transformed parenchyma. Endothelial cells lining the lymphatic and blood vessels, immune infiltrates, and stromal cells, e.g., fibroblasts, mesenchymal stem cells, and pericytes, constitute the recruited stromal cellular component of the TME. By-products of the cells in and around the lesions, like exosomes, metabolites, cytokines, chemokines, hormones, growth factors, etc., form the extracellular matrix (ECM) and signify an essential aspect of the TME, which influence the evolutionary selection of tumor cells. [24-25]

Viral Stratagems for multiplication, persistence, and induction of Core Cancer hallmark Capabilities (detailed in Table 3)

(a) Insertional Mutagenesis and cellular entropy:

One of the mechanisms by which oncogenic viruses aid oncogenesis is by integrating their genetic material – wholly or partly into the infected cells' genome (stated under section 2 above). Thus, such inclusions of viral genetic elements into the host genome may alter the structure and function of both host and viral genes. Integrating foreign genetic material into the cellular genome imparts genetic diversity to the cell, causing genomic instability and raising the possibility of stimulation of novel oncogenic pathways, thus contributing to the state of "biological entropy."." Simultaneously, viral integration into the host genome also deregulates the expression of viral genes. [21,26]

(b) Aiding cell immortalization:

Oncogenic viruses can transform cells into malignant phenotypes. Viral gene products activate the expression and function of the enzyme telomerase –also called human telomerase reverse transcriptase (hTERT) resulting in cell immortalization during cell division.[26]

(c) Activation of cell cycle pathways:

Many oncogenic viruses can turn on genes regulating the cell cycle. Inducing cell proliferation, one or more of the viral proteins activate one of the following targets: protooncogene *MYC,* cyclins, *E2F, and mTOR* genes in infected cells.[26]

(d) Inhibition of tumor suppressor genes:

Triggering tumor suppressor pathways is a natural protective mechanism in a cell during transformation. Activation of this pathway checks the initiation of tumorigenesis by arresting the cell cycle, repairing DNA damage, and suppressing the replication of the virus. This pathway has two primary gatekeepers: tumor suppressor protein p53 and retinoblastoma (pRB) protein. Oncogenic viruses have various unique means of deregulating these proteins: by repression, degradation, dissociation from associated functional partners, or inactivation - thus, an effective form of cellular defense is overcome, pushing the cells into persistent aberrant S phase wherein synthesis of DNA occurs, facilitating viral nucleic acid synthesis as well. Other targets for tumor suppression are inhibiting cyclin inhibitors and other tumor suppressor genes like *ATM and DLG.* [26-27]

(e) Inhibition of apoptosis:

A series of molecular events leading to the death of abnormal cells is called apoptosis or programmed cell death, is a protective mechanism of the host. There are two apoptotic pathways: the intrinsic pathway, which comes into play in oxidative stress, and the extrinsic pathway which is immune-mediated via various death receptors: Fas/FasL, TNFR/TNF and, TRAIL-R/TRAIL pathways. Intrinsically, a decrease inpro vs. anti-apoptotic proteins (e.g., p53 vs. BCL2) helps Cancer cells evade apoptosis, and extrinsically altered death receptor signaling and defective caspase signaling aid the process. Oncogenic viruses have adopted varied mechanisms for overcoming apoptosis: e.g., inducing over-expression of anti-apoptotic proteins like A20, BCL2, etc., and suppressing pro-apoptotic genes like *BIM*.[26]

(f) Induction of chronic inflammation:

When specific PAMPs interact with their corresponding PRRs on or within the cells, inflammatory signaling pathways get stimulated. This leads to the activation of various transcription factors like NFχB, which initiates the transcription of numerous NFχB-responsive genes. The net result is the production of proteins that negotiate an inflammatory response (e.g., IL-6, TNFα, COX-2,etc.). Oncogenic viruses adopt chronic activation of NFχB signaling as a means "to keep the fire burning," - contributing to oncogenesis. Besides, chronic inflammation also generates reactive oxygen species (ROS), which could drive mutagenesis.[26]

(g) Immune evasion:

Avoiding being killed by the host immune responses is another strategy oncogenic viruses adapt for survival. They achieve this using one or more of the viral products to interfere with TLR signaling pathways, regulate immune cell infiltration into the lesions, inhibit cytotoxic killing by NK and CTLs, downregulate HLA I and II antigens and adhesion molecules, alter the epigenetic landscape of immune response genes, counter apoptosis etc.[26-27] Viral oncogenes also interfere with autophagy - a catabolic innate immune response of the cell and, in the bargain, promote oncogenesis.[28]

(h) Induction of angiogenesis:

Activation of the vascular growth pathway is one of the critical steps in oncogenesis. Oncogenic viruses promote angiogenesis by inducing Hypoxia Inducible Factor 1 alpha (HIF1α)/Vascular Endothelial Growth Factor (VEGF)/Platelet-Derived Growth Factor (PDGF)/angiopoietin and inhibiting antiangiogenic pathway, e.g., thrombospondin (TSP1) etc. [26]

(i) Reprogramming host cell metabolism:

Malignant cells often reprogram various metabolic pathways like glucose, amino acid, fatty acid, and nucleotide metabolism to suit their growing energy demands. A change in glucose metabolism from oxidative phosphorylation to aerobic glycolysis in Cancer cells is known as the "Warburg effect" after the Nobel Laurette Otto Heinrich Warburg (1931). Using several factors and dynamics, oncogenic viruses alter the energetics of infected cells to mirror that of Cancer cells: by inducing mTORC1 signaling, increasing glucose uptake through the activation of glucose transporter I (GLUT1), binding and suppressing pyruvate kinase M2 and altering the amino-acid metabolism by using alternative substrates like serine and glutamine. Besides, the limited availability of oxygen and glucose in the TME promotes immunosuppression. Oncogenic viruses also regulate methylation and acetylation of host cell genes, e.g., promote methylation of tumor suppressor genes, thus blocking their expression.[26]

(j) Aiding invasion and metastasis:

Polarity complexes and junctions (cell-cell and cell-ECM) are gatekeepers protecting against Epithelial Mesenchymal Transformation (EMT). Altered cell polarity influences cell mobility and EMT - a crucial point in the initiation of invasion and metastasis and, thus, malignant progression. Oncogenic viruses regulate the expression of adhesion molecules (EpCAM, E-cadherins), stem cell markers and enzymes like matrix metalloproteinases (MMPs) which digest the ECM, thus paving the way for the invasion of Cancer cells.[26]

Co-factors modulating Viral Oncogenesis

(co-infections, hormones, metabolites, microbiomes, etc.)

As stated earlier in the chapter, infections by oncogenic viruses necessarily deliver only one hit but cannot transform a cell into a malignant phenotype. Various other additional factors aid multistep carcinogenesis. Some of these are viral subtypes, immune deficiencies, age, environmental factors, host genetics, hormones, co-infections, gut and tissue microbiomes, etc.

Vaginal dysbiosis and other sexually transmitted infections like *Chlamydia trachomatis,* Human Immunodeficiency Virus (HIV), HHV2 (Human Herpes Simplex 2), and *Neisseria gonorrhoeae* induce inflammation, thereby promoting the establishment and/or persistence of HPV infections and progression to malignant disease, hence are co-factors in HPV mediated CxCa.[29] Likewise, the interaction of *Plasmodium falciparum* erythrocyte membrane protein (PfEMP1) with B cells harboring latent EBV reactivates the virus, expands these B cells, suppresses EBV-specific T cell immunity, induces Activation-Induced cytidine Deaminase (AID) mediated genomic translocation and activation of oncogenes (*c-MYC*). Hence, the increased incidence of childhood BL in sub-Saharan Africa – region holoendemic for malaria.[30]

Somatic mutations in the host genome also act as a co-factor, e.g., chromosomal translocations often between chromosomes 8 and 14 [t(8;14)] is an impelling feature of EBV-induced BL. This translocation causes the re-positioning of a protooncogene - *c-MYC* downstream of the highly active immunoglobulin promoter resulting in upregulation of *MYC* and subsequent increase in cell growth. Dietary nitrosamine, salted fish, tobacco, etc. are some environmental cofactors in EBV-associated Nasopharyngeal Carcinoma (NPC). While infection with specific genotypes of HPV (vide **Table 2**) poses a higher risk of CxCa, low-risk genotypes (HPV6/11) cause anogenital warts and laryngeal papillomatosis, HBV genotypes C or D have a greater predilection for producing Hepatocellular Carcinoma (HCC) than genotypes B or A. Also, variants of the virus at *X*/pre *S1*/ pre-core/basal core promoter have a varying relationship with HCC causality.[14] People with HLA gene polymorphisms and those with inborn errors in immune response genes have been recognized to be more prone to the persistence of oncogenic viral infections, e.g. HPV, HHV-8, and EBV.[31]

Immunosuppression caused either by therapeutic drugs or HIV infection too can influence the promotion of Cancers. Similarly, immunosenescence is one of the reasons for the reactivation of latent viral infection-induced malignancies in the elderly, and neonates easily fall prey to chronic infections due to their immature immune systems.

Sex steroid hormones like 17-β Estradiol have long been declared human carcinogens, posing a risk for certain Cancers.[32] While Estradiol is a co-factor promoting CxCa, the hormone is protective in HBV and HCV-mediated viral hepatitis and HCC. Both hormone concentrations and Estrogen Receptors (ER) statusare crucial role in modulating carcinogenesis.[33-34] Conversely, Androgens (testosterone)/Androgen Receptor (AR) complexes promote transcription of the HBV genome yielding higher viral load and HBx protein levels, furthering HCC.[35] Estrogen-ERα / testosterone-AR signaling downregulates/upregulates occluding and scavenger receptors – entry receptors for HCV and suppresses synthesis of mature virion particles, explaining the worse prognosis of HCV infection and higher incidence of HCC in men and post-menopausal women.[35]

Normal gut flora and the gut epithelium steer the development and functioning of the immune system. Diet and gut microbiota are interconnected: nutrients and metabolites govern the composition and function of the gut flora and their dialogue with the immune system, and microbes, in turn, regulate the absorption of nutrients by the gut epithelium. Thus, changes in the types and abundance of normal gut microbial flora can control inflammation and immunity in organs distal from the intestine. The microbiome-gut-liver axis - a reciprocal relationship between the gut, its microbial flora, and the liver- is another relevant aspect increasingly recognized in promoting liver diseases. Gut dysbiosis, represented by alteration of the gut's normal flora (e.g., increase in gram-negative bacilli like *E. coli*), causes a rise in gut permeability (leaky gut) and the subsequent movement of bacteria to the liver. Bacterial lipopolysaccharide binding to TLR4 on the hepatocyte surface is one of the critical proinflammatory signaling pathways involved in HCC pathogenesis. Thus, in the liver, as a result of a conglomeration of signals generated from multiple sources: dietary substances, their metabolites, genetic factors like PRRs and PAMPs, etc. inflammation occurring on the background of viral hepatitis (HBV and HCV infections) further gets advanced, leading to fibrosis and HCC.[36-37] Dietary exposure to aflatoxin - a type I carcinogen, is an environmental co-factor that promotes HBV-mediated HCC.[38]

Prevention and Management of chronic Viral infections

Tumors of viral origin are a substantial public health liability in the developing world. Southeast Asian countries have a very low prevalence of both Kaposi Sarcoma (KS) and KSHV; however, they have vast burdens of EBV-associated NPC and gastric Cancers, HBV-associated HCC, and HPV-associated Cancer Cervix. Sub-Saharan Africa, which has high endemicity of KSHV, witnessed a massive increase in KS cases following the HIV pandemic. Other geographical areas with a high prevalence of endemic KSHV are Western China and Andean South America.[7]

Raising awareness is a fundamental step towards WHO's call for the global eradication of hepatitis by 2030, mainly since currently, rates of detection and treatment of HBV and HCV are dismally low. The risk of progression of HBV infection in children <5yrs is high. Vertical transmission of HBV from mother to child, horizontal transmission of the virus amongst children - within the family/household and child-to-child transmission, emergence of HBsAg escape mutants, the rapid increase in occult HBV infections (OBI), and the possibility of its spread in the vaccinated population are issues requiring attention by public health authorities.[39] Testing blood and blood products, safe injection practices, proper healthcare waste management, scaling up detection and treatment of HBV and HCV infections, and increasing safety in the high-risk population – a person who injects drugs (PWID) would further help prevent transmission of these blood-borne viruses. Likewise, HCV too could be transmitted vertically from mother to child.

(a) Vaccines for the prevention of infection

Primary prevention of Cancers having an infectious etiology is through prophylactic vaccination. Intramuscular injections of vaccines against significant HPV genotypes [bi (HPV16/18), Quadri (HPV16/18/6/11),and nonavalent(HPV6/11/16/18/31/33/45/52/58) vaccines are L1 capsid proteins assembled into Viral Like Particles (VLPs)] that have proven to be an efficient public health policy to curtail the spread and establishment of chronic infections, thereby reducing the incidence of the CxCa etiologically associated with them.[40] The vaccines generate high titers of neutralizing antibodies, which offer protection against the targeted genotypes in virus naïve subjects and partial cross-protection against related genotypes. Additional offshoots are herd immunity which also protects against other HPV-mediated Cancers like oropharyngeal Cancer and anogenital warts caused by low-risk genotypes - HPV 6/11 in the case of the quadrivalent vaccine. While adolescent girls (9 to 14 years) should receive two intramuscular injections of HPV VLP vaccines (0, 6 months), those older (>15 years) / immunocompromised should be given three doses.[41] Post-vaccination screening of women is recommended for detecting infection with non-vaccine types (**Table 4**). Thus, a combination of HPV vaccination and screening is the need of the hour to reduce the incidence of CxCa in the world today. HBV vaccine (recombinant HBsAg) is recommended at $10\mu g/20\mu g$ per dose for children (<18yrs)/adults, respectively. Vaccination should cater to neonates within 24 hrs of birth (to prevent infection during the perinatal period/early infancy), health care workers, and high-risk groups. Immunocompromised patients should receive $40\mu g$. The recommended schedule of HB vaccination is either at 0,1 and 2 months or 0,1 and 6 months. The injection site is the anterolateral aspect of the thigh/deltoid in neonates. For passive protection against perinatal transmission of HBV infection - hepatitis B immunoglobulin (HBIG) could be administered simultaneously with the HBV vaccine but in the contralateral thighs. The protective titer of anti-HBV antibodies is $\geq$10IU/ml. Antiviral agents like tenofovir can further help reduce the risk of perinatal transmission.[40]

(b) Treatment and monitoring of chronic infections and premalignancy

Recent WHO guidelines for secondary prevention of CxCa among women in the general population are detailed in **Table 4**.[41] Women in the age range of 30-49 years should be given preference for screening considering that the occurrence of Precancerous lesions - Cervical Intraepithelial Neoplasia (CIN) 2/3 is the highest in this age group. The upper age limit could be extended to 50-65 years in women who have never been tested and should be prioritized. The guidelines for screening HIV-positive women are slightly different in some aspects.[41] Since sexually transmitted organisms *C.trachomatis* and HIV enhance the pathogenicity of HPV, screening for these co-pathogens is helpful for strategic triaging for follow-up of such patients.[29] Employing HPV VLP vaccines to reduce the risk of cervical dysplasia in the adjuvant setting post-treatment of ≥CIN 2 lesions is an attractive approach too.[42] Systemic immunization with HPV 16 E6/E7 DNA vaccines and vaccines using viral vectors are still at the stage of clinical trials, although they produce efficient mucosal immune responses. An interesting pointer, although preliminary, is the administration of oral probiotics (*L. crispatus* strain) to influence HPV clearance from the cervix.

Acute HBV infection naturally resolves within six months post-infection. Consensus WHO guidelines for treating Chronic HBV infection are provided in **Table 5**.[43] However, to encompass patients within the immunotolerant (IT) phase having mild inflammation and prevent them from progressing to HCC, these guidelines may require modifications on several fronts: gender-based definition of average values of serum ALT, the need for better markers indicating active transcription of intrahepatic ccc DNA, e.g., HB core related antigen (HBcrAg)/HBV RNA etc.[44] Currently, treatment with Directly Acting Antivirals (DAA) inhibits viral replication: nucleos(t)ide analogues (Entecavir) or those inhibiting DNA polymerase (Tenofovir) combined with/without IFNα to prevent severe consequences of liver cirrhosis and HCC in later years. While intrahepatic ccc DNA and integrated forms of the virus are formidable targets for elimination, aiming at a functional cure that arrests replication and spread of the virus is considered achievable. And accordingly, these patients should be followed up regularly to detect the possibility of reactivation (**Table 5**). [43-45]

Screening for HCV infection should primarily be based on detecting antibodies to the virus in the blood and confirmatory nucleic acid testing for detecting viral RNA. The absence of HCV RNA in serum-reactive patients indicates past infection, and those positive for HCV RNA are currently considered to harbor the virus. Similar to acute HBV infections, about 20-25% of acute HCV infections get cleared naturally. The presence of HCV RNA in blood for >6 months indicates chronic HCV infection, and such patients are eligible for treatment. Non-structural proteins NS3, NS5A and NS5B are good targets for antivirals: protease inhibitor NS3/4 and NS5A and RNA-dependent RNA polymerase (RdRp) inhibitor encoded by *NS5B*. Velpatasvir and sofosbuvir – are examples of NS5A protease and RdRp antagonists, respectively, that are effective against all the virus genotypes. Sustained virological response (SVR) is defined as no traces of the virus in the blood after 24 weeks of treatment. Protease inhibitors can achieve SVR within 8 to 12 weeks of treatment. PEGylated IFNα/Ribavirin increase the SVR to 40-50% in HCV genotype 1 and ~80% in genotype 2 and 3.[46-47] For decades, Alpha-fetoprotein (AFP)-L3, AFP, and des-gamma-carboxy prothrombin have been used as biomarkers for diagnosing HCC in patients with chronic HBV and HCV infections. Aldo-keto reductase family 1 member B10 (AKR1B10) is one of the newer potential prognostic markers. Likewise, the gut microbial ecology may serve as a potential diagnostic (e.g., elevated *E. coli* abundances in the feces, degree of dysbiosis etc.), prognostic and therapeutic target in chronic liver disease and HCC. Accordingly, prebiotics, probiotics, postbiotics, synbiotics, antibiotics and fecal microbiota transplantation have been recommended for resetting the flora for the prevention and treatment of HCC.[37]

Table 1: Oncogenes identified in Oncogenic Viruses

No.	Virus	Oncogene
1.	High-risk genotypes of Human Papilloma Virus (hr-HPV)	*E6* and *E7*
2.	Hepatitis B Virus (HBV)	*HBX* and *PreS/S*
3.	Epstein Barr Virus (EBV)	*LMP1* and *LMP2A*
4.	Human T Cell Lymphotropic Virus – 1 (HTLV-1)	*TAX* and *HBZ*
5.	Kaposi Sarcoma Herpes Virus (KSHV)	*LANA*
6.	Merkel Cell Polyomavirus (MCPyV)	*EVGR*

Table 2: Association of Human Cancers with Viruses [4,12]

No.	Virus	Type	Cancer (Association with viral etiology)	Global Prevalence (Total number)
1.	Human Papilloma Virus (HPV)	Small dsDNA virus; 8kbp; 50-60nm; nonenveloped; icosahedral symmetry. Discovered in 1983 Kingdom: *Shotokuvirae* Phylum: *Cossaviricota* Class: *Papovaviricetes* Order: *Zurhausenvirale* Family:*Papillomaviridae;* Genus: *Alphapapillomavirus* Clades A9, A7, A5, A6. High risk genotypes: 16,18,26,31,33,35,45, 51,52,56,58, 59, 68, 73.	Cervical Cancer (CxCa) (>99.7%)	570,000
			Oropharyngeal Cancer (OPC) (33%).	140,000
			Anal Squamous Cell Carcinoma (~100%).	29,000
			Penile Squamous Cell Carcinoma (53%).	34,000
			Vaginal Squamous Cell Carcinoma (78%).	18,000
			Vulvar Squamous Cell Carcinoma (25%).	44,000
			Oral Cavity Cancer (2.1%).	280,000

			Larynx Cancer (2.2%).	180,000
			Breast Cancer*# (sporadic, non BRCA1) (~2%).	2,089,000
2.	Hepatitis B Virus (HBV)	ds DNA Virus (short ss segment) with reverse transcriptase; 3kbp; 52-55nm; enveloped; icosahedral symmetry. Discovered in 1965 Kingdom: *Pararnavirae.* Phylum: *Artverviricota.* Class: *Revtraviricetes.* Order: *Blubervirales.* Family: *Hepadnaviridae.* Genus: *Orthohepadnavirus.*	Hepatocellular Carcinoma (HCC) (55%)	660,000
			Non-Hodgkin Lymphoma * (12%[a])	480,000
			Cholangio-carcinoma* (Not known)	Unknown
			Pancreatic Cancer* (Not known)	458,918
3.	Hepatitis C Virus (HCV)	+ss RNA Virus; 9.5 - 12.5kb; 40-60nm; enveloped; icosahedral symmetry. Discovered in 1989 Kingdom: *Orthornavirae.* Phylum: *Kitrinoviricota.* Class: *Flasuviricetes.* Order: *Amarillovirales.* *Family: Flaviviridae.* Genus: *Hepacivirus.* Genotypes: HCV 3,6,1.	HCC (21.2%)	660,000
			Non-Hodgkin Lymphoma (3.3%)	480,000
			Cholangio-carcinoma* (Not known)	Unknown
4.	Epstein Barr Virus (EBV)	Large linear ds DNA Virus; 200nm; 170kbp; enveloped; icosahedral symmetry.	Nasopharyngeal Carcinoma	130,000

		Discovered in 1964 Kingdom: *Heunggongvirae.* Phylum: *Peploviricota.* Class: *Herviviricetes.* Order: *Herpesvirales.* Family: *Herpesviridae.* Subfamily: *Gamaherpesvirinae* Genus: *Lymphocryptovirus.* Species: *Humanherpesvirus* 4.	types II and III (NPC) (84.6%)	
			Hodgkin Lymphoma (HL) (~50%)	80,000
			Endemic Burkitt Lymphoma (BL) (55%)	12,000
			Gastric Carcinoma* (7.7 to 10.4%)	82,800-116,400
			Non-Hodgkin Lymphoma (3.6–12.8%)	480,000
			Breast Cancer* (sporadic, non BRCA1) (Unknown)	2,089,000
5.	Human Herpes Virus 8 (HHV8) or Kaposi's Sarcoma Herpes Virus (KSHV)	Large circular ds DNA Virus; 100-150nm; 170kbp; enveloped; icosahedral symmetry. Discovered in 1994 Kingdom: *Heunggongvirae.* Phylum: *Peploviricota .* Class: *Herviviricetes.* Order: *Herpesvirales.* Family: *Herpesviridae.* Genus: *Rhadinovirus.* Species: *Humangammaherpesvirus 8.*	Kaposi Sarcoma (KS) (>99%)	42,000
			Primary effusion lymphoma (>99%)	Data not availabl e
			Multicentric Castleman's Disease (50%)	3,000 to 30,000 (for the US, not availabl e for the rest of the

29

				world)
6.	Human T Cell Lymphotropic Virus – 1 (HTLV 1	Retrovirus +ss RNA with reverse transcriptase;100nm; 9kbp; enveloped; icosahedral symmetry. Discovered in 1980 Kingdom: *Pararnavirae*; Phylum: *Artverviricota;* Class: *Revtraviricetes;* Order: *Ortervirales;* Family: *Retroviridae;* Subfamily: *Orthoretrovirinae;* Genus: *Deltaretrovirus.* Species: Primate T-lymphotropic virus 1	Adult T cell Leukemia (ATL) (>99%)	3600
7.	Merkelcell polyom avirus (MCPyV)	ds DNA Virus; 5.4kbp; 40-55nm; nonenveloped; icosahedral symmetry. Discovered in 2008 Kingdom: *Shotokuvirae.* Phylum: *Cossaviricota.* Class: *Papovaviricetes.* Order: *Sepolyvirales.* Family: *Polyomaviridae.* Genus: *Alphapolyomavirus.* Species: *Human polyomavirus 5.*	Merkel Cell Carcinoma (80%)	1600 (for the US), not availabl e for the rest of the world

*Limited evidence.

a Based on seropositivity, true association may be much higher if HBV DNA is tested, considering OBI.

Exosomes from HPV infected cervices have been shown to induce HPV mediated Breast Cancer.

ds- double stranded; ss-single stranded.

Table 3: Activation of Core Hallmark capabilities Of Cancer by Oncogenic Viruses [26]

No.	Hallmark of Cancer	Virus	Viral product	Pathway
1.	Insertional Mutagenesis	HPV	Break in *E2* ORF; *E6* inserted.	Non-random insertion, common fragile sites: *PTPN13/ERBB2*.
			Break in *E2* ORF; *E7* inserted.	*NR4A2, RAD51B* (DNA break repair response pathway), *MACROD2, TP63, LRP1B, DLG2* and c-*MYC* loci.
		HBV	*HBx*	Non-random insertion, common fragile sites: *KMT2B (MLL4)/TERT* (telomerase), near proto-oncogenes/tumor suppressor genes/loci.
		HTLV-1	*TAX*	NF-kB, PI3K, CREB, DDR.
		KSHV	*LANA*	pRB, p53, HIF, Wnt, Notch.
			vIRF-1	p53, IFNα, Bim, Atm.
		MCPyV	LTT (truncated Large T antigen)	Random insertion; linear ds DNA – LTT, LT-pRB-E2F.
			sT	Random insertion linear ds DNA, p53, LSD-4E-BP1, sT-MYCL-EP400.
		EBV	*EBNA1,*	Non-random, with

			EBNA2, LMP1	involvement of bands 1p31, 1q43, 2p22, 3q28, 4q13, 5p14, 5q12, and 11p15.
2.	Aiding cell immortalization	HPV	E5	EGFR signaling, Prevents differentiation of epithelial cells.
			E6	hTERT.
		HBV	HBx	HBX gene is inserted near hTERT promoting its over expression, also HBX protein induces hTERT.
		HTLV-1	TAX	hTERT
			HBZ	hTERT
		KSHV	LANA	hTERT
			vGPCR	VEGFR2, alternative lengthening of telomeres (ALT)
		MCPyV	sT	LSD-4E-BP1, sT-MYCL-EP400
		EBV	LMP1	hTERT
		HCV	NS3, Core, NS5A	hTERT
3.	Activation of cell cycle pathways	HPV	E6	mTOR
			E7	E2F
		HBV	HBx	WNT, DNMTs, SRC, RAS, JNK, PI3K-AKT,

				NFκB, TGFβ, ERK1/2, HDACs, JAK/STAT, Hedgehog.
		HTLV-1	TAX	NFκB, PI3K-AKT, CREB, DDR, CDK, REL, MYC, IL2/IL2R.
			HBZ	E2F, c-jun
		KSHV	LANA	HIF, Wnt, Notch, MYC
			vGPCR	Erk, PI3K-Akt-mTOR, p38, NFκB, JNK
			v-cyclin	Homolog of cyclin-D
		MCPyV	LTT	LT(LXCXE)-pRB-E2F
			sT	sT-MYCL-EP400
		EBV	EBNA2 protein	*CD21, CD23, c-FGR, c-MYC*
			LMP2A	ERK, PI3K-AKT-mTOR
		HCV	NS3, Core, NS5A, NS5B, NS2, E2	PARP, p53, h*TERT.* HDACs, TGFβ, cdk2, cyclin E, *MYC*
4.	Inhibition of tumor suppressor genes	HPV16/18	Oncoprotein E6	Ubiquitination mediated proteasomal degradation of p53
			Oncoprotein E7	calpain-mediatedproteasomal degradation of pRB; proteasomal degradation of PTPN14
		HBV	HBx	Induces phosphorylation

				of pRB, directly binds p53 TGFβ
		HTLV-1	TAX	Inhibit p53 by modulating p300/CBP or through phosphatase Wip-1, and Inhibits DLG tumor suppressor
		KSHV	LANA	pRB, p53
			v-cyclin	Suppresses p27^{KIP1} – a CDK2 inhibitor.
			vIRF-1	Homolog of IRF1 suppresses p53, Atm
		MCPyV	LTT	LT-pRB-E2F
			sT	p53
		EBV	EBNA2	Suppresses CDK2 inhibitors p21^{CIP1} and p27^{KIP1}
		HCV	NS3, Core, NS5A	p53
LMP 2 EB NA1 NS3 Core NS5	Inhibition of apoptosis	HPV	E6 (intrinsic pathway)	Targets proapoptotic proteins p53, Bax, Bak for proteolytic degradation.
			E6 (extrinsic pathway)	Inhibits TNF-mediated apoptosis: TNFR1, Fas, TRAIL.
			E7 (intrinsic)	Targets proapoptotic protein pRB for

A				degradation.
E6, E7 E5 HBx (mai nly in the mito chon dria)			E5 (intrinsic pathway)	Targets proapoptotic protein Bax for proteolytic degradation.
			E5 (extrinsic pathway)	Downregulates Fas thereby reducing FasLand TRAIL-mediated apoptosis.
		HBV	HBx (intrinsic)	Targets proapoptotic proteins pRB, p53.
			HBx (extrinsic)	Prevents TNFα, TGFβ, Fas mediated apoptosis by blocking caspases-8 and -3
		HTLV-1	TAX	NFκB antiapoptotic signaling – XIAP, survivin, BCL2, Bcl-xl, stabilizes MCL1, inhibits caspase 3,7,8,9
			HBZ	Impairs binding of AFT3 to p53; inhibits transcription of *BIM* and Fas Ligand, induces survivin promoter, stabilizes MCL1
		KSHV	LANA	pRB, p53
			vFLIP	NFκB antiapoptotic signaling
			vIRF-1	Inhibits p53 via p300/CBP; inhibits proapoptotic *BIM*

			vGPCR	Inhibits p53, Activates PI3K/Akt and NFkB antiapoptotic pathway
		MCPyV	LTT	LT-pRB-E2F
			sT	p53, LSD-4E-BP1
		EBV	miRNA	Inhibit transcription of pro-apoptotic genes *PUMA* and *BIM*
			BALF1	Viral homolog of BCL2
			LMP1	NFκB, A20, BCL2
				inhibits proapoptotic *BIM*
				Upregulates Survivin - a member of the inhibitor of apoptosis protein family
		HCV		Blocks caspase 3 mediated cleavage and stabilizes PARP-1
				Inhibits caspase 8
				Blocks caspase 3 mediated cleavage and stabilizes PARP-1
6.	Induction of chronic inflammation	HPV		EGFR-Ras-MAPK-COX2-PGE2 pathway
				EGFR- NFκB-AP1-COX2-PGE2/caspase I
		HBV		1. Suppresses

				COX2, SOD, increases IL6, IL18, IL1β, NF-κB, malondialdehyde, phospho-AKT 2. Increases expression of TNF-α 3. Chronic necro-inflammation - resulting in mutagenic ROS
		KSHV	vFLIP + cell surface molecules	JAK2/STAT3, NFκB
			vIL6, vCCLs(virokines) + cell surface molecules	JAK2/STAT3, NFκB
			vGPCR, K15	JNK, NFκB
		EBV	EBER	TLR3 - proinflammatory cytokines, IFN
			LMP1+ cell surface molecules	JAK2/STAT3, NFκB
			BILF1+ cell surface molecules	JAK2/STAT3, NFκB
		HTLV1	vFLIP	JAK2/STAT3, NFκB

			HBZ+ cell surface molecules	JAK2/STAT3, NFκB
			TAX+ cell surface molecules	JAK2/STAT3, NFκB
		HCV	HCV RNA	TLR3, IL-8, CCL-5, MIP-1 and CXCL-10
			NS3, Core	TLR2, STAT3, NFκB
			NS5A	TLR4 promoter, My88, IRF3, NFκB, IL6, IFNβ
7.	Immune evasion	HPV	Unique life cycle - mature viral particles formed only in the topmost epithelial layer and shed by sloughed epithelium.	Escapes recognition by low density intraepithelial antigen presenting cells and Langerhans cells.
			E6/E7 proteins	Downregulate TLR9, repress expression of IFN β, IFNα, STAT1; block NFκB signaling, reduces intraepithelial expression of CCL20 – reducing influx of LCs.
			E6 protein	Blocks transactivation domain of IRF3 protein.
			E7 protein	Blocks transactivation domain of IRF1 protein;

					inhibits Granzyme B expression in NK and CTLs
				E5 protein	downregulate MHC class I expression
			HBV	HBx	1. Inhibits TLR9 hence IFNα. 2. Blocks RIG-I -TLR3 - IRF3 -abolishing IFN-β. 3. Inhibits NEMO mediated nuclear translocation of IRF 3,7 – blocking IFNα,β. 4. Competitive inhibition of MAVS-TRIF and IRF3, blocking TLR3 signaling -IFNα,IFNγ. 5. Blocks Smc5/6 mediated transcriptional repression of HBV ccc DNA. 6. Promotes transcription of HBV cccDNA by reversing its epigenetic changes.
				HBV polymerase	Blocks RIG-I-TLR3-IRF3 -abolishing IFN-β;
				HBeAg	Binds MyD88, TIRAP, inhibiting TLR2 signaling.

			HBsAg	Blocks TLR3 signaling – inhibiting IFNα.
			HBeAg and HBsAg	1. Inhibit MVP-MyD88 interaction, preventing IFNα. 2. Inhibit ISG tetherin, promoting virion budding.
		HTLV-1	TAX	Highly immunogenic protein – cell senescence
			HBZ	1. Inhibits TAX activity. 2. Poorly immunogenic. 3. TAX⁻HBZ⁺ATL cells immune evasion.
		KSHV	vFLIP	Resists Fas induced apoptosis.
			K3, K5 ubiquitin ligases	Downregulate ICAM, MHC-I and NK receptors.
			vIRF-1 to 4	Suppress IFNα
			ORF 63	Viral homolog of NLRP1- Prevents activation of inflammasome.
		EBV	BGLF5	Downregulates TLR2 & 9, degrades HLA I & II.
			LMP1	Reduces TLR9, regulates

				STAT1.
			LMP2	Inhibits JAK/STAT, NFκB signaling, downregulates HLA I increases IFNR turnover.
			EBNA1	Inhibits STAT1, NFκB signaling, peptide transport and presentation.
			BZLF1	Inhibits IRF7 expression, inhibits NFκB & IFNγsignaling.
			BRLF1	Inhibits IRF3,7.
		HCV	Replication of viral RNA	Occurs in membranous web, concealed from the host.
			NS3/4A serine protease	Cleave MAVS & TRIF - blocking TLR3 signaling - IFNα, IFNγ.
			NS3	Binds TBK1 – inhibiting IRF3 – IFN production.
			Core	Inhibits JAK/STAT signaling – IFN production.
			NS5A	Binds Myd88 and PKR thereby inhibiting TLR signaling.
			E2	Binds PKR thereby inhibiting TLR signaling.
8.	Reprogramming	HPV	E5	Initiates PI3K-AKT-

host cell metabolism			mTORC1 signaling.
		E6	Activates GLUT I, initiates PI3K-AKT-mTORC1 signaling.
		E7	1. Activates GLUT I. 2. Binds and suppresses pyruvate kinase M2 – boosting glycolysis. 3. Initiates PI3K-AKT-mTORC1.
	HBV	HBx	1. Reduces intracellular citrate – affecting acetyl co A – epigenetic modulation of host genes. 2. Suppresses miR-205 - a rise in ACSL1-increase in triglycerides.
	HTLV-1	TAX	Initiates PI3K-AKT-mTORC1.
		HBZ	Initiates PI3K-AKT-mTORC1.
	KSHV	K1	Initiates mTORC1 signaling, miRNAs induce a metabolic shift from OXPHOS to aerobic glycolysis.
		vGPCR	Initiates PI3K-AKT-mTORC1 signaling and PDGF, VEGF.
		ORF 45	Initiates mTORC1

				signaling through ERK2/ RSK.
		MCPyV	sT	Induces a proglycolytic state and increases lactate synthesis.
		EBV	LMP1	Initiates PI3K-AKT-mTORC1-NFκB signaling- GLUT1-glycolysis.
			LMP2A	downregulates adipose triglyceride lipase (ATGL) – increases lipid droplets - growth of NPC.
			EBNA2	MYC- activation of nucleotide and amino acid metabolism,SREBP2 -increases fatty acid metabolism and lipid biosynthesis.
		HCV	Core	Dysregulated lipid metabolism – promotes steatosis.
9.	Inducing angiogenesis	HPV	E6	Decreases TSP1 and induces *HIF1α/VEGF*, Stabilizes HIFα.
			E7	Induces *HIF1α/VEGF*.
		HBV	HBx	1. Stabilizes, nuclear translocates, phosphorylates HIF1α.

				2. Increase transcription of the *HIF1α*. 3. Activates *ANGPT2*, *VEGF*, *cMET* (HGFR).
			K1	VEGF
		KSHV	vGPCR	PI3K-AKT-mTORC1,ANGPT2, HIF1α/VEGF/VEGFR, IL6, PDGF/PDGFR
			LANA	HIF1α/VEGF, IL6, PDGF
			vFLIP	NFκB/IL6, PDGF
			vCCLs, vIL6	Homolog of chemokines and cytokines - proangiogenic
			miRK1-5	Downregulates antiapoptotic TSP-1
		EBV	LMP1	PI3K-AKT, HIF1α/VEGF, FGF, IL8
			LMP2A	PI3K/AKT/mTOR/HIF-1α vasculogenic mimicry
		HCV		ROS via several signaling pathways stabilize HIF1α
			Core	VEGF
10.	Aiding invasion	HPV	E6	AKT phosphorylation -

and metastasis			AP1,Sp1,ETS,NFκB -– MMP1 – metastasis
		E7	AKT phosphorylation - AP1,Sp1,ETS,NFκB - MMP1 – metastasis
	HBV	HBx	1. Beta catenin – adherens. 2. Alters global epigenetics of the cell e.g. EpCAM, MTA1- metastasis. 3. cMET. 4. Induces NANOG. 5. Expression of MMP-10. 6. AFP/AFPR-Src-PI3K/mTOR-metastasis. 7. TGFβ.
	KSHV	K1	MMP9, EMT.
		vGPCR	Degradation of VE cadherins.
	MCPyV	sT	MMP9
	EBV	LMP2A	MMP9 via ERK/Fra-1
	HCV	Core	Inhibits JNK/pSmad3L signaling – EMT, TGFβ, delocalizes "Scribble".

				NS5A	EMT: by NANOG, TWIST, TGFβ, TLR4, activation of hepatic stellate cells, Steatosis.
				E1	EMT: by NANOG, TWIST, TGFβ, TLR4.
				E2	EMT: by NANOG, TWIST, TGFβ, TLR4.
				E2A	Suppresses E-cadherin, EMT.
				NS4	Alters cell polarity, EMT.

Table 4: Routine screening guidelines for CxCa[40]

1.	Samples	Self-collected/clinician collected cervical brushing samples.
2.	Age For Starting, Stopping screening	Primary screening should start at the age of 30 years and continued up to 50 years - provided two consecutive screening results performed at regular intervals are negative.
3.	Screen and treat approach	In this approach, the decision to treat is based on a positive primary screening test only.
		1. Visual inspection with acetic acid (VIA) as the primary screening test, followed by treatment. HPV DNA (self- or clinician-collected) as the primary screening test, followed by treatment.

4.	Screen, triage and treat approaches:	2. In this approach, the decision to treat is based on a positive primary screening test only.
		3. Cytology as the primary screening test, followed by colposcopy triage, followed by treatment.
		4. HPV DNA as the primary screening test, followed by HPV16/18 triage (when already part of the HPV test), followed by treatment, and using VIA triage for those who screen negative for HPV16/18.
		5. HPV DNA as the primary screening test, followed by VIA triage, followed by treatment.
		6. High-risk HPV DNA as the primary screening test, followed by colposcopy triage, followed by treatment.
		7. HPV DNA as the primary screening test, followed by cytology triage, followed by colposcopy and treatment.

Table 5: Modified Guidelines for The Management of Chronic HBV Hepatitis [43,44]

Parameters	Immune tolerant (Chronic Infection)	Immune Active (Chronic Hepatitis)	Immune Control	Functional Cure#	Reactivation
HB DNA Viral Load	High[1]	Moderate	Low	Negative	Low/Moderate
Serum HBeAg	+	+/-	-/+	Negative	-/+
Serum Anti HBe Abs	-	-/+	+/-	+/-	+/-
Liver enzymes (ALT/SGPT)	Normal or Mildly elevated	High	Moderate	Normal	Low/Moderate
Immune Response to HBV, Liver tissue	Weak, No to minimal necro-inflammation	Strong, Biopsy evidence of necro-inflammation	Strongest, Regeneration of liver tissue	Intrahepatic ccc DNA and integrated HBV may still be present	Weak
Antivirals	Not required*	Required especially if age >30 to 40 years, family h/o HCC.	Not required*$	Not required	Required Entecavir for 2 to 17 years and tenofovir for 12 to 18

		Entecavir for 2 to 17 years and tenofovir for 12 to 18 years			years with/witho ut IFNα.

* Required if cirrhosis is present as evidenced by raised liver enzymes.

\$ To evaluate after 6 months after completion of a defined course of treatment to assess functional cure.

\# Indicated by loss of HBsAg and viral DNA. To be kept on regular follow-up to check for recurrence especially in patients on immunosuppressive therapy.

[1] May need close monitoring with better markers of active cccDNA replication - which best reflects the risk of HCC development.[44]

3

STRESS, IMMUNITY AND CANCER

Dr. Nanda Rajaneesh, Dr. Anagha

Although the term stress has been used extensively in the psychological literature for several decades, a precise definition of the term has proven to be elusive. Stress is a psycho-physiological response of our body to external stressors, usually experienced as a negative emotional state. [48] Stressors can be biological or chemical agents, environmental conditions, external stimuli, or events that cause stress. It can be real or imaginary, internal or external.

Stressors can be acute or chronic. Acute stressors are time-limited stressors that occur within minutes of stressor onset- the flight/fight response. E.g., Mental arithmetic and public speaking. Chronic stressors are prolonged-lasting stressors that last for months or years, E.g., traumatic injury, marital discord, and poverty.

What is Anxiety?

Anxiety is a feeling of worry, nervousness, or unease about something with an uncertain outcome. Extreme stress can have an accumulative effect on the body's physiology. Exposure to an aversive stimulus typically results in behavioral and physiological changes to meet environmental demands. Although this physiological phenomenon is fundamental to survival, it is also strongly related to several brain disorders, including depression, anxiety, and post-traumatic stress disorder,[49] according to the International Classification of Diseases, 10th edition (ICD-10). There is also evidence suggesting that physical and social stressors may be contributing to carcinogenesis. The contribution of psychological factors to the neoplastic disease was considered as early as the second century by Galen, who believed that melancholic women were more likely to develop cancer than those who were more confident and vital.[50]

Stress Neurobiology

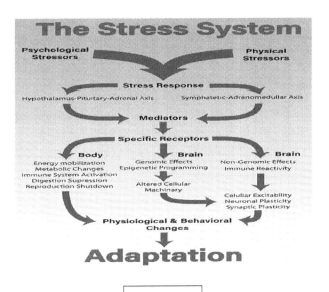

Figure 1

Complex mechanisms integrate the brain and body by processing and coping with stressful situations.

Step 1: Detect or interpret events as actual or potential threats (stressors).

Step 2: Activate two significant constituents of the stress system and release its final mediating molecules.

1. Sympathetic-adreno-medullar axis- noradrenaline and norepinephrine.

2. Hypothalamus-pituitary-adrenal (HPA) axis- glucocorticoids.

Step 3: Generating a coordinated response that starts within seconds and might last for days.

These body-brain effects collectively mediate physiological and behavioral alterations that enable adaptation and survival.[51] Distressed persons sleep less, exercise less, have poor diets, smoke more, and use alcohol and other drugs more often than distressed persons. These behaviors have all been shown to alter the immune system.

Effects of Stress on the Body

Substantial nutritional raw material utilization and indigestion because of stress affect the immune system.

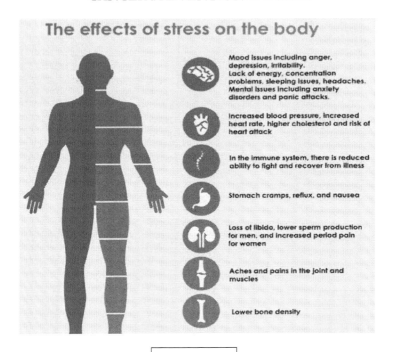

The effects of stress on the body

Mood issues including anger, depression, irritability. Lack of energy, concentration problems, sleeping issues, headaches. Mental issues including anxiety disorders and panic attacks.

Increased blood pressure, increased heart rate, higher cholesterol and risk of heart attack

In the immune system, there is reduced ability to fight and recover from illness

Stomach cramps, reflux, and nausea

Loss of libido, lower sperm production for men, and increased period pain for women

Aches and pains in the joint and muscles

Lower bone density

Figure 2

How stress affects the Immune System?

Immunity can be defined as all the physiological mechanisms that enable an individual's body to recognize materials as foreign and neutralize, eliminate, or metabolize them without injury to its tissue.

The difference in immune alteration may depend on the duration of the stressor.

Neuro-immune connection: A bidirectional relationship exists between the nervous and immune systems in health and disease. The same molecules mediate in both directions, including cytokines, neurotransmitters, and trophic factors. [52]

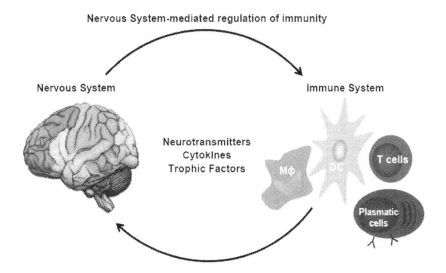

Nervous System-mediated regulation of immunity

Nervous System

Immune System

Neurotransmitters
Cytokines
Trophic Factors

Mφ

DC

T cells

Plasmatic cells

Immune system-mediated regulation of nervous system function

Figure 3

Influence of the Nervous system on the Immune system

T cells and dendritic cells (DCs) express receptors for neurotransmitters classically seen in the nervous system. They are glutamate receptors (GluRs), acetylcholine receptors (AChRs), serotonin receptors (5-HTRs), dopamine receptors (DARs) and adrenergic receptors. Hence, it is clear that CNS and PNS influence immune cells. The autonomic nervous system innervates the Lymphoid tissue through the above neurotransmitters. [52] By innervating the Primary lymphoid organs(Bone marrow, thymus), the ANS regulates the generation and differentiation of new lymphoid and myeloid cells. Innervating the secondary lymphoid organs (Lymph nodes, spleen) influences antigen presentation and T-cell differentiation and affects immune response initiation and development.

Theory 1: Hans Selye suggested that stress globally suppressed the immune system and provided the first model relating stress and immune response. (6). He described three stages of General Adaptation Syndrome in response to stress:

ALARM STAGE: The body prepares for fight-or-flight in response to a threat (Acute manifestations).

RESISTANCE STAGE: The body channelizes all its resources by secreting other hormones and blood sugar to sustain energy to fight.

EXHAUSTION STAGE: When the stressor remains long, the body runs out of reserve energy and immunity. Due to this depletion of body resources, one may fall ill or die.[54]

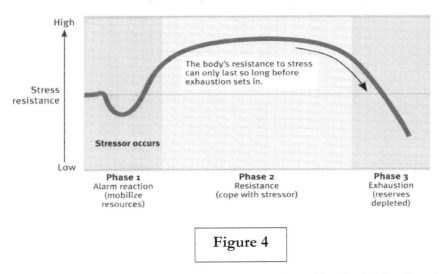

Our stress response system defends, then fatigues.

Figure 4

Theory 2: Stress and the immune system are activated by the HPA axis and Cortisol (anti-inflammation theory). [55]

Stress causes dysregulated Cortisol response- Recent research suggests that hormones are responsible for the adverse effects of stress. Their secretion increases upon activation of the HPA axis and sympathetic branch of ANS.

Both neuroendocrine and behavioral mechanisms provide plausible explanations for stressor exposure and immune alteration. Stress is associated with the activation of the neuroendocrine system, including the hypothalamic pituitary adrenal axis and the sympathetic nervous system. Activation of these two pathways results in elevated serum cortisol and catecholamine levels. The immune cells have receptors for these hormones, implying that these hormones have a role in modulating the immune system. Recent evidence suggests that SNS activation alters immune function even before the HPA axis has enough time to increase serum cortisol. In the case of specific immune responses (e.g., Lymphocyte proliferation), SNS plays a more significant role in stress-induced immune alteration than the HPA axis. It is also possible that the other endocrine systems activated by stressors play a role in altering the immune responses. These systems include prolactin, growth hormone, opioids, etc.

Short-term stress raises cortisol levels.

Long-term stress might result in too low cortisol levels- flattening out the daily cycle of cortisol production.

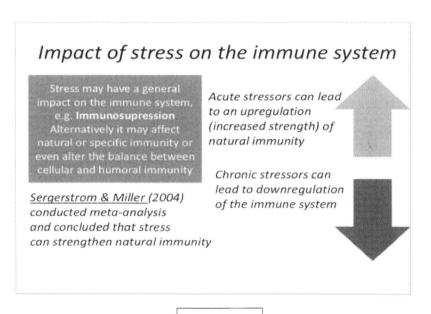

Impact of stress on the immune system

Stress may have a general impact on the immune system, e.g. **Immunosupression** Alternatively it may affect natural or specific immunity or even alter the balance between cellular and humoral immunity

Sergerstrom & Miller (2004) _conducted meta-analysis and concluded that stress can strengthen natural immunity_

Acute stressors can lead to an upregulation (increased strength) of natural immunity

Chronic stressors can lead to downregulation of the immune system

Figure 5

Studies relating stress and cancer: Several studies have pointed to the possibility that cancer incidence is marked among individuals who expressed a sense of loss, hopelessness, and inability to cope with the stress of separation. Schmale and Iker [58] were able to predict cancer development among asymptomatic women predisposed to cervical cancer who were unable to cope with stress and responded with feelings of hopelessness. Moreover, cancer relapse after surgical removal of malignant melanoma was more frequent, with individuals unable to adjust to the disease and the surgery than individuals who could accept the condition. [59]

Phases of Tumor Development

Stress can affect different stages of tumor development.

The first phase is tumor induction, which is the appearance or induction of a tumor cell. Although cancer may be a spontaneous mutation or due to genetic inheritance, many types of cancers in humans are caused by environmental factors. All the tumor stimuli can be divided into carcinogens and anticarcinogens. Carcinogens include direct-acting carcinogens, cocarcinogens, and procarcinogens. Studies have shown that stress can act as a promoter or enhancer of direct-acting carcinogens. [60,61]

The second phase is tumor growth, influenced by various stimuli and host reactions. The immune system has been thought to play a central role as a natural defense against neoplasia during tumor development through immune surveillance. [62]

The third and last phase is metastasis, which is the development of secondary neoplasms in areas of the body not directly adjacent to the primary. If stress affects metastasis, it will likely be through alteration in circulation, selection factors, and hormonal and immunological mechanisms that may be involved in inhibiting secondary tumor spread.

Keeping the body in good physical and mental condition by staying positive and maintaining a good diet, exercise, and yoga helps promote immune function and combat the effects of stress. There is preliminary evidence that relaxation therapy may influence endocrine function and counterbalance stress-induced endocrine changes. [63]

How do we boost our immunity?

1. Physical activity- Pranayama, Yoga, Meditation.

2. A Healthy and nutritious diet- increases the raw materials for the immune system.

3. Good sleep.

4. Positive attitude.

5. Social interactions.

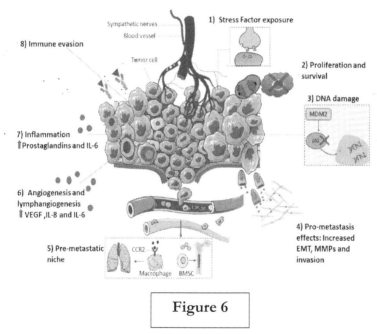

Figure 6

Immunology in Cancer

Evidence of tumor immunity:

The effect of the immune system on tumors is evident by the regression of some tumors spontaneously (Eg. Melanoma, Lymphoma), regression of metastases after the removal of the primary tumor (Eg. Pulmonary metastases from renal cancer), infiltration of tumors by lymphocytes and macrophages (Eg. Melanoma, Breast cancer), lymphocyte proliferation in draining lymph nodes and higher incidence of cancer after immunosuppression, immunodeficiency (AIDS), children and elderly (less immunity).

Immuno-Oncology Theories

• **Cancer Immunosurveillance Theory:**

Burnet proposed this theory in 1957, which states that tumors produce antigens that may evoke an immune response. Lymphocytes act as sentinels in recognizing and eliminating nascent transformed cells. Immunosurveillance Inhibits carcinogenesis and maintains cellular homeostasis.[48]

• **Cancer Immunoediting Theory:**

Novel theory (Theory of 3 E's) by R.D. Schreiber and Dunn implies that while the immune system protects from cancer, it also drives the development of tumors that undergo immunogenic "sculpting" and may survive immune cell attacks. It comprises 3 phases-

PHASE 1- ELIMINATION

Tumors arising in tissue are recognized and eliminated early on by immune cells (innate + adaptive).

PHASE 2- EQUILIBRIUM

Cancer remains clinically undetectable and dormant; cells that survive elimination can replicate with newer resistant variants.

PHASE 3- ESCAPE

Cancer cells escape the killing mechanism or recruit regulatory cells to protect it, eventually replicating into clinically detectable tumors. [49]

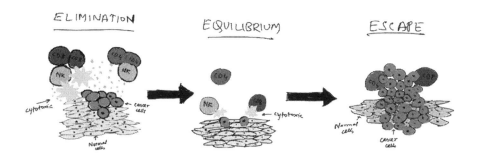

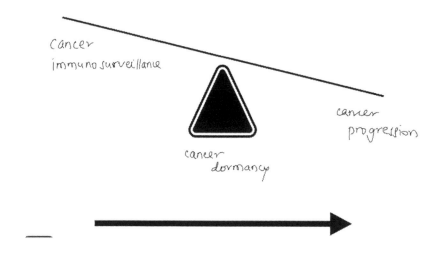

Tumor Antigens

Tumor antigens are of 2 types: Tumor Specific Antigens (TSA) and Tumor Associated Antigens (TAA).

Tumor Specific Antigens (TSA):

1. Unique to tumor cells.

2. Never in normal cells.

3. The result of mutations in normal cellular genes.

e.g., BCR/ABL fusion in CML, Mutant p53 protein.

Tumor-associated antigens (TAA):

1. Not unique to tumor cells.

2. Normal cellular proteins aberrantly expressed.

3. The reactivation of embryonic genes increases their expression. e.g., Tyrosinase in melanomas (enzyme in melanin biosynthesis).

4. Antigens of oncogenic viruses- DNA viruses- EBV, HPV; RNA viruses- HTLV-1 (infects CD4).

5. Oncofetal antigens- expressed in cancer and normal fetal tissues.

CEA in the colon and other cancers, AFP in HCC, and inflammatory conditions.[50]

Tumor Surveillance-Effectors

Detection of tumors is undertaken by the following cells in the body- Macrophage/ Dendritic cells, CD8+ cell (cytotoxic T-cell) mediated cytotoxicity, Natural killer (NK) cells, Antibody-dependent cell-mediated cytotoxicity (ADCC) and Miscellaneous- inflammation, neutrophils, eosinophils, complement system, cytokines.

Macrophage/ Dendritic Cell

Dendritic cells and macrophages can attack the tumor cell phagocytosis and release lytic molecules (free radicals and TNF-α). In other cases, they present tumor antigens by processing them into peptides and expressing them using MHC class II. TCR recognizes this in T-helper cells, which release cytokines and activate other immune cells (NK, CTL), thereby killing the tumor cell.

CD8+ Cell (Cytotoxic T-Cell) Mediated Cytotoxicity

Tumor cells present their antigens using MHC class I receptors on their surface, which are then recognized by T-cell receptors (TCR) on cytotoxic T-cells. They release cytolytic granules (perforins, granzyme B), which cause necrosis/apoptosis of tumor cells. Ligation of Fas on the target cell can initiate apoptosis. Apart from these, CD4+ T cells (Th cells) also release cytokines that activate CTL.[51]

Natural Killer (NK) Cells

Natural killer cells recognize tumor cells via receptors that recognize the loss of expression of MHC-I molecules, detecting **"MISSING SELF"** common in cancers. Upon recognition of cancer cells, they secrete pore-forming granule perforin into the immunological synaptic region, causing tumor cell lysis. They also activate dendritic cells by producing IFN-γ and increase their access to tumor antigens, thus enhancing tumor immunogenicity. [52]

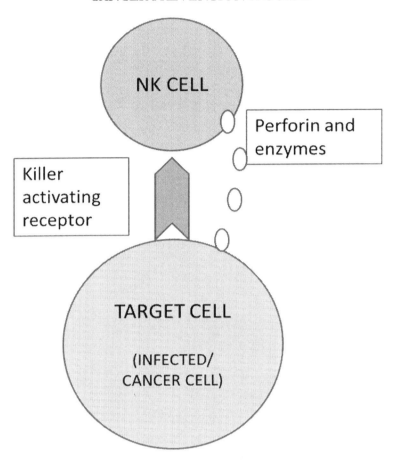

Antibody-Dependent Cell-Mediated Cytotoxicity (ADCC)

B-cells can recognize specific antigens on tumor cells and produce antibodies against them. As part of the humoral immune response, these antibodies can limit and contain infection and tumors. A typical effector cell is the NK Cell, which interacts with IgG antibodies via Fc receptors (CD16), which bind to the Fc region of the antibody. Other cells known to mediate ADCC include macrophages, eosinophils, and neutrophils.[53]

Immune Evasion

Tumors can evade the immune system because even though immune responses kill tumor cells, tumors proliferate. Often, the growth outstrips immune defenses. Immune response against tumors may be weak because many tumor antigens are weakly immunogenic or differ very slightly from self-antigens. Growing tumors also develop specific mechanisms to evade the immune response. [54]

Mechanisms of Immune Evasion

Loss of T-Cell recognition: Antigens sometimes lose variants. Or else, the loss of transporter-associated proteins (TAPs) and other molecules involved in antigen processing and tumor cells stopping the expression of class I MHC molecules can cause the loss of T-cell recognition.

Tumor antigens may be inaccessible to the immune system: Tumor cells express more glycocalyx molecules than normal cells, leading to 'Antigen Masking' because cell surface antigens are hidden from the immune system by glycocalyx molecules.

Tumor may engage molecules that inhibit immune response: Involvement of PD-L1, CTLA-4.

Secreted products of tumor cells may suppress anti-tumour immune response: TGF-β secreted significantly by the tumor inhibits proliferation and effector functions of lymphocytes and macrophages.

Tumor-associated macrophages (TAMs): These create an immunosuppressive tumor microenvironment by producing cytokines, chemokines, and growth factors, increasing angiogenesis and recruitment of T-reg cells.

Increased regulatory T-cells: T-reg cells regulate activation and effector function of other T-cells and maintain tolerance to self-antigens; express CD4+ and CD25. Excess T-regs in the tumor microenvironment allow tumor cells to escape.

Fas counterattack: Tumors may over-express Fas ligand and induce the apoptosis of infiltrating lymphocytes, allowing immune escape.

Cancer Immunotherapy

Cancer Immunotherapy uses the body's immune system to reject cancer. It can be passive or active, specific or non-specific. The following are the immunotherapy types in use-

1. Monoclonal Antibodies, naked vs. conjugated Mabs; e.g., Anti-Her2 Mab= Traztusumab.
2. Oncolytic Virus Therapy.
3. Therapeutic cancer vaccines.
4. Cytokines, e.g., Interleukins, interferons.
5. Checkpoint inhibitors.

4

ROLE OF NUTRITION IN PREVENTION OF CANCER

Ms. Sharanya Shastry

"Health" is an extensive term used by fitness enthusiasts and social media influencers in every lecture and literature. However, the experts (nutritionists and medical professionals) cannot provide an exact definition of the word "health."

Per our science textbook, health is an individual's mental, social and physical well-being. But off late, everything associated with "health" is directly connected to weight loss, weighing a particular number on the weighing scale, fitting into specifically sized jeans, losing weight for a special event, or impressing our partner. Hence the majority have a notion that whenever a doctor or nutritionist advice a better diet/ asks to be healthy, it is taken as "dieting" or "cutting down on food" or "deprivation of something" or, in simple terms, "shed weight in some way or the other – either by hook or by crook." In the whole process of weight loss, people tend to ignore the role of nutrition in preventing diseases like Cancer.

How poor nutrition leads to Cancer?

Understanding how a nutrient deficit poor diet can cause Cancer is essential before moving into the preventive methods.

a) It has been estimated that 30–40 percent of all Cancers can be prevented by lifestyle and dietary measures alone.

b) **We know that India is leading in obesity, and according to the WHO, the global prevalence of obesity has almost tripled in the last 40 years.** There is strong evidence from the World Cancer Research Fund that consumption of fast or refined foods can lead to being overweight or obese, leading to at least 12 types of Cancers.

c) Hence, it is essential to maintain a healthy weight, but it is also vital to have good health, which gives weight loss as a by-product; however, the vice versa is not valid!

d) Obesity is directly linked to nutrient sparse foods like the consuming of concentrated sugars and refined products consisting of hormonally injected plant sources and meat, low-fiber diets, and artificially flavored drinks and beverages, which increase **cellular inflammation** causing a mutation or a mitotic condition like Cancer. Hence, antioxidant diets and moderate exercise decrease inflammation in the body, thus, preventing you from Cancer.

But yes, prevention starts from the day you are born and what you've been following for years. A quick diet followed for a month or two will not give quick results or prevent Cancer.

Talking about diets that help in the prevention of Cancer, as a nutritionist, there are numerous messages and articles that get forwarded in multiple group messaging platforms that talk about the consumption of a particular fruit, vegetable, or spice in some form or the other (a juice or a concoction), which can protect against various diseases. Very few people verify the authenticity or scientific evidence behind such claims.

The most important factors in Cancer prevention are nutrition discipline, sleep patterns, exercise, and eating right, but they are often neglected in the face of 'fancy diets' or 'superfoods. Other lifestyle factors such as erratic sleep patterns, consumption of alcohol and, smoking increase the risk of Cancer.

There are no fixed or specific answers to commonly asked questions such as "What is eating right," "how much to eat," "What to eat," "How to eat," "Which food prevents Cancer" or "Which fruit/leaf has anti-Cancer properties." These questions have nuanced answers. However, some basic rules may be followed as there are numerous unverified unscientific claims and advice by unqualified people.

In a nutshell,

a)   How much to eat? – Start mind mapping.

b)   What to eat? – Anything fresh, local, and home-made preferably.

c)   How to eat? – in the way your ancestors have asked you to eat.

These are simple solutions for complex questions. Hence professional guidance is always advisable.

Go Indian

Indian diets are naturally anti-Cancer in nature. The staple food that is chosen, irrespective of the region, consists of complex carbohydrates, protein in the form of lentils/dals (pulses) or animal protein, fiber and vitamins-minerals in the form of fruits and vegetables (curries/subzis/dals/sambars), probiotics, (khadi/buttermilk/curd/fermented foods) and, majorly spices. Although these diets are nutritionally balanced, here are a few places we go wrong.

a)   **The ingredients used** (most of the ingredients are ready to eat or ready-made or hormonally injected, especially with the animal products – milk, eggs, chicken).

b)   **The cooking method** (most of us do not cook, and we end up ordering foods online or we have someone else cook for us who use an excess of oil/dalda/vanaspati or even as simple as using baking soda to ferment the idli/dosa batter).

c) **Using of ovens frequently or lack of fresh** home-made **food** (we are so used to heating- reheating food or food packets proven to be carcinogenic in the long run. Also, using of plastic and polyethylene-like materials for sauteing, frying, and cooking is known to be carcinogenic since they are made of PVCs and Teflon. Hence, using iron vessels for cooking (like in the olden days) and using earthen metal pots (matkas) for storing water is beneficial.

d) An advantage of storing water in earthen pots is that it saves you from micro-nutrient deficiency like Selenium, Copper, and Zinc. Cooking in iron vessels helps absorb iron, giving you better Hb levels.

e) **Usage of ready-to-eat or processed foods/fast foods.**

A few corrective/preventive actions that can be included in our diet are:

f) **Include a fruit (at least a min of 2) daily.**

Any local, seasonal fruit can be consumed, "a fruit over a juice" is recommended. Also, remember to include fruits that do not have an English equivalent (which is grown exclusively in your region) Ex: Lakshmanphal, Ramphal.

g) **Include a serving of vegetables (more dark-colored vegetables) in every meal, preferably in the cooked form (a dal/a subzi/a soup/stir-fried form).**

Avoid having raw salads because the nutritional value of a vegetable is best extracted only when a vegetable is treated with a tadka and when it is cooked at a decent (medium flame) temperature. Cooking at a very high temperature can hamper the B vitamins. Also, when consumed raw, these vegetables can cause food poisoning.

Include spices in every form of cooking (in the form of a dal/subzi/chutney) – Ex – turmeric milk, turmeric in dal and subzi, cinnamon in sweets, cardamom in tea/coffee, ginger in chutney or ginger in tadka, coriander seeds in the form of any home-made concoction or any other local spice that is native to your cuisine. These spices are anti-inflammatory, help lower the LDL and Triglycerides, aid in weight loss, and have anti-Cancer properties. Example – Curcumin of turmeric(To boost the myth – lemon-ginger-honey water doesn't aid in weight loss; in the long run, it changes your pH. Hence, read about the scientific benefits and research about it before you start any fad).

h) **Include hand-pound rice or rice that is single polished or millets that are not refined/processed.**

Most of the time, the flour we use (wheat/ragi) is mainly refined, and they are also adulterated with maida, which is nutritionally poor. It is also seen that "gluten" based products are pro-inflammatory (cause inflammation) in the body. It could result in bloating, muscle catch, acidity, and skin rashes in some people. Hence, it is advisable to reduce the consumption of refined wheat flour, or anything processed; instead, substitute it with healthy alternatives like a barnyard, Kodo, proso, foxtail millet, finger millet, jowar, or bajra. Example: 1. A pizza with a Wheat/Maida-based crust can be replaced with Ragi/finger millet as a base. 2. A millet-based biryani is a better alternative than rice-based biryani. Millets keep you full for an extended period and prevent you from over-eating.

i) **Including a wholesome, balanced meal.**

There is a lot of "nutritionism" (like racism) in the country. Fitness enthusiasts and the so-called "certified nutritionists" have started addressing food in the name of Protein, Fats, and Carbohydrates. Many people have concluded that by cutting down on one food group and increasing the other food group on your plate, you gain benefits concerning weight and health. I also know many people who weigh their food, thinking about calorie counting and calorie deficit. I am not against it, but counting calories or weighing food doesn't help you prevent Cancer. You need to consider the quality of the food, if the food is fresh or home-made. If the food is local, regional, and traditional to our cuisine, and most importantly, food that takes time to reach you always loses its nutritional value. So folks, eat a good masala dosa in Bangalore, have a gud-ghajak in Lucknow, or have broccoli in California or pizza in Italy.

Also, keep in mind that just increasing the portion size of a particular food group doesn't prevent you from Cancer. What matters is consuming a "balanced" meal where the pulses (lentils, dals), cereals, and vegetables along with probiotics (home-set curd/buttermilk) are in equal proportion without over-eating/overdoing and, of course, at the same time, meeting the daily requirements of the RDA (Recommended Daily Allowance).

(**NOTE:** The above advice is written keeping only the preventive actions for Cancer in mind. Other co-morbidities like Hypothyroidism, Diabetes Mellitus, Renal conditions, Pregnancy-lactation, or any of the heart conditions are not considered).

RDA gives different recommendations based on age, gender, physical activity levels, and physiological condition.

j)   The USDA recommends that 45 to 65 percent of your total daily calories come from carbohydrates. Make sure that it comes from complex carbohydrates.

k)   The American Dietetic Association (ADA) recommends daily protein intake for healthy adults as 0.8-1.0 g of protein/kg body weight. However, it is subject to change when the person is involved in sports or any physiological condition.

l)   Fat intake should equal 30% of your total daily calories.

It is advisable to modify your diet based on these recommendations.

The right type of nutrition prevents Cancer, helps combat infections and diseases, improves immunity, lowers blood cholesterol, improves insulin resistance, and aids in weight loss and fertility.

Conclusion

Writing about Cancer exclusively, we need to understand that like Rome wasn't built overnight, it takes consistent effort, nutritional discipline, and patience to maintain good health nutritionally and lifestyle, preventing us from developing a condition like Cancer.

After doing much research and going through the literature, I want to tell all the readers the harsh truth that there is no magic pill, superfood, or magic recipe for preventing Cancer.

It entirely depends on the foundation that you've constructed your diet upon.

Indicators that one needs to look for are:

a) How many times/week do you order fod through an online platform?

b) How many times/week do you tend to binge eat or overeat?

c) How many times/week do you indulge yourself in a party that contains alcohol?

d) How frequently do you eat fresh- home-made food without re-heating?

e) How often have you carried the previous night's dinner for the next day's lunch?

f) How compliant are you with your exercise?

g) Mainly, how energetic are you in a day without depending on a sweet/smoke/chocolate?

If you tick these boxes, I guess you're always in the pink of your health.

5

ROLE OF YOGA IN PREVENTING CANCER

Ms. Ruchika Dawar

Yoga means union. It is the union of body, mind, and soul. Yoga is that which joins the three. Yoga helps deal with various health issues like obesity, fatigue, hypertension, autoimmune diseases, etc. There is no scientific proof that yoga can cure Cancer. However, it helps prevent Cancer, and plays a significant role there.

Big C Cancer is a greatly feared disease by humanity. Carcinogenic substances, radiations, diet, environment, genetics, and most importantly, the mental and emotional factors form the etiological factors for Cancer. Expensive and extensive Cancer research has pointed to the same culprit, STRESS, as one of the major etiological factors in the causation. Cancer causes about 13% of deaths in the world. The rate at which Cancer spreads – one in three persons will develop Cancer in the developed world.

Until a few decades ago, contagious diseases were the main culprit both in terms of their impact and variety. Non – communicable Diseases (NCD) are now creating havoc. They are also called Psycho-somatic Diseases whose cause is now within, and so is the cure. NCDs are generally slow in progression. The four main NCDs are –

1.   Cardiovascular diseases (CDV).

2.   Cancers.

3.   Chronic Respiratory Diseases.

4.   Diabetes.

NCDs have been labeled as idiopathic, meaning "a condition that arises spontaneously or for which the cause is unknown." What is treated is only the symptom of the disease, but not its roots. The two main factors for the development of NCD are- wrong lifestyle and stress.

A wrong lifestyle includes sedentary work – routine, lack of physical exercise, bad food habits, smoking and alcohol, lack of exposure to nature, etc. Stress is not in the situation outside but in our response to it. "Stress is Response," not the problem itself.

Bhagavad-Gita shloka 5.23

śhaknotīhaivayaḥsoḍhuṁprākśharīra-vimokṣhaṇāt

kāma-krodhodbhavaṁvegaṁsayuktaḥsasukhīnaraḥ

Meaning- He who can withstand before the liberation from the body(death), the speed born of desire and anger, is Yogi, a happy man. The key word here is "speed." Stress is the form of unrestrained psychological momentum that forcefully drags us along with it. This refers to the mental distress born out of seriousness in worldly pursuits. But "speed" can also refer to the general working of the mind. When we play a sport, the mind is to be fast. This speed is good. It makes our transactions productive and efficient. Speed without brakes is life-threatening.

An episode of stress response like anger or grief triggers physiological arousal in the body. The stress response is a necessary emergency mechanism to activate when survival is at stake.

Yoga has three main elements:

1.   Physical yoga or Asanas.

2.   Breathing techniques.

3.   Meditation or Mindfulness.

There is a strong connection between the body and mind and the disease it causes in the body. According to yoga, the human body is divided into five sheaths of existence or koshas.

1.   Annamaya kosha- The physical body.

2.   Pranamaya kosha- The pranic energy.

3.   Manomaya kosha- Mental body.

4.   Vijnanamaya kosha- Wisdom body.

5.   Anandmaya kosha – Bliss body.

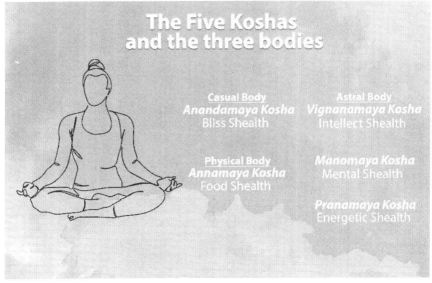

Figure 1

These layers range from the gross to the most subtle. These sheaths are not independent of the other. These are interdependent, interrelated, and interpenetrable from each other. If one of these layers is disturbed, it affects the different layers.

Cancer is a mind-body disease. Cancer is an imbalance at different levels-

a) At the physical level- An imbalance between naturally existing protectors of healthy cells and promoters of unhealthy cell production.

b) At the psychological level- Negative emotions, anger, fear, depression.

c) In the social group- Loneliness, rejection.

d) At the Genetic level- Mutated genes.

e) Immune system- Chronic inflammation.

f) Mechanical carcinogens- Repeated injuries.

g) Physical carcinogens- Nuclear radiation, microwave, radiations from mobiles.

We will look at an integrated approach to yoga therapy for Cancer prevention and treatment.

1. Annamaya kosha practices- We are what we eat. "Food is thy medicine"-Socrates.

    Eating a sattvic diet is very important. A diet with loads of fresh fruits, vegetables, greens, whole grains, nuts and seeds, legumes, etc. High fiber, anti-oxidants (Vitamin C&E), and Phytochemicals in plant products have a protective effect. Foods to be avoided are- red meat, processed foods, meat and fish cooked at high temperatures, and all junk foods.

As per yogic philosophy, we have three types of foods:

a) Saatvik food- foods that nourish the body and provide strength and purity to the mind. – all fresh fruits and vegetables.

b) Rajasic food- foods that stimulate the nervous system.

c) Tamasic food – foods that make the mind lazy and dull. Stale food; non-vegetarian foods.

2. Asana and kriya practice – These practices aim to give deep rest to the sick organ or to the part of the body where the imbalance has settled down, cleanse the inner passages, remove tardiness of cellular activities by opening up blocked channels, and build up stamina.

Kriyas are cleansing practices that help cleanse the inner passages. – egjal neti, sutra neti.

3. Pranayama Kosha- Prana is the basic fabric of the whole creation. Nothing is more essential to our health and well-being than breathing- take in air- let it out, repeat 25000 times daily. Modern research shows that by making slight adjustments to how we inhale and exhale, we can rejuvenate internal organs, allergies, asthma, autoimmune diseases, etc. Breathwork is needed like-Breath awareness, anulomvilom, nadishuddhi, kapalbhati.

4. Manomaya Kosha- "You are what you think"-Swami Vivekananda.

According to psychologists mind is the total of all the cognitive functions carried out by the wakeful mind. Maintaining silence, Mind sound resonance technique, Chanting mantras.

5. Vijnanmaya Kosha- In humans, the intellect has reached such a level that we Cn do introspection.

6. Anandmaya Kosha- The search for happiness forms the basis of yoga. Happiness is silencing the mind.

6

HOLISTIC THERAPIES TO PREVENT A CANCER RELAPSE

Dr. Samara Mahindra

What are integrative and holistic therapies?

Integrative and holistic therapies inculcate a multidisciplinary approach focusing on a patient's overall well-being. This could include psycho-social, physical, nutritional, emotional, and spiritual factors, and mainstream medical treatment. Conventional forms of medical therapy provide a symptomatic approach, analyzing the patient's symptoms and evaluating the correct treatment methodology to treat those symptoms and heal the patient effectively. Today, however, research is pointing towards the importance and effectiveness of a holistic approach that integrates conventional medical treatment with other factors, as listed above, to provide complete therapy and treatment for the patient.

About Integrative Oncology

Integrative oncology is a form of integrative therapy specific for Cancer and is the diagnosis-specific field of integrative medicine, addressing symptom control with non-pharmacologic therapies. Known commonly as "complementary therapies," these are evidence-based adjuncts to mainstream care that effectively control physical and emotional symptoms, enhance physical and emotional strength, and provide Cancer patients with skills enabling them to help themselves throughout their Cancer journey.

Integrative oncology focuses on building a comprehensive, evidence-based approach to Cancer care that combines standard Cancer treatments and integrative therapies to improve patient clinical outcomes.

These integrative oncology therapies mainly focus on managing treatment side-effects, improving recovery rates, quality of life, and survival, and decreasing side effects of conventional therapies that may be toxic. Research has shown that such treatments may be essential to effectively manage pain, fatigue, stress, neuropathy and malnutrition.

Sometimes the side effects from the treatment are so extreme that the treatment needs to be halted for a while until the patient recovers. To help reduce or avoid those interruptions, many oncologists are turning to an integrative approach to care. This approach involves using supportive care therapies to help Cancer patients manage their side effects while treating the disease with surgery, chemotherapy, radiation therapy, immunotherapy, or other conventional methods.

With increasing education, awareness and acceptance by healthcare providers, and traditional institutions, integrative modalities could be equally valued between patients and providers. Furthermore, increased availability, and utilization of integrative oncology modalities at tertiary hospitals could improve patient satisfaction, quality of life, and other clinical endpoints.

Components of integrative therapies

Integrative therapies are often called non-clinical and non-medical treatments that contribute to a patient's healing. Integration oncology promotes the integration of conventional, nutritional, lifestyle and complementary medicine to improve the lives of people affected by Cancer. These can encompass multiple elements that can impact a patient on some level. Standard integrative therapies include mind-body methods (meditation, yoga, music therapy, spirituality, and art therapy), herbs and supplements, and other therapies such as massage therapy and acupuncture. Along with this, nutrition and physical therapies are essential in integrative therapies. There is growing evidence of the effect of physical therapy on managing Cancer patients' symptoms and the role nutrition plays in improving the nutritional deficiencies caused by Cancer treatment. All of which contribute to expediting the recovery of the patient.

How do integrative therapies relate to Cancer?

Cancer is a complex disease that affects multiple facets of a person. Cancer impacts the body, mind and spirit of any individual. While Cancer or tumor makes itself evident through the body and the physical symptoms caused to the individual, Cancer also affects the nutritional status of the person, as well as their psychological and spiritual well-being. Therefore, just treating the physical body or physical symptoms is not enough. The side effects of treatment can also cause considerable discomfort through pain, fatigue, weight loss, nausea, digestive issues, anxiety, fear, and stress. All of which need a multidisciplinary approach to be treated. Hence integrative therapies are implemented for treating Cancer. This treats patients as a whole, and all aspects of healing are considered, including food, body and mind.

Nutrition and Cancer

When it comes to nutrition and Cancer, much research has pointed toward certain foods and nutrients that may help prevent or, conversely, contribute to certain types of Cancer. While there are many factors you can't change that increase your Cancer risks, such as genetics and environment, there are others you can control. Estimates suggest that less than 30% of a person's lifetime risk of Cancer results from uncontrollable factors. The rest you can change, including your diet, improves your quality of life.

Over the last 25 years, science has shown that diet, physical activity, and body weight, especially being overweight or obese, are major risk factors for developing certain Cancers. Your body's ability to resist Cancer may be helped by following a healthy diet, staying physically active and avoiding excess body fat. Study after study suggests that a healthy diet is rich in a variety of vegetables, fruits, whole grains and legumes (beans) and low in red and (especially) processed meat, which can fight Cancer. This will ensure our immune system works efficiently to fight harmful Cancer cells.

When you are healthy, eating enough food is often fine. But this can be a real challenge when dealing with Cancer and Cancer treatment. A Cancer diet might require extra protein and calories. More liquid or semi-liquid nutritional recommendations are provided for chewing and swallowing obstructions. Sometimes, one might need to eat low-fiber foods instead of those with high fiber. Therefore, following a customized and personalized Cancer diet is essential. Research suggests that eating well benefits people during and after Cancer treatment.

The nutrition needs of people with Cancer vary from person to person. A Cancer care team often helps identify nutrition goals and plan ways to achieve them.

Below are a few ways a Cancer nutrition diet can benefit a patient:

1. Management of nutritional deficiencies due to Cancer or Cancer treatment.

2. Improvement in gut health.

3. Decrease collateral damage the treatment can cause.

4. Management of blood counts, which can dramatically decrease due to Cancer treatment.

5. Improvement in fatigue, energy, and strength.

6. Maintain weight and the body's store of nutrients.

7. Better tolerate treatment and side effects.

8. Lower the risk of infection.

9. Expedite healing and recovery.

10. Improve immunity.

11. Improve overall quality of life.

Good nutrition should be implemented as the following practice for healing and recovery. It's the foundation of health and contributes towards building a robust immune system and, as a result, effectively managing the side effects of treatment and improving quality of life during and post-treatment.

Physical therapy and Cancer

Exercise is an integral part of a Cancer treatment plan. A growing amount of research shows that regular exercise can significantly improve physical and mental health during every phase of treatment. Exercise has been shown to improve cardiovascular fitness, muscle strength, body composition, fatigue, anxiety, depression, and several quality-of-life factors in Cancer patients and survivors.

Following a well-designed exercise plan during and after treatment will help Cancer patients reduce the chance of having physical side effects, such as fatigue, neuropathy, lymphedema, osteoporosis, and nausea. Exercise helps to reduce the risk of depression and anxiety and also keeps a patient as mobile and independent as possible. Moreover, exercise helps to prevent weight gain and obesity, which are linked to increased Cancer risk and improved quality of life.

Taking precautions while exercising is essential if a patient has side effects from Cancer or its treatment. One may have to change an exercise plan depending on specific side effects. Even if a patient was physically active before Cancer treatment, the activity level must gradually be built post-treatment. If treatment has weakened the immune system, large and crowded gyms must be avoided, where germs can spread quickly. If energy levels are low, an adjustment must be made on how long or strenuous the exercise should be. The right foods, significantly high in protein, help the body recover after a workout.

As we all know, Cancer has major physical strains on the body, and loss of muscle mass, and range of motion might be affected due to surgery and the treatment side effects. There are tried and tested movement patterns that have improved functional mobility, hormonal levels, pain, strength, and physical and mental symptoms of patients.

Therapeutic yoga practices, physiotherapy and functional movement exercises help patients with the physical and mental strains of Cancer. The focus is on stretching and strengthening muscles, pain management, stimulating the digestive, lymphiatic, circulatory system and breathing techniques that help balance the body and mind.

Mental well-being and Cancer

A patient's psychological well-being is integral in managing the disease and coping with Cancer treatment. As Cancer affects the mind, causing substantial emotional and mental distress, working the reason appropriately is essential. Fear, anxiety, stress, and depression are all everyday psychological stresses regularly felt and can hinder healing and recovery. Some patients lose faith in their ability to recover, negatively impacting their treatment response.

Here are a few points to keep in mind when a patient is on Cancer treatment:

1. Understanding and accepting the diagnosis.

2. Knowing the side effects and contacting therapists who can guide and handhold the patient.

3. Finding support programs and services.

4. Balancing your food, body, and mind and paying attention to each.

Here are some of the ways that can help manage the mind:

1. Having a consistent support system (Family, friends, pets).

2. Being organized with time and medical information.

3. Spending time with loved ones.

4. Embracing one's passion.

5. Remembering to pay attention to the breath and practicing meditation.

6. Listening to and reading inspiring stories.

7. Connecting with other Cancer patients or survivors who have experienced a similar situation.

There are many emotions to process during a Cancer diagnosis. Not only is it emotional and exhausting, but it can be stressful as well. It's surprising to what extent diet, exercise and sleep affect one's stress levels. Meditation is highly effective and has been proven to affect stress and the physiological state of being profound. Breathing and pranayama are also very effective at low anxiety and stress levels.

As stress plays a significant factor during and after Cancer treatment, below are a few ways to manage stress better:

1. **Spending time outdoors.**

    Getting fresh air and a dose of greenery can be incredibly relaxing and refreshing. Outdoors is an excellent remedy for depression, anxiety, and stress. Walking in nature can be therapeutic and can substantially improve mental health.

2. **Limiting alcohol, caffeine and nicotine.**

    Though often considered a stress-relieving vice, alcohol, nicotine, and caffeine cause sleeplessness and anxiety, contributing to the body's stress response.

3. **Asking for and accepting assistance.**

    Many people will offer to help in various ways. While it might be awkward or uncomfortable for some to accept help, it can sometimes be highly beneficial in calming the mind.

4. **Exercise.**

    Physical activity will help a patient stay in better shape, keep the body active and energized, and is known to improve mental health and eliminate stress. Exercise is one of the essential tools in the fight against stress during Cancer treatment.

5. **Joining a support group.**

    Sometimes, even when friends and family have the best of intentions, they cannot understand what a Cancer patient is going through undergoing Cancer treatment. A support group can alleviate stress because one can talk about Cancer-related issues with people who genuinely understand.

Why does Cancer reoccur, and how can we use integrative therapies to manage a recurrence?

Cancer recurrence can contribute to many factors. It's often difficult to pinpoint one definitive cause for a Cancer recurrence, as they are usually related to multiple reasons. One of the contributing factors can be a lifestyle that predominately involves nutrition, a sedentary lifestyle or high-fat percentages, chronic stress, hormonal disruptions, excessive alcohol, smoking, and other environmental factors that can suppress the immune system. With suppressed immunity, Cancer can develop once again, as the mainline of defense cannot fight off or eradicate the harmful effects of free radicals caused by these poor lifestyle habits. In this case, integrative therapies play an imperative role in reducing risks associated with Cancer recurrence. While integrative therapies cannot guarantee to stop a Cancer recurrence, they most definitely can decrease the possibility of it and help the body withstand the side effects of a Cancer relapse.

How do integrative therapies impact a Cancer recurrence?

As explained earlier, integrative therapies mainly include lifestyle mechanisms, or broadly put, food, body, and mind in managing Cancer and the side effects of Cancer treatment. While lifestyle can contribute to Cancer relapse, integrative therapies can control and reduce the risk. Suppose a person were to manage their lifestyle efficiently. Eat nutritious foods, maintain a healthy weight, manage stress and live an overall healthy lifestyle that boosts immunity and health; the possibility of Cancer relapse is less. Integrative therapies promote a holistic approach to overall health and well-being.

How can integrative therapies be implemented into a daily routine to decrease the chances of a Cancer relapse?

Food

Many studies help us find a link between diet and Cancer, either from a preventive approach or by associating the consumption of certain food products with tumor generation and growth. However, with the development of holistic therapies in treating and recovering from Cancer, nutrition is an emerging science that relies on well-established factors such as genetic and epigenetic variations and the microbiome. It has recently been shown that treating human cell lines with different bioactive foodstuffs influences their physiological attributes depending on their ability to control the expression of other genes. The possibility of using nutritional therapies against Cancer as a complementary medicine is internationally accepted due to its advantages of less toxicity and better acceptance by patients. It's found to be easy and accessible by patients as they feel comfortable with the food.

Specific side effects like Nausea, weight loss or weight gain, loss of appetite, changed taste, etc., are nutrition-related issues that develop due to Cancer treatments like chemotherapy, radiation, etc. These deficiencies can lead to other health-related problems and weakened immune systems. To avoid this or minimize the nutritional deficiencies that might occur due to the Cancer treatment or Cancer itself, here are a few areas to focus on post-Cancer treatment.

Gut health

Gut health is essential when considering rebuilding the immune system and avoiding a Cancer relapse. Our gut contains certain beneficial bacteria that help us to fight multiple illnesses. These bacteria, termed 'Microbiome', support us in better nutrition absorption. Our body has trillions of such microbiomes.

We can provide these bacteria through food in the form of Probiotics to our bodies. Probiotics, thus, help us maintain a healthy gut. It also helps in maintaining intestinal homeostasis. Probiotics are live microorganisms that are administered through food in our bodies. The sources of probiotics are generally fermented foods like yoghurt, sauerkraut, kimchi, kefir, etc. However, for these probiotics to survive, we need to give them food. The food that these organisms survive on is called prebiotics. The sources of prebiotics are vegetables such as cabbage, broccoli, cucumber, etc. There is much of evidence that using probiotics can be essential in Cancer prevention and support anti-Cancer therapies. As a result of laboratory research, many promising results were obtained, indicating probiotics' anti-tumor effect.

Antioxidants

Antioxidants are the compounds that neutralize free radicals in our bodies. Free radicals, when combined with carcinogenic compounds, initiate tumor growth. Hence to avoid relapse, antioxidants do play a significant role. Antioxidants include Vitamin E, Vitamin C and many phytochemicals. Antioxidants are majorly found in colorful fruits and vegetables. Studies suggest that people who eat more vegetables and fruits, which are rich sources of antioxidants, may have a lower risk for Cancer. Because Cancer survivors may be at increased risk for second Cancers, they should eat various antioxidant-rich foods daily. Hence, it is advisable to make the plate colorful by adding different fruits and vegetables to your diet.

Exercise

Many studies show active movement and physical exercise during, and post-treatment are beneficial in keeping the side effects of treatment to the minimum and expediting recovery post-Cancer. Re-building the immune system, increasing strength, stamina, and muscle mass, and reducing fatigue are achieved primarily through physical movement and exercise.

Here are some tips for Cancer survivors:

a) Avoid inactivity.
b) Any physical activity helps, even if it is not moderate or vigorous. More studies are showing that being inactive increases the risk of some Cancers. Being passive, or sedentary, means you spend most of your time sitting without physical activity.
c) Try to get at least 150 minutes of moderate or 75 minutes of vigorous activity each week. Try spreading these activities throughout the week. However, getting this much exercise over 1 to 2 days also helps. Try to include some exercises to help you keep lean muscle mass and bone strength, like exercising with a resistance band or light weights. It would be best if you consisted of exercises that will increase your flexibility and control the range of motion in your joints.
d) Include strength training.
e) Lift weights and do other muscle-building exercises at least two days a week. Strength or resistance training helps you maintain and build strong muscles. Increasing muscle mass can improve your balance, reduce fatigue, and make it easier to do daily activities.
f) If you do not have time or energy for long exercise sessions, go for shorter periods. The health benefits of several short, 10-minute segments are similar to those of 1 more extended exercise session. Try short periods of exercise with frequent rest breaks. For example, walk briskly for a few minutes, slow down, and walk briskly again until you have done 30 minutes of brisk activity. You can also divide your workout into three 10-minute sessions. You'll still get the benefit of the exercise.
g) If you are new to exercise, slowly increase the length and intensity of your physical activity. An exercise regime must be implemented based on your current physical activity level and expert advice. What may be a low- or moderate-intensity activity for a healthy person may seem like a high-intensity activity for some Cancer survivors. Take your time and patience as you gradually increase your activity.

Components of an Effective Exercise Program for Survivors

A. Relaxation breathing

Research shows that relaxation breathing can help reduce stress and anxiety during recovery. During relaxation breathing, the goal is to breathe slowly and deeply. Being aware of your breath can have a calming effect and allow you to focus your energy on s healing.

B. Aerobic exercise

i) Aerobic exercise is essential to good health. Any movement that elevates your heart rate and breathing counts as aerobic.

ii) Walking is one of the easiest ways to get aerobic exercise. You might be able to walk for only a few minutes at first, but you'll gradually get stronger. Try to walk farther each session until you can walk for 30 to 45 minutes daily. Aim for 15 minutes 1 to 3 times daily if this isn't possible.

C. Stretching

Stretching regularly can gradually improve your posture, range of motion, and flexibility. The older you are, the more critical daily stretching is to maintain flexibility. You may need to do each stretching exercise 2 to 5 times daily at the beginning of your recovery.

D. Strength training

1) Improve your balance and posture by strengthening your core.
2) Improve your quality of life by making activities more accessible and enjoyable.
3) Empower you physically and mentally.
4) Restore strength.
5) Through strength training, you can gain muscle. Strength training helps build bone density. That's important because many Cancer treatments can increase the risk of osteoporosis which causes weak and brittle bones.

Mind-Body Therapies

Mind-body practices can be defined as techniques to help modify biological, physiological, or psychosocial processes and improve quality of life outcomes. Mind-body therapies can make a substantial impact by helping patients. Families reduce anxiety and depression, manage their emotions, engage in decision-making, reduce adverse effects of Cancer treatments and procedures, manage pain, stimulate an immune response, deal with loss, plan for the future, support the will to live, and, if necessary, come to terms with end-of-life issues.

People's daily choices concerning diet, physical activity, and how they deal with stress are the most prominent domain of influence over health prospects. A growing body of research indicates that mind-body therapies are safe and effective ways of mitigating physical and emotional symptoms.

Meditation

Meditation is not forcing your mind to ignore or mitigate thoughts that might appear while you sit in silently, focusing on your breath. Most people cannot meditate because they find it difficult to do so. It's impossible to eradicate thoughts from your mind; during meditation, you must allow your ideas to flow in and out; the difference is that you shouldn't react to them or be emotionally stimulated by them. This enables one to enter into a relaxed state of being, in which the mind rests and the body is not physically stimulated or charged. The outcome is the release of endorphins and where the parasympathetic nervous system kicks in. This has proven to have an incredible impact on the body and its healing. Meditation comes in many forms, chanting, visual meditation, guided meditation, deep breathing, sound therapy and even, at times, gardening and cooking, which can be highly relaxing and therapeutic to many people. Indulging in some form of meditation can profoundly impact stress levels, inflammation, gut health, and immunity. Cancer survivors, while clearly from the disease, still suffer significant stress and anxiety. Fear of relapse, finding a new normal, returning to work, retaining and strengthening personal relationships, etc. Meditation must become an integral part of your healing journey. It helps manage unwarranted stress and anxiety and improves the overall quality of life.

Sleep

Often sleep is overlooked as a crucial part of a Cancer patient's overall treatment plan. According to The National Sleep Foundation, sleep is a significant component in boosting the immune system. "Without sufficient sleep, your body makes fewer cytokines, a protein that targets infection and inflammation, effectively creating an immune response. Cytokines are produced and released during sleep, causing a double whammy if you skimp on shut-eye." Sleep deprivation prevents your immune system from building up its forces. If you don't get enough sleep, your body may be unable to fend off invaders, and it may also take longer to recover from illness. Lack of sleep can also create digestive havoc and release the hormone Ghrelin (hunger hormone) that will invariably result in you reaching out for junk food while the assimilation or absorption of nutrients is compromised.

7

MUSIC THERAPY TO PREVENT THE RECURRENCE OF CANCER

Ms. Sujatha Visweswara, Mr. Sridhar Pallia

The risk of Cancer is relatively well-known to the general public. Besides being life-threatening and complex in diagnosis & treatment of Cancer; the emotional upheaval it causes to individuals and their unprepared families is enormous. A Cancer diagnosis generates a higher sense of distress than non-neoplastic diseases with poorer prognoses. High levels of mental distress for sustained periods in Cancer patients may lead to anxiety, depression, or both. This mixed symptomatology is very common, with two-thirds of Cancer patients with depression expressing clinically significant anxiety levels. Depression leads to a poorer quality of life (QOL) and compromises patient outcomes, with depression resulting in higher rates of mortality in Cancer. This also has a higher chance of recurrence of Cancer.

The Cancer burden continues to grow globally, exerting tremendous physical, emotional, and financial strain on individuals, families, communities, and health systems. Stress can be caused by daily responsibilities and, recurring events, and more unusual circumstances, such as a trauma or illness in oneself or a close family member. People are distressed when they feel unable to manage or control changes caused by Cancer or normal life activities. Distress has become increasingly recognized as a factor that can reduce the quality of life of Cancer patients. There is even evidence that extreme distress is associated with poorer clinical outcomes. [115,116]

People with Cancer may find the disease's physical, emotional, and social effects to be stressful. Those who attempt to manage their stress with risky behaviors such as smoking or drinking alcohol or who become more sedentary may have a poorer quality of life after Cancer treatment. In contrast, people who can use effective coping strategies to deal with stress, such as relaxation and stress management techniques, have been shown to have lower levels of depression, anxiety, and symptoms related to Cancer and its treatment.

Emotional and social support can help patients learn to cope with psychological stress. Such support can reduce depression, anxiety, and disease- and treatment-related symptoms among patients.

They are permanent, leave residual disability, are caused by non-reversible pathological alteration, require special training of the patient for rehabilitation, or may be expected to require a long period of supervision, observation, or care.

Achievements have not matched the remarkable advances in biomedical care for Cancer in providing high-quality care for the psychological and social effects of Cancer.

According to National Institute of Health findings, numerous Cancer survivors and their caregivers report that their psychosocial needs were not understood, nor adequately addressed depression and other symptoms of stress, were unaware of or did not refer them to available resources, and generally did not consider psychosocial support to be an integral part of quality Cancer care.

Due to the nature of the disease, its risk of life or residual disabilities, the financial burden, and the need for long-term rehabilitation, the quality of life of the Cancer survivors and their caregivers/families quality of life is significantly impacted. Long-term Cancer survivors' main problems are Cancer social/emotional support, health habits, spiritual/ philosophical view of life, and body image concerns.

The challenge for doctors is to improve the quality of life without any additional pharmacological burden to the patient and also help patients improve QOL post-recovery lead a. Their constant endeavor is to minimize the dependency on medicines wherever possible. This is where using frequency-moderated music comes as a savior for patients to help manage their recovery, and this would aid them in non-occurrence to a great extent.

The Science behind Music Therapy

The auditory sense is one of the basic human senses. In utero, our hearing ability develops by about eighteen weeks, making it one of the earliest senses to develop. By the end of the second trimester, research has shown that a fetus responds specifically to the sounds of the mother's voice. Once out in the world, babies demonstrate a continued preference to the maternal tone. Sound is an essential aspect of our daily lives, playing a role in everything from communication to entertainment. It can affect people differently on people, from calming and relaxing to exciting and energizing.

In its basic form the sound is the vibrations passing through matter through waves. Vibrations transmitted as sounds are measured in hertz (Hz), which captures the frequency with which vibrations occur every second. Om chanting, for instance, is at a frequency of 432 Hz. Similarly, the middle C note on a piano is 262 Hz, meaning there are 262 vibrations every second when that note is struck. By contrast, the fundamental frequency of a typical adult female voice is 165 to 255 Hz, whereas a typical male voice is 85 to 180 Hz. The human auditory system can perceive sounds between of 20 to 20,00 Hz frequencies.

We perceive sounds in a variety of forms. We hear sounds in the form of people speaking, sounds of machines, and sounds of animals, and sounds from nature, such as rain, thunder, water flowing, or the breeze. We also listen to the sound of music or movies. Each type of sound has a range of frequencies and power, affecting listeners positively or negatively. Some sounds are soothing, while others may be irritating or even hazardous. There are also emotions and moods associated with different types of sounds. We associate Music to be the most pleasing form of sound. Unwanted sounds are unpleasant to humans and may cause stress and hypertension [91] as well as affect the cognitive function of children.[92]

What makes music pleasing to the ears that elicit a positive reaction most often? Music is a complex and multi-disciplinary field combining elements of physics, mathematics, physiology, and psychology to create unique and powerful effects. Music is sound that follows certain grammar and syntax. Music is based on the principles of sound waves, including frequency (measured in hertz), amplitude (measured in decibels), and wavelength.

The frequency of a sound wave determines its pitch, while the amplitude determines its volume. By manipulating these properties, musicians can create various sounds, from whispers to powerful crescendos. In addition to the physics of sound, the science of music also includes the study of musical scales, harmony, and rhythm. These elements of music are based on mathematical ratios and principles, such as the relationship between the frequencies of different notes in a scale. The human brain is wired to respond to these patterns in music, which is why it can evoke such strong emotional responses.

The effect of music on the mind is best measured using EEG (electroencephalogram machine). Sound waves are usually visualized as sine waves and have fixed frequencies and amplitudes, perceived as pure tones. EEG and a computer record the subject's brainwave activities in three phases; before, during, and after listening to music to compare the subject's brainwave reaction during these three phases/conditions. The fundamental brain patterns of an individual are obtained by measuring the subject's brain signals during his/her relaxed condition. Brain patterns usually form sinusoidal waves that range from $0.5\mu V$ to $100\mu V$ peak-to-peak amplitude.[97] During the activation of a biological neuron, this complex electrochemical system is able to generate electrical activity, represented in terms of waves comprising of four frequency bands, namely, Delta, Alpha, Theta and Beta.[94] Previous studies have determined that among these four groups, the Beta band has the highest frequency with the lowest amplitude while the Delta band has the lowest frequency with the highest amplitude.[94] The Alpha and

Beta waves reflect a conscious or awake state of mind while Delta and Theta waves indicate the unconscious state. Table below illustrates the brainwave bands and their relation to amplitude, frequency, and functions. [93,94]

Table

Brain wave bands and relation to frequency, amplitude, and function.
[82,93,94]

Brainwaves	Frequency (Hz)	Amplitude (μV)	Functions
Delta	0.1-3	Highest	**Instincts:** Survival, Deep, Sleep, Coma, Dreaming
Theta	4-7	High	**Emotions:** Feelings, Dreams, Drowsy, Idea-ling
Alpha	8-12	Low	**Consciousness:** Awareness of body, Integration of feelings, Relax
Beta	13-40	Lowest	**Concentration:** Thinking, Perception, Mental Activity, Alert

The Delta band, with its lowest frequency (0.1 – 3Hz) and highest amplitude, is particularly active in infants during the first few years of life.[95] It is also known as a key state for healing, regeneration, and rejuvenation. The Delta state, often referred to as being in 'deep sleep,' stimulates the release of human growth hormones, which heightens the synthesis of proteins and mobilizes free fatty acids to provide energy. Delta brainwave conjures an anaesthetic pseudo-drug effect.[96] Theta (4 – 7Hz) is sometimes said to have the same anaesthetic pseudo-drug effect as the Delta band during its lowest frequency (example, 4Hz). [96] It is a state when a person is having a daydream or a short break after a certain task or is unable to recall their short-term memory. Unlike Delta and Theta, the Alpha (8-12Hz) band usually appears when a person is in a conscious condition, such as when a person takes a break after completing a certain task.[93,94] The Alpha state is activated during a calm and relaxed condition.[83] The brain can easily interpret and absorb most data during this state because of the relax-but-aware brain mode.

Sounds of different frequencies have shown to be beneficial in certain conditions. For instance. Historically, a popular finding called Solfeggio frequencies is a set of nine musical frequencies supposedly used in ancient Gregorian chants and said to have spiritual and healing properties, although not empirically tested. The frequencies are: 396 Hz, 417 Hz, 528 Hz, 639 Hz, 741 Hz, 852 Hz, 963 Hz, 174 Hz, and 285 Hz.

Music and Mind-The Relationship

The human nervous system processes music in different ways - perceptual processing, emotional processing, autonomic processing, cognitive processing, and behavioral or motor processing.

Perceptual processing

Although music stimulates some skin receptors by changes in local pressure, it is primarily made of sound waves that enter the primary acoustic circuit through the outer ear. The human primary acoustic circuit involves the auditory nerve, brainstem, medial geniculate body of the thalamus, and the auditory cortex. The auditory brainstem processes the neural signals from the cochlea and sends them to the thalamus, which projects them into the auditory cortex. [103]

Emotional processing

The amygdala, cingulate gyrus, and medial orbitofrontal cortex are involved in the processing of emotional behaviors. Hence, as these structures are found to have auditory projections, these are proposed to be involved in the emotional processing of music. There is evidence also to suggest that music activates these regions. [104,106]

Autonomic processing

Music has been found to induce relaxation and alter pain perception, blood pressure, and respiratory and, heart rates.[107,108] Soft, slow, non-lyrical music significantly decreased systolic blood pressure, heart rate, respiratory rate and oxygen saturation.[108] Music with a faster tempo significantly increased heart rate, minute ventilation, blood pressure, and sympathetic nervous activity, and that music with complex rhythms grew , though insignificantly, the same parameters.[109]

Cognitive processing

The cognitive processing of music is hypothesized under two mechanisms: Affective or indirect mediation and non-affective or direct mediation. Affective mediation basically refers to the activation of specific cognitive networks by means of the activation of emotional music-processing networks.[110]

Behavioral or motor processing

Behavioral response to music is most evident in the form of dancing. Functional brain imaging has shown that music activates the cerebellum, basal ganglia, and motor area. These areas are reported to coordinate motor movement in response to music. [111,112] Activation of the mirror neurons, the praecuneus region of the parietal lobe, the pre-supplementary motor area, the supplemental motor area, the dorsal premotor cortex, the dorsolateral prefrontal cortex, the inferior parietal lobule, and lobule VI of the cerebellum is seen during dancing or tapping to musical beats.[113]

Hemispheric heterogeneity

Although music is traditionally thought to be mainly processed (i.e., perceptually) in the right hemisphere, according to the modular theory of music perception, different aspects of music are processed in distinct, although partly overlapping, neuronal networks in both cerebral hemispheres with considerable subjective variability. Melody processing is proposed to specialize the right hemisphere, whereas the left hemisphere is postulated to be specialized in rhythm processing.

Neurochemistry

Dopamine is postulated to be involved in the enjoyment of music.[104] It is demonstrated to be released from the ventral striatum and in the ventral tegmental area in subjects listening to pleasant music.[114] In addition, role of endorphins/endocannabinoids and nitrous oxide in emotional perception of music and in producing physical effects such as vasodilatation, local warming of the skin and, a reduction in blood pressure as a response to listening music respectively are described.[104]

How Does Therapeutic Music help Cancer patients?

A Cancer diagnosis generates a higher sense of distress than non-neoplastic diseases with poorer prognoses.[117] High levels of mental distress for sustained periods of time in Cancer patients may lead to anxiety, depression, or both.[118] This mixed symptomatology is very common, with two thirds of Cancer patients with depression also expressing clinically significant levels of anxiety.[119]

Depression leads to a poorer quality of life (QOL) and compromises patient outcomes, with depression resulting in higher rates of mortality in Cancer.[120,121] A meta-analysis revealed that minor or major depression increases mortality rates by up to 39% and that patients displaying even few depressive symptoms may be at a 25% increased risk of mortality.[122] The impact of mood and mental well-being on Cancer progression is considered important by doctors and patients, with >70% of oncologists and 85% of patients believing that mood affects the progression of Cancer.[123]

Music energizes mood, music is a great stress buster, music drives away blues, and music soothes souls. Music therapy is increasingly being used to address the physical, emotional, cognitive, and social needs of individuals. Music therapy has been used to improve various diseases in different research areas, such as rehabilitation, [85-90] public health, clinical care, and psychology. There are studies that show a positive effect of music on common conditions of a patient undergoing chemotherapy such as reducing the severity of pain, anxiousness, nausea, and stress.[98,99] Music can decrease preoperative anxiety, reduce intraoperative sedative and analgesic requirements, and increase patient satisfaction.[100,102] Active music engagement allowed the patients to reconnect with the healthy parts of themselves, even in the face of a debilitating condition or disease-related suffering. The safety and efficacy of Music and its ease of adoption make it a compelling proposition to adopt in the Cancer risk spectrum of people both as a preventive measure and the recovery phase for a healthier lifestyle.

8

PRE-CANCEROUS CONDITIONS – A RADIOLOGIST'S PERSPECTIVE

Dr. Govindarajan MJ

Cancer is the final stage of prolonged abnormal cell division, eventually leading to malignant tissue. Pre-Cancerous condition, as the name implies, is a stage before Cancer development; a stage of a lesion involving abnormal cells with an increased risk of malignancy [124] before actual malignancy emerges. Generally, converting a Precancerous condition to Cancer depends on the potential risk of the lesion becoming Cancer; the conversion percentage varies for different conditions, as does time taken to become Cancer. However, a Precancerous lesion will be Cancerous even when the carcinogenic agent is withdrawn.

Some relatively common examples of Precancerous conditions are colonic polyps developing into colon Cancers, hepatic adenomas developing into hepatoma, cervical dysplasia developing into cervical carcinoma, intraductal papillary neoplasm of pancreas developing into pancreatic Cancers, etc. Even though many known Precancerous conditions can be diagnosed pathologically, only a few can be detected by imaging; those which can be identified on imaging are relatively well documented with a few specific features attributing to frequent detection across various imaging modalities; also, many of these are identified in patients at risk of developing Cancers, like heavy smokers, familial history of Cancer (breast and colon). Identifying a target population to implement imaging modalities for identifying Precancerous lesions is imperative if the tests are efficient. A thin line exists between 'early diagnosis of Cancer' and 'detecting the Precancerous condition.' Early diagnosis is probably the most practical imaging methodology for reducing the morbidity and mortality from Cancer, whereas detecting a Precancerous lesion is perhaps the ideal way of preventing Cancer, though the latter is more challenging and easier said than done; as mentioned earlier, imaging plays only a minor role in the latter as only a tiny percentage of Precancerous lesions are detectable on imaging. A radiologist, being a specialist in medical imaging, needs to know these limited conditions to make a proper identification resulting in appropriate treatment.

"this will inevitably become cancer"

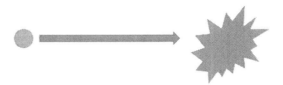

Fig. 1. Precancerous lesion eventually developing into Cancer.

Causes and Process: There are several unknowns concerning the process of carcinogenesis; the three integral components are the carcinogenic agent, the actual pathological process of carcinogenesis, and the host, which is the susceptible tissue /cell/organ. The susceptible host has to get exposed to a sufficient quantity of the carcinogen for a minimum amount of time to start the process of carcinogenesis. This process begins at the intracellular level by changing the genes responsible for the division of cells. The agents are either ionizing radiation, chemicals, toxins, or chronic irritation/inflammation.

Once the process starts, the cells are diverted to the path of carcinogenesis; then it is only understandable that these cells eventually result in Cancer even when the carcinogen is removed from their milieu; however, the time required varies for different Cancers and depends on other extrinsic factors like concentration of the carcinogen, susceptibility of the host, type of cell, etc. It can be argued then that detection of the Precancerous condition is nothing but early detection; the fact of the matter is that Cancer, by pathological definition, is a tumor having components of infiltration of the basement membrane with neoangiogenesis (development of new defective capillaries to feed its cells), which is when the potential of the tumor to spread across the body becomes exponential. In other words, imaging in the above context focuses on detecting pre-invasive Cancers.

In general, there are only a handful of conditions where imaging is used as a screening tool for identifying early Cancers and Precancerous conditions, namely, breast, lungs, and colon; even these are not well accepted as standard screening methods in India and maybe barring breast Cancer screening to a certain extent, as the cost of mass screening may be prohibitive, given the lower prevalence of these Cancers in India, as compared to the developed countries. Hence, a radiologist may occasionally come across a Precancerous condition as an incidental finding on an imaging study performed for other clinical indications; it is in this setting that a "don't miss" approach needs to be adhered to as identification of these lesions can save lives and reduce mortality, morbidity, and financial burden to that particular individual.

Precancerous conditions in the breast: Breast Cancer screening is possibly one of the most effective Cancer screening programs globally and undoubtedly the most efficient method of reducing the breast Cancer burden among humans. There are different imaging modalities for the breast, including Mammography, Ultrasound, Magnetic Resonance Imaging (MRI), Positron Emission Tomography, Computed Tomography (PET CT), thermography, and Computed Tomography (CT) scan. Generally accepted screening protocols include annual mammography after the age of 40 years. However, earlier commencement of the yearly screening is recommended for high-risk groups with MRI added to specific risk types (like BRCA mutation-positive individuals).

Even though screening targets early detection of breast Cancer, along the process, it identifies many Precancerous conditions, namely in situ Cancers like ductal and lobular carcinomas (DCIS and LCIS), atypical ductal hyperplasia (ADH), papillary neoplasms, radial scar, etc.

DCIS is typically identified as clustered pleomorphic microcalcifications that X-Ray mammography can identify; it is also the most common Cancer detected in breast Cancer screening programs, amounting to almost 25% of all breast Cancers in the screening setting;[125] more than 50% of patients of high-grade DCIS progress to invasive carcinoma in less than five years if left untreated while this percentage is significantly less for low-grade DCIS, which is about 35–50%, and also in a more prolonged time course, up to 40 years; this distinction between high and low grade is possible by histopathological examination of the tissue.

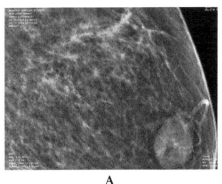

A

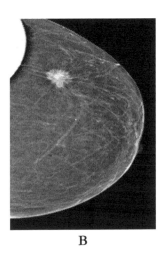

B

Fig.2.

A. Mammogram demonstrating clustered pleomorphic microcalcifications, biopsy suggestive of DCIS.

B. Spiculated density with architectural distortion typical of invasive Cancer, biopsy confirming IDC.

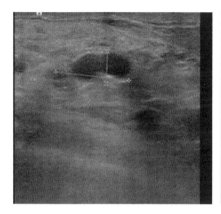 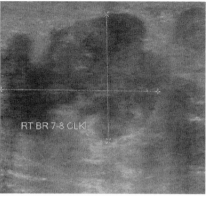

Fig. 3.

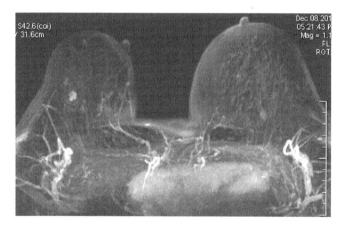

Ultrasound of axillary metastatic node with irregular thickened hypoechoic cortex and the primary breast Cancer demonstrates irregular margins. Ultrasound is insensitive to microcalcifications and DCIS.

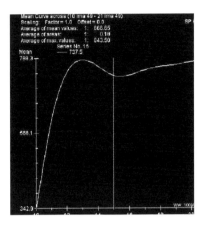

Fig. 4.

Screening MRI breast (patient had BRCA mutation-positive first-degree relative) demonstrating small irregular enhancing nodule, the kinetics showing an indeterminate curve; biopsy confirmed invasive ductal carcinoma.

The radial scar mimics invasive Cancer on mammography and needs an image-guided biopsy for confirmation. However, other Precancerous conditions, like ADH, papillomas, etc., do not have specific or pathognomonic imaging features on mammography and are identified variably across other modalities, including ultrasound and MRI. A biopsy is the only method of confirming any of these Precancerous conditions of the breast. Other common breast conditions are not genuinely Precancerous, like fibroadenomas, phyllodes tumors, etc., though they are rarely associated with Cancer; Cancer may develop along the margin of a fibroadenoma, which is otherwise a benign lesion; similarly, a phyllodes tumor may be benign or Cancerous (sarcomatous); these lesions are identified clinically and on imaging, but diagnosis rests of biopsy. There are counterarguments about breast Cancer screening using mammography and other imaging modalities, particularly in countries like India, where it is estimated to over-diagnose breast Cancers up to as much as 25%; these breast Cancers would have otherwise been undiagnosed in the woman's lifetime, and hence the diagnosis of such Cancers may make the woman unnecessarily worried and increase the cost of healthcare; instead, there is a strong argument that a clinical breast examination is as much accurate in identifying the clinically significant breast Cancers, particularly in the mid – low-income countries.[126]

110

Precancerous conditions in the lung

These lung lesions are not Cancerous yet but can potentially progress to Cancerous. WHO has defined three categories in this group, viz.

1. Squamous dysplasia (SD) of the lungs, which can progress from squamous cell carcinoma in situ (CIS) lung to squamous cell carcinoma.

2. Preinvasive adenocarcinoma of the lung, which includes atypical adenomatous hyperplasia (AAH) and adenocarcinoma in situ of the lung (AIS), which can progress to minimally invasive adenocarcinoma (MIA),[127] and

3. Diffuse idiopathic pulmonary neuroendocrine cell hyperplasia (DIPNECH).

A High-resolution CT scan is a significant modality for identifying these lesions through differentiation between each other is not always possible on imaging alone. While AAH has a typical appearance of a slight ground glass opacity measuring 5 mm or less on high-resolution CT scans, persisting for a longer time (as opposed to infectious alveolar opacity), AIS appears as a ground glass opacity of up to 30 mm or can appear as a solid nodule in an otherwise ground glass nodule, and measures up to 30 mm; however, there is significant overlap among the imaging features of these entities and biopsy may be necessary for further confirmation. An MIA can similarly appear as a mass of 30 -50 mm on CT scan images through differentiation from invasive adenocarcinoma is possible only on biopsy. F18 FDG PET CT is less useful in identifying these lesions and can lead to false negative results.

Screening programs for lung Cancer are not well accepted in India, though there are well-documented methods of and benefits from these programs; it is particularly applicable to the at-risk population, i.e., heavy long-term smokers. While a chest radiograph is used for general screening in regular health check-ups, its poor sensitivity in detecting sub centimeter-sized and, at times, even bigger nodules has rendered them less effective for identifying early lung Cancers and Precancerous conditions. Low-dose CT scan is generally used for these purposes to identify lung nodules that otherwise go unnoticed; there are specific protocols to be followed for the follow-up of these nodules depending upon the size, number, and risk category of the individual and other morphological and functional parameters.[128] However, given highly prevalent conditions like tuberculosis and other granulomatous diseases in India, the false positive results of this test have made it an unpopular screening method. No specific standardized screening protocol exists for the Indian population. Hence, a radiologist needs to have a higher level of suspicion of identifying such lesions in an imaging study performed for an otherwise unrelated clinical indication. Awareness of the imaging features and the patient profile needs to be emphasized for optimal results.

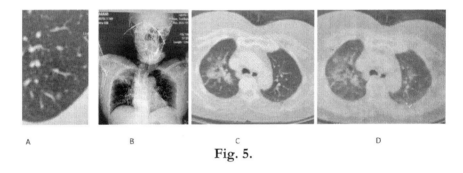

A   B   C   D

Fig. 5.

A. Small soft nodule in the right lung and a biopsy demonstrated AAH.
B. Ill-defined larger area of patchy opacity on the radiograph in the right lung,
C. Irregular ground glass opacity in the upper lobe of the right lung on CT scan,
D. Showing mild FDG uptake on PET CT scan and biopsy, demonstrating invasive adenocarcinoma of the lung.

Precancerous conditions in colon and rectum: A CT colonography is a wonderful non-invasive tool for screening colonic polyps; a proper preparation with bowel cleansing is all that is required, and the entire process is relatively simple; the post-processing by the computer applications provides exquisite details about the location and size of the polyps in the whole colon; a screening colonoscopy though indicated in people after the age of 50 years, conventional colonoscopy being invasive is less popular; a CT colonography serves an almost similar purpose with additional information being available about rest of the abdomen including any extra-luminal pathology, which cannot be assessed by conventional colonoscopy;

however, conventional colonoscopy and biopsy may be required if CT colonoscopy reveals a significant sized polyp; also, CT colonoscopy involves ionizing radiation whereas conventional colonoscopy does not involve radiation. Irrespective of the method used, a screening test is designed to identify a suspicious lesion, i.e., a polyp in the colon or rectum. If necessary, this needs to be biopsied. However, another non-polypoidal Precancerous condition, inflammatory bowel disease, can also be identified by CT colonoscopy or conventional colonoscopy screening. However, many patients with this disease often present with symptoms related to the condition.

Polyps appear on CT scan and CT colonography as small intraluminal projections along the wall of the colon or rectum, which can be either sessile or pedunculated; the surface may be smooth or corrugated; MRI helps in better characterization of larger polyps; PET CT demonstrates significantly increased F18 FDG uptake in these polyps even when they are benign, and the malignant differentiation cannot be identified accurately by PET CT.

Polyps can be neoplastic adenomas like tubular, tubulovillous, and villous; the size of the polyp is vital as any polyp of 10 mm or larger needs to be biopsied. Hereditary syndromes, such as familial adenomatous polyposis, Peutz-Jeghers syndrome, and juvenile polyposis, often demonstrate multiple polyps and generally have an increased risk of developing invasive Cancers.

Chronic inflammatory bowel diseases (UC, Crohn's) can be identified as diffuse circumferential wall thickening of the bowel on CT scan with loss of haustra in the colon, which may be characterless on CT scan and other investigations like barium enema studies. A conventional colonoscopy with biopsy is needed for confirmation of diagnosis.

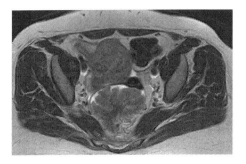 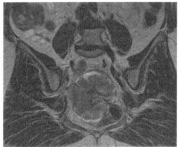

Fig. 6.

MRI of a villous adenomatous polyp in the lower rectum seen as an irregular surfaced intermediate signaled lesion arising from the left posterolateral wall of the rectum, nearly occluding the lumen, proctoscopy and biopsy confirming the diagnosis.

Pancreatic Precancerous conditions are most commonly identified as incidental findings on CT, MRI, or PET scans performed for other abdominal clinical indications. No specific screening imaging tests exist today, although many follow-up or work-up protocols exist once such lesions are identified on imaging. The Precancerous conditions in the pancreas can be cystic or solid and may include:

a) **Mucinous cystic neoplasm (MCN)** is commonly found in the body and tail of the pancreas, most often in women of about 40 - 50 years of age and has a 10 -15% risk of developing malignancy; it appears as a prominent unilocular fluid containing lesion often in the body or tail of pancreas with occasional peripheral calcifications; it can be characterized on CT scan or MRI.

b) **Intraductal papillary mucinous neoplasm (IPMN)** usually occurs in the head of the pancreas, is found in older individuals, both men and women, and appears as a fluid-containing lesion generally communicating with the duct, either the main duct or the side branch. It has a variable risk of malignancy, ranging between 10% for the side branch lesion and up to 80% for the main branch lesion. MRI is the ideal imaging modality to characterize and follow up on these lesions.

c) **Solid pseudopapillary neoplasm (SPN)**, also known as the Hamoudi

114

tumor, occurs most often in the tail of the pancreas with a predilection to affect young women in their 20s and 30s; it appears as a solid mass with cystic and papillary foci and has about 15% malignant potential; MRI can be helpful for characterization and follow-up, although histopathological evaluation is required for diagnosis.

d) **Neuroendocrine tumors** can be either Precancerous or Cancerous; larger tumors are more likely to be malignant, with a size more than 50 mm most commonly malignant. These tumors can also be secretory when the symptoms depend mainly on the hormones secreted. In general, these tumors have about 20% malignant potential. Diagnosis largely hinges on histopathological examination, although many demonstrate characteristic imaging findings in appropriate clinical settings; most of these are hyper vascular and hence appear to be intensely enhancing well-defined lesions, well seen on multiphase contrast CT and MRI as well as in the contrast-enhanced ultrasound images; they also commonly express somatostatin receptors (mainly type 2), which can be imaged using DOTANOC PET CT scan, which is one of the most accurate non-invasive diagnostic methods available. These lesions are often incidental to cross-sectional imaging performed for other clinical indications. Still, awareness about them and their imaging appearance can allow specific curative treatments in these patients.

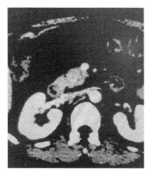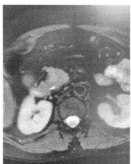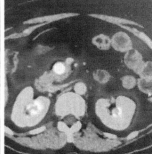

Fig. 7.

CT scan, MRI, and DOTANOC PET CT fused image of a neuroendocrine neoplasm of the head of the pancreas, which was incidentally detected on contrast-enhanced CT scan performed for acute pain abdomen due to appendicitis (not demonstrated in these images); CEMRI attempted specific imaging characterization; however, DOTANOC PET CT scan shows an avid tracer nodule which is typical for somatostatin receptor-expressing tumors; histopathology post-surgery demonstrated NET grade 1.

Various Precancerous conditions detected on imaging are borderline ovarian tumors, Barrette's esophagus, hepatic adenomas, and Menetrier's disease.

Borderline ovarian neoplasm is a lesion of varied types with uncertain malignant potential; they are treated with surgical excision using all oncological principles followed by long-term surveillance. They can be small or large; when large, they can cause a pressure effect on the adjacent structures resulting in associated symptoms. However, smaller lesions may not be clinically detected and are usually identified incidentally during imaging performed for unrelated clinical indications. Preoperative diagnosis is difficult though the IOTA study demonstrated more than 90% sensitivity for identifying malignant lesions by experienced Sonologists; however, the accuracy is only around 60% across the globe. A conclusive diagnosis is mainly by histopathological examination after surgical excision. Solid components in a predominantly cystic lesion, with postcontrast enhancement or increased vascularity on color Doppler, are signs of malignancy in these lesions. High F18 FDG uptake on PET CT favors a diagnosis of malignancy. In general, they have an excellent overall survival rate.[129]

Barrette's esophagus is a condition in which the lower esophageal mucosa demonstrates intestinal metaplasia, seen in 3 to 15% of patients with gastroesophageal reflux disease (GERD) and has a malignant potential ranging between 0.1 to 1% and progress to esophageal adenocarcinoma. A double contrast barium enema is the best available non-invasive imaging modality to diagnose this condition. However, endoscopy is frequently required for histopathological confirmation and minimally invasive treatment procedures, including endoscopic resection or ablation.[130]

Hepatic adenomas are rare neoplasms of the liver arising from the hepatocytes, mostly seen among women of the childbearing age group, particularly on oral contraceptive medications; most of the literature suggests a 5 – 10% malignant transformation to hepatocellular carcinoma from hepatic adenoma, with more prominent lesions at relatively higher risk of transformation to malignancy.[131]

Menetrier's disease is a rare condition demonstrating hypertrophic gastropathy involving the body of the stomach, which is characterized by the thickening of the mucous membrane in the form of giant rugal folds, hypochlorhydria, and protein loss. They are seen either incidentally on cross-sectional imaging performed for other clinical indications or specifically when symptomatic, present with hypoproteinemia and hypochlorhydria when a CT scan may be requested to look for changes in the stomach; on CT scan images, these appear as thickened gastric rugae, often with entrapped air loculi in between the folds, even in a well-distended stomach; often they are misdiagnosed as gastric Cancers (linitis plastica or lymphoma); however, F18 FDG PET CT scan demonstrates no abnormal FDG uptake and endoscopy with biopsy may be required for final diagnosis. The malignant potential of these lesions remains controversial, although many cases of these patients developing gastric adenocarcinoma have been reported.[132] This condition is often treated with gastrectomy.

Conclusion

The carcinogenesis pathway and the causes are poorly understood for most Cancers; the carcinogens are known only to a handful of Cancers. Imaging diagnosis of a Precancerous condition is often by identification of lesions incidentally on studies performed for other clinical indications though increased screening may be required for specific Cancers like breast, lung, and colon; identification of at-risk populations is necessary to optimize the screening programs. However, essential requirements by the radiologist are being aware of the imaging characteristics of these otherwise 'not expecting' lesions, possessing a high index of suspicion, appreciating the individual to be in the 'at risk' bracket for particular Cancer, and being diligent in evaluating the stack of images. Having a checklist while generating a report on any imaging modality and avoiding "search satisfaction" often help to minimize missing these lesions, which are often subtle. Most imaging screening studies are directed at early Cancer diagnoses Cancer like breast, lung, etc., although Precancerous lesions are sometimes detected during this process. Most Precancerous conditions have imaging features overlapping with those of Cancers; hence, specific radiologic features need to be identified and defined. Biopsy and follow-up are indicated in many of these conditions.

9

EARLY DETECTION OF PRECANCEROUS CONDITIONS - A PATHOLOGIST'S PERSPECTIVE

Dr. Malathi M

Benjamin Franklin famously wrote, "An ounce of prevention is worth a pound of cure."

Introduction

Cancer in a simplistic way, Cancer is defined as the uncontrolled and disordered growth of cells that invade adjacent tissues. This means to say that the irreversible changes have already occurred in the cells; the disease has set in. Whereas Precancerous or Cancer precursor lesions are defined by localized morphologic changes that identify a field of epithelium that is at increased risk for malignant transformation.[133] Otherwise, also Precancerous lesions are called morphologically altered tissue, in which Cancer is more likely to occur than in its normal counterpart. At the beginning of twentieth century, George Papanicolaou and Aurel Babes first published terminology of dysplasia, which is the early changes of carcinoma cervix.[134] In 1958,

Foulds stated, 'Lesions described as "Precancerous" are visible steps in a dynamic process of neoplasia; these lesions may or may not undergo progression to a more advanced stage of neoplasia'.[135] Initially, the use of this terminology for Precancerous lesions was much confined to the cervix, and colon lesions later for oral lesions. But nowadays this terminology is also used for fields of epithelial cells in the mucosa that are not visible clinically too.[136-138]

Many new methodologies/technologies exist for screening and early detection of Cancer. Advances in imaging technology, many innovations in genetic abnormalities, Cancer biomarkers, and developing proteomic fields are progressively evolving in the early detection and management of Cancer. Progressive scientific studies are going on in this field to find a technology that could be at a molecular level that can detect small Precancerous lesions and/or high Cancer-risk individuals.[139]

Identifying clearly defined precursor lesions provides scope for primary and secondary Cancer prevention Cancer. Early detection, surveillance, and management of these lesions in any anatomical site will reduce mortality and morbidity. Above all these, molecular and genetic studies of precursor lesions provide insight into the process of pathogenesis.[137-141]

With this background, the National Cancer Institute and The George Washington University Cancer Institute convened a 'Precancer' Conference on November 2004. The main objective was to have an appropriate definition of 'Precancer' regardless of the detection method. Following the definition was to establish Precancer as a formal area of research based on its own set of biological principles, fundamental research questions, and clinical goals. It's said that all these discussions were on histopathology findings because that is the current method of diagnosis. In brief, the results of this meeting were as follows:[139]

1. Overall conference participants aimed to develop a general definition of Precancerous lesions, which could apply to multiple disciplines and provide common terminology for clinical and experimental studies. They developed and agreed on a set of defining criteria for Precancer and suggested how pathologists, oncologists, and Cancer researchers can determine when these criteria are satisfied.

2. Terminology: Premalignant, Precancer premalignancy, potentially malignant lesions, dysplasia, atypical hyperplasia, preinvasive lesion/Cancer, Cancer precursors, incipient neoplasia, intraepithelial neoplasm, carcinoma in situ are the existing terminologies. The commonly used term 'Intraepithelial Neoplasia' should be replaced by 'Precancer.' By this includes non-epithelial Lymphoid, hematologic, and soft tissue Precancerous lesions and entities diagnosed by non-morphologic methods, e.g., pre-dysplastic molecular lesions. One should note that Precancer does not imply that Cancer is the ultimate.

3. Definition: One must include five criteria to define a Precancer. They are pieces of evidence should exist that the Precancer is associated with an increased risk of Cancer, resulting Cancer arises from cells within the Precancer, a Precancer is different from the normal tissue from which it arises, a Precancer is different from the Cancer into which it develops. However, it has some, but not all, of the molecular and phenotypic properties that characterize Cancer and lastly there is a method by which Precancer can be diagnosed.

4. Discussion on the selected five criteria of definition, regression and progression of Precancer, non-epithelial Precancer, multiplicity of lesions and chronology of progression.

It is said that identification of precursor lesion helps to identify the etiological factor if it is an intermediate stage between exposure and development of Cancer. More studies are focused on Cancer precursors to know whether this is an intermediate stage in the Cancer development. For this repeated tissue samples are required to study as well as for the diagnosis of the lesions. An alternative method for this is cytopathology e.g., Cervical cytology-PAP test. As we all know histological examination is gold standard, errors can occur due to inadequate sampling and microscopic interpretation.[138] A good clinical history and examination is also essential, adding to the correct histological diagnosis.

Lack of awareness about the signs and symptoms of Precancerous lesions in the general population and even healthcare providers is believed to be responsible for these entities' diagnostic and management.

Etiopathogenesis: Description of etiological factors and the process of carcinogenesis by molecular alteration are beyond the scope of this context. Several studies and researches documented that carcinogenesis is a multistep process and these multistep processes reflect genetic alterations that drive the progressive transformation of normal human cells into Cancer cell.[133] Availability of advanced methods in the basic research on cellular and molecular mechanisms in the development of Cancer has helped us to understand this multistep process of carcinogenesis.[138] The genetic alteration occurs mainly in growth-promoting proto-oncogenes, growth-inhibiting tumor suppressor genes, genes that regulate programmed cell death (apoptosis), and genes that are responsible for DNA repair. There is accumulated mutational changes by repeated cell injury induced by risk factors causes cellular changes which transforms cell into dysplasia and neoplasia.[133,142] Because of multiple mutation of one or more of these genes, a study model has documented that six essential alterations are required in a cell for a malignant growth. These are self-sufficiency in growth signal, insensitivity to growth- inhibitor signals, evasion of programmed cell death (apoptosis), limitless replicative potential, sustained angiogenesis and tissue invasion and metastasis.[142] Pathological analyses of a number of organ sites, reveal lesions that appear to represent the intermediate steps in a process through which cells evolve progressively from normalcy via a series of premalignant states into invasive Cancers.[135]

Documented mechanism of multistep process of carcinogenesis are initiation, promotion and progression. An irreversible carcinogen interaction with tissue DNA and damages it in the initiation process, which not pathologically visible but essential for the next action of promotion. Tumor promotion is a reversible process wherein the initiated cellular changes are expressed and leads to precursor lesions and development of benign tumors. During the progression benign tumor becomes malignant. [133-138]

There are two predicted distinct pathways between an exposure and Cancer. In the direct pathway Cancer directly develops without passing through a known Precancer step. Whereas in the indirect pathway, develops a Precancer stage that may then progress to Cancer. Precancer is a causal mediator between exposure and disease but also a pathogenic state.[137]

Pathological studies from different anatomic sites reveal lesions that appear to represent the intermediate steps in a process through which cells evolve progressively from normalcy via a series of premalignant states into invasive Cancers.[142] Progression or regression of this can occur and both are equivalent. It's said that factors most likely external to the biology of the Precancer will determine this process.[139]

Pathology: "What mind does not know eyes can't see," are the apt words for a pathologist. A pathologist may miss diagnosis and documentation of precursor if he/she is unaware of such an entity.

To understand the Precancerous lesions, one should know the meaning and definitions of neoplasia-related terminologies like hypertrophy, atrophy, hyperplasia, hypoplasia, aplasia, metaplasia, dysplasia, and desmoplasia, including neoplasia. As the classification of the tumors is based on the cell of origin, pathologists should learn about normal histology, development, and renewal of body tissues. To predict the biological behavior of the tumor, histopathological diagnosis and classification of tumors as benign and malignant is essential.[133]

Understanding and identification of characteristics of benign and malignant tumors helps to diagnose the Precancerous lesion. Carcinomas are the malignant tumors of the epithelium, and sarcomas are malignant tumors of mesenchymal tissue – supporting soft tissue. These are commonly called as Cancers means to say malignant tumors. Invasion is the characteristic feature of Cancer which differentiates Precancer from the well-established Cancer. Epithelial tumors are example of this, i.e., carcinoma in situ tumor- a Precancerous lesion, cells limited to basement membrane, does not metastasize. Whereas in adenocarcinoma, tumor cells invade beyond basement membrane of epithelium and metastasize.[133]

Similar to the grading of tumors, Precancerous lesions are also graded qualitatively as grades of dysplasia. Due to intra and inter-observer variability, usually accepted two-tiered grading system as low or high grade, examples being in cervix and urinary bladder.

In hematopoietic neoplasms, as the cells are circulating via lymphatic and/or blood vasculature throughout the body, the concept of Precancerous lesion is not applicable to these neoplasms. However, identification of molecular abnormality in a few benign proliferations helps to assess the increased risk of development of malignancy in some of the benign conditions.[138]

But in mesenchymal tumors, the transition from the benign to malignant tumor is reflected by the quantitative assessment of mitotic count, and there is no barrier to assess the invasion like basement membrane as in the epithelium. Though progression of benign to malignant tumors noted, Precancerous lesions are not much documented in mesenchymal tumors.[138]

With this background in pathology, silent features of some of the site-specific, well documented common Precancerous will be highlighted in this section. In depth description of these Precancerous lesions are difficult to cover in this short note.

Female Genital System

Uterine Cervix: Cancer Cervix (Ca Cx) is the fourth most common Cancer in women. About 5 decades back, Ca Cx was the first common Cancer in occurrence and mortality rates. Cervical Cancer is one of the very few Cancers where a precursor stage lasts many years before becoming invasive Cancer. The natural history of Precancerous lesions of the cervix well documented, providing ample opportunity for detection and treatment. The remarkable benefits of effective screening, early diagnosis, and curative therapy for cervical precursor are well recognized too. George Papanicolaou, is the pioneer who found Pap test in detecting cervical precursor lesions, some of which would have progressed to Cancer if not treated and low-stage Ca Cx which are highly curable Cancers. Other added factors to this is that the accessibility of the cervix to Pap testing, visual examination and the slow progression of the precursor lesions to invasive carcinoma, provides sufficient time for screening, detection, and preventive treatment. After the discovery of Human Papilloma Virus (HPV) as the etiological factor it is considered nearly completely preventable by primary prevention (HPV vaccine) and secondary prevention by screening measures. Though HPV infection is necessary for cause of cervical Cancer, but alone not sufficient. Association of HPV with other important cofactors like some sexually transmittable infections (HIV and Chlamydia trachomatis), smoking, a higher number of childbirths, and long-term use of oral contraceptives add to the causative risk factors. With all this, it has been noted that though majority of women infected with HPV during the reproductive period, only a few will have persistence of infection and develop Cancer. So, exposure to co-carcinogens and host immune status, may influence whether an HPV infection regresses or persists and eventually leads to Cancer. These precursor lesions are asymptomatic and do not produce any visible lesions or alterations in the cervix which can be seen by the naked eye.[143]

A few points to note here about HPV is that there are more than 70 types of HPV which are sequentially numbered by an international agreement as HPV1, HPV2, HPV3 and so on. Among these HPV16, 18, 31, 33 and HPV 35 are identified as high risk and HPV 6 and 11 are low risk for the causation of cervical precursors and Cancer.[143]

Classification of the precursor lesions of the cervix is evolved from the cytologic nomenclature of Papanicolaou's Classes of atypical cells, WHO accepted Reagan's designation of the degree of dysplasia, Richart's cytohisto correlated grades of Cervical Intraepithelial Neoplasia (CIN) and carcinoma in situ to The Bethesda system (TBS) of Surface Intraepithelial Lesions (SIL) over a period of six decades. (Table 1). TBS is mainly aimed to give uniformity in the reporting format of cervical cytology for the management of the lesions. [143-144]

Table 1: Classification Systems for Squamous Cervical Precursor Lesions

Papanicoloau class system	Dysplasia/CIS (Reagan 1953)	CIN (Richart 1968)	Modified CIN (Richart 1968)	SIL terminology (TBS)
Class I - No evidence of disease.	-	-	-	Within normal limits.
Class II - Atypia not further defined.	-	-	-	ASC
Class III- Suggestive of, but not conclusive of malignancy.	Mild dysplasia*	CIN I	CIN-Low grade	LGSIL
Class IV- Strongly suggestive of malignancy.	Moderate and severe dysplasia, carcinoma in situ.	CIN II CIN III	CIN-High grade	HGSIL
Class V- Conclusive of, malignancy.	Invasive Cancer	Invasive Cancer	Invasive Cancer	Invasive Cancer

(TBS-The Bethesda System: ASC-Atypical Squamous Cell; CIN-Cervical Intraepithelial Neoplasia; SIL-Squamous Intraepithelial Lesion; LSIL- Low grade SIL; HSIL-High grade SIL)

As per the widely used TBS, the cytology findings of a SIL are identified based on nuclear atypia in the form of nuclear enlargement, darkly stained nucleus, i.e. hyperchromasia, coarse chromatin granules, variation in nuclear size and shape with changes in the nuclear membrane. In LSIL, nuclei often vary up to three-fold in size and have quite variable staining patterns, and histology usually has minimal nuclear atypia in the epithelial cells residing in the lower third of the epithelium. Koilocytosis is the appearance of perinuclear cytoplasmic cavitation or halos that is accompanied by thickening of the cytoplasmic membrane, best appreciated in cytology specimens, is pathognomonic of a productive HPV infected (fig). In HSIL, the cell size is smaller than the LSIL, cells in singly/sheets/syncytial, nuclear abnormalities resemble parabasal/metaplastic cells, coarse granular chromatin, no nucleoli, irregular nuclear margin, decreased cytoloplasm, increased N/C ratio. (Fig). It is documented that SIL is associated with high-risk HPVs, that is, HPV-16 being the most common HPV type and seen in about 80% of LSILs and 100% of HSILs. Once SIL can regress or persist or progress, it is observed that the majority of LSIL will regress, and a minority of cases progress to HSIL, whereas majority of HSIL progress to Cancer and a minority of cases regress. And about a third of LSIL and about two thirds of HSIL cases may persist. The progression period observed being two to ten years. [133,138,143,144]

Atypical Squamous Cells (ASC) are the cellular changes that are more marked than those attributable to reactive changes but that qualitatively and quantitatively fall short of a definitive diagnosis of SIL. This has two categories; one is Atypical Squamous Cells – Undetermined Significance (ASC-US), and the second is Atypical Squamous Cells – a high-grade squamous intraepithelial lesion cannot be excluded (ASC-H). This is based on the understanding of LSIL being transient and regressing in the majority of cases, and HSIL is a Precancerous lesion. (Fig…) ASC includes not only the cellular changes not related to HPV infection and carcinoma, but also it may be a clue to the possible presence of underlying SIL and carcinoma very rarely. There are many mimickers of ASC, like cellular changes due to inflammation, air drying, atrophy with degeneration, hormonal effects, and other artifacts. To avoid the overuse or underuse of this category to maintain the quality assurance of ASC, the recommended laboratory thresh hold is the [144] ASC/SIL ratio, which should not exceed 3:1, and HPV test.[143-144]

Endocervical adenocarcinoma (ECA) is less common than squamous carcinoma. Endocervical adenocarcinoma in situ (AIS) is glandular precursor of EAC, similar to HSIL precursor of SCC. One can identify these lesions in pap smears which needs experience in interpretation. In glandular cytology, Low sensitivity is seen due to sampling errors as the location of glandular neoplasia high in the endocervical canal rather than at the transformation zone, interpretive errors due to misinterpretation of preneoplastic/neoplastic glandular epithelium as a normal lower uterine segment, tubal metaplasia or reactive endocervical cells. Above all these, it has been noted that the cytologic features are poorly reproducible, with no unanimity, and purely based on individual experience. There is recorded evidence that the endocervical AIS is preceded by glandular cell abnormalities, which can be identified in cytology and biopsy samples of the uterine cervix. [138,143,144]

Precancerous lesions of the cervix can be detected early and treated, so invasive Cancer can be prevented. This is substantiated by primary and secondary prevention. Primary prevention can be done by providing Cancer awareness to the community people. Another step in this is HPV vaccination for the target individuals. Secondary prevention is by screening the target women population.

Detection of cervical precursors is regular PAP tests, HPV tests, and Colposcopy examinations. WHO announced that every country in the world should reach the target of 90-70-90 by 2030, which means 90% of girls fully vaccinated with the HPV vaccine by the age of 15; 70% of women screened using a high-performance test by the age of 35, and again by the age of 45; 90% of women with pre-Cancer treated and 90% of women with invasive Cancer managed and hence to achieve the goal to eliminate the Cancer cervix.

Endometrium: Endometrial carcinoma (EC) is the sixth most commonly diagnosed Cancer in women as per Globocon 2020 statistics, and incidence rates vary across world regions by 10 folds.[146] Endometrioid carcinoma is known to arise from endometrial hyperplasia (EH), a precursor lesion. The risk factors recognized for both EH & EC are obesity, anovulatory cycles, and exogenous hormones with increasing body mass index (BMI) and nulliparity added risk factors for EH. All these risk factors are the cause of an unopposed estrogen stimulation of the endometrium in turn development of EH and EC. The usual symptom is abnormal bleeding, and in some cases, the lesion is detected in an endometrial biopsy performed for other causes, like in pre or postmenopausal women before starting hormonal therapy.

EH is classified into EH without Atypia and EH with atypia/Atypical EH by World Health Organization (WHO) and the International Society of Gynecologic Pathologists (ISGYP). The term 'Endometrioid intraepithelial neoplasia (EIN) is considered synonymous with Atypical EH. Histologically

EH without atypia (simple), minimal abnormal glandular architecture with cystically dilated glands with abundant cellular stroma, occasional epithelial outpouchings, and minimally dilated glands. In progressive process- complex hyperplasia consisting of proliferating crowded complex glands, back-to-back arranged, lined by columnar stratified epithelium, nuclei perpendicular to the basement membrane, branched with irregular outlines and papillary infoldings into the lumens, and absence of nuclear atypia. (Fig....) Whereas EH with Atypia/EIN shows features of complex glandular hyperplasia with scanty stroma with nuclear atypical features and loss of cell polarity (Fig..). The risk of EC is 1-3% with EH without Atypia, whereas in atypical EH has 45-fold. The only methodology to diagnose EH is by endometrial biopsy by curettage in a woman who has abnormal uterine bleeding.[133,147]

Breast: Female breast Cancer ranking first for incidence and the fifth leading cause of Cancer mortality as recorded by global Cancer incidence in 2020; [146] it accounts for 1 in 4 Cancer cases and for 1 in 6 Cancer deaths. Hence it is important to recognize its precursors and treat breast Cancer at an early stage. Etiological factors of precursor lesions are said to be the same as the risk factors of Invasive Breast Cancer (IBC).

Breast precursor lesions are discussed under benign intraductal proliferative lesions of the Terminal Ductal Lobular Units (TDLU). These include Usual Ductal Hyperplasia (UDH), Atypical Ductal Hyperplasia (ADH), Flat Epithelial Atypia (FEA), and Columnar Cell Lesions (CCLs) like columnar cell change and hyperplasia, lobular neoplasia (LN)-Atypical Lobular Hyperplasia (ALH) and Lobular carcinoma in Situ (LCIS), papillary lesions, radial scar and Ductal Carcinoma in Situ (DCIS). These have different levels of risk for progression to invasive breast carcinoma (IBC), mainly low-grade carcinoma. UDH has 1.5- 2-fold, ADH has 3-5-fold, and DCIS of 8-10-fold risk of malignancy. There is a complex interrelationship between these and the progression to IBC. Available molecular evidence with the morphological and immunohistochemistry (IHC) finding suggests that these lesions have a low risk of progression to IBC. As UDH is a precursor of ADH and DCIS, included in this category, though by itself is not a precursor lesion. DCIS is graded as low and high grade, but interobserver variability is seen in reporting of ADH and low-grade DCIS. Molecular studies have also shown that CCLs and FEA are not only precursors of ADH and DCIS but also can progress to IBC. (Fig...) Sclerosing adenosis, apocrine adenosis and adenoma, microgladular adenosis, and radial scar/complex sclerosing adenosis are the other benign proliferative breast lesion which may have ADH and has a very low risk of malignancy.[133,148,149,150]

The majority of these lesions are not detected by mammography, except often, some may show micro-calcification. These lesions are identified accidentally during the histological examination of the core biopsies of suspicious lesions on screening programs.[133,148]

Diagnosis is by correlation of clinical history and examination with tissue biopsy. The Histomorphological evaluation of tissue architectural pattern, nuclear Atypia, and proliferation rate with added immunohistochemistry markers studies like High and low molecular weight cytokeratin's, E catherdin, ER and PR will help in the definitive categorization of the precursors. Molecular studies of these lesions have revealed that the development and progress of precursors are due to the acquisition of genetic instability and the accumulation of random genetic events, [148-150] One has to note and weigh all available information like clinical findings, lesion size, lesion extent, percentage of lesion removal, representative sampling, biological and individual risk factors, and the possibility of surveillance in the management of these lesions.

Detection of breast Cancer susceptibility genes 1 and 2 (BRCA1& BRCA2) are the strongest risk factors for the development of breast and ovarian Cancer, and breast Cancer cases account for approximately 6% and up to 20% of ovarian Cancer cases. [133,148]

Preventive measures are disease awareness education and screening programs. In breast screening, one can adopt a triple test methodology which includes clinical examination, breast imaging- mammography with/and ultrasonography, and biopsy/cytology study for early detection of the lesion.

Upper Aerodigestive Tract: Oral cavity, Pharynx, and Larynx – Precursors in these sites are the most common clinically defined entities, especially in the oral cavity. 90% of the Cancers in these sites are squamous cell carcinoma. GLOBOCON 2020 survey documented that lip and oral cavity Cancers are a highly frequent and leading cause of Cancer death among men in India.[146]

The Centre for Oral Cancer and Precancers Cancer in the UK, in collaboration with WHO, did the first workshop in Landon 2005 and the second in March 2020.[151-152] Precancerous lesions and conditions of the oral mucosa were discussed regarding the current concepts, terminology, classifications, natural history, pathology, and of molecular markers, and to critically analyze the evolution of knowledge and practice concerning diagnosis and management. As not all the precursors' lesions progress to malignancy, in 2005 terminology of Potentially Malignant Disorders/ Lesions of oral cavity- PMD was renamed as Oral Potentially Malignant Disorders – OPMD in 2020, which includes a group of lesions and conditions characterized by a variably increased risk of developing Cancers of the lip and the oral cavity [151] Table -2.

Table-2: List of Oral Potentially Malignant Disorders (OPMDs)

List of OPMDs – 2007	Newly added OPMDs - 2020
Leukoplakia,	Oral lichenoid lesions.
Erythroplakia	Oral manifestations of chronic graft-versus-host disease.
Proliferative verrucous leukoplakia,	Oral exophytic verrucous hyperplasia.
Oral lichen planus	Oral manifestations of chronic graft-versus-host disease.
Oral submucous fibrosis,	**Disorders with Limited/insufficient epidemiological evidence.**
Palatal lesions in reverse smokers,	Oral epidermolysis bullosa.
Lupus erythematosus	Chronic hyperplastic candidosis (CHC).
Epidermolysis bullosa	
Dyskeratosis congenital	

WHO incorporated these in the latest 2017 edition of the classification of Head and Neck tumors as Oral Potentially Malignant Disorders, Oral Epithelial Dysplasia, and Proliferative Verrucous Leukoplakia.[153] Discussion and description of these individual entity are very vast to include here; hence the most common and important word, leukoplakia, will be covered in brief.

So, the term oral leukoplakia is defined as *'The term leukoplakia should be used to recognize white plaques of questionable risk having excluded (other) known diseases or disorders that carry no increased risk for Cancer.'* It is accepted that it is a clinical term with no specific histology and is generally asymptomatic.[151] Oral leukoplakia is the most common OPMD and has a prevalence rate of 1% and malignant transformation rates of 2-5% over a follow-up period ranging from 12 months to 20 years. It can occur anywhere in the oral cavity, and distribution depends on specific etiological factors and to some extent, patient age and sex. Erythroplakia is most frequently seen on the soft palate, floor of the mouth, and buccal mucosa. Tobacco (smoking and/or chewing), alcohol consumption, and areca nut, with or without tobacco, are the main causes of leukoplakias and submucosal fibrosis. For many cases of OPMDs, no etiological factors are known. Till now high-risk HPV infection very rarely seen in OPMDs.[152-154]

Based on the color and surface texture, leukoplakia is typed as homogeneous, which is uniformly white, flat, and thin, with a smooth surface that may exhibit shallow cracks, cannot be rubbed off, circumscribed area, and has well-demarcated borders. And non-homogeneous type will have more diffuse borders, which include nodular showing small polypoidal or rounded outgrowths, red or white (erythroleukoplakia) speckled excrescences, and verrucous showing nodular, raised, exophytic, wrinkled or corrugated surface. There should not be any evidence of chronic traumatic irritation to the area, and it is not reversible on the elimination of apparent traumatic causes. The risk of malignant transformation is high in non-homogeneous type as compared to the homogeneous type, which is relatively low.[136,151]

Histologic findings vary from atrophy or hyperplasia (acanthosis), and epithelial dysplasia may or may not be present. (Fig..) Both architectural and cytologic changes are utilized for grading oral epithelial dysplasia. Because of inter and intra-observer variability in pathology reporting leukoplakia, it is recommended that a pathology report of a leukoplakia should be in the format as "keratosis with no/mild/moderate/severe dysplasia, consistent with oral leukoplakia" to achieve uniformity in the report. Dysplasia is reported as mild, moderate, and high grade and/or low grade and high grade.

Grading of dysplasia should be done considering the histopathological features.(Table 3) Dysplasia is seen in a minority of leukoplakias and is usually seen in erythroplakia and erythroleukoplakia.[138,153] Added to this, the word keratosis should not be used clinically as a synonym for leukoplakia.[151,155]

Table 3: Histological features to consider oral epithelial dysplasia.

Architectural Features	Cytological Features
Irregular stratification of epithelium.	Abnormal variation in nuclear size.
Loss of polarity of basal cells.	Abnormal variation in nuclear shape.
Drop-shaped rete ridges.	Abnormal variation in cell size.
Increased number of mitotic figures.	Abnormal variation in cell shape.
Abnormally superficial mitotic figures.	Increased N:C ratio Atypical mitotic figures increased number and size of nucleoli.
Premature keratinization in single cells.	
Keratin pearls within rete ridges.	Hyperchromasia.
Loss of epit11elíal cell cohesion.	
The cut-off point between low-grade and high-grade dysplasia is four architectural and five cytological changes, [156] irrespective of the level within the epithelium. According to Nankivell P et al. 2019, [156] a cut-off point of tour architectural and four cytological changes may improve the correlation between the operators with regard to dysplasia.	

Palatine erythroleukoplakia, which occurs in reverse smoking, keeping the burning end of a cigarette or cigar inside the mouth, is a precursor of 50% of cases of malignancies of the hard palate.

Among the OPMDs, Oral submucosal fibrosis (OSF) well-recognized precursor of oral SCC, which is a chronic condition caused by the habit of chewing gutkha/ areca nut. Clinically OSF presents with a burning injury sensation for spicy food and a gradual inability to open their mouth.

Histologically shows atrophic epithelium with submucosal diffuse fibrosis, loss of tissue pigmentation and localized taste papillae, leathery mucosa, restricted tongue mobility due to tissue stiffness, muscle, and vascular changes, which may progress to dysplasia and malignancy.[138,155] Precursors of the oropharynx and hypopharynx include erythroplakia or in the process of OSF and Plummer-Vinson syndrome. The latter condition is associated with iron deficiency anaemia causing post-cricoid or upper oesophageal webs and glossitis, in turn, dysphagia. Improvements in nutrition have decreased the incidence of this syndrome and malignancy. Laryngeal keratosis is a precursor of laryngeal Cancer, similar to oral leukoplakia, and tobacco smoking and alcohol being the risk factors. Other lesions like erythroplakia with keratosis are also the precursors of laryngeal Cancer including recurrent papilloma's. Malignant transformation is documented in the range of 5.6% to 40% in laryngeal keratosis with dysplasia compared to 16% in keratosis without dysplasia [138]

OPMDs being asymptomatic, the oral exam is of upmost importance in the prevention, diagnosis and clinical monitoring of these lesions. Clinically a through visual oral cavity inspection in high-risk individuals and palpation of the intraoral region is the most important step for early detection and management of OPMDs. A lot of techniques with low diagnostic accuracy and high rates of false positive results available, but a lesion biopsy and histopathological examination is the gold standard for diagnosis.[154-155] But careful selection of these lesions for biopsy by the clinician, proper handling and process of the biopsy tissue and interpretation of biopsy are critical for an accurate diagnosis. These steps are explained in detail by Kumaraswamy et al.[157] Primary prevention of OPMDs is by controlling the risk factors like use of tobacco and alcohol drinking.

Early recognition and treatment of OPMDs may help to prevent malignant transformation in oral lesions. It is said that classification of OPMDs is not only an academic interest but essential for clinicians to plan for an evidence-based management decisions of these lesions, in turn this will help in patient's quality of life.

Lungs: There are four types of morphologic precursor epithelial lesions are recognized in the lungs. They are atypical adenomatous hyperplasia ($\leq$5 mm), adenocarcinoma in situ ($\leq$ 3cm), squamous dysplasia and carcinoma in situ, and diffuse idiopathic pulmonary neuroendocrine cell hyperplasia. It is not possible to detect and distinguish these lesions regarding the progression or regression. A linear correlation between the intensity of exposure to cigarette smoke and the worrisome epithelial changes is seen. The sequence is the same like initial innocuous-appearing basal cell hyperplasia, squamous metaplasia to dysplasia and carcinoma in situ, finally to the Cancer.[133]

Gastrointestinal Tract

Esophagus: Esophageal Cancer ranks seventh in terms of incidence and sixth in overall mortality.[146] The most common histologic types esophageal Cancers are squamous cell carcinoma [ESCC] and adenocarcinoma [EAC]), which have quite different etiologies and ESCC constituting 80% of all esophageal Cancers particularly in developing countries. It has the poorest survival of all Cancers. Documented evidences shown that esophagitis causing dysplasia is a precursor for ESCC. In the regions of high incidences of ESCC, prevalence of esophageal dysplasia is 25%. One of the largest study shown squamous dysplasia and carcinoma in situ were associated with a significantly increased risk of developing ESCC within 13.5 years after endoscopy.[158] Histological features of esophagitis showed either, elongation of lamina propria, papillae into the upper third of the epithelium together with basal cell hyperplasia (BCH) and epithelial infiltration by neutrophils or eosinophils or dense lymphocytes or neutrophils in the lamina propria and/or dysplasia. [138,159]

Whereas esophageal adenocarcinoma (EAC), arises in the background of Barrett esophagus and long-standing chronic Gastro Esophageal Reflux Disease (GERD). Barrett esophagus is a complication of GERD characterized by intestinal metaplasia of esophageal squamous mucosa, progressing to dysplasia and with an increased risk of Cancer of gastro esophageal junction (GEJ). Hence Barrett esophagus is a precursor lesion of EAC. Endoscopic examination in GERD patients helps in the diagnosis of Barrett esophagus. Biopsy of this altered mucosal membrane seen by endoscopy at GEJ will help to identify the features of Barrett esophagus. The histologic features include metaplastic columnar mucosa of intestinal-type replacing the squamous esophageal epithelium with goblet cells. Goblet cells are diagnostic of Barrett esophagus which will have a distinct mucous vacuoles and stain pale blue, shape of a wine goblet in the cytoplasm (Fig.).

Though the non-goblet columnar cells, like gastric-type foveolar cells seen, it is not accepted as sufficient criteria for the diagnosis of Barrett esophagus.. Features of dysplasia of low or high grade with atypical glandular architecture may be seen. With progression, epithelial cells may invade the lamina propria, a feature that defines progression to intramucosal carcinoma. [133,138,158]

Remarkable advances are being done and in progress too in identifying the biomarkers by minimally invasive methods for early detection of these lesions. A validated biomarker for clinical use is not available till date. [160]

It is suggested that early detection of precursor lesions and planning subsequent preventive measures like chemoprevention or endoscopic therapy helps the patients in reduction of Cancer mortality.[158]

Stomach: Stomach Cancer ranks fifth for incidence and fourth for mortality.[146] Chronic Helicobacter pylori infection is considered as the principal cause of a gastric Cancer. The recognized Precancerous lesions of the stomach are chronic atrophic gastritis, intestinal metaplasia due to Helicobacter pylori infection, autoimmune gastritis of pernicious anemia, peptic ulcer disease, gastric stump after partial gastectomy and gastric polyps. The process of gastric carcinogenesis is known to be a multistep process. The progression is that normal mucosa due to chronic inflammation- chronic gastritis – mucosal atrophy/adenoma- intestinal metaplasia- dysplasia (intraepithelial neoplasia)-carcinoma. The diagnostic features of dysplasia are cellular atypia, abnormal differentiation, glandular architectural atypia and increased mitosis. Endoscopic examination of the dysplasia appears as a flat or depressed or polypoidal lesion which may be intestinal type and foveolar type of adenoma, histology resembling a colonic adenoma.[133,138,161] Detection of Precancerous lesions of stomach is by endoscopic examination and biopsy study. In 2012 a European group association of Endoscopists, pathologists and gastroenterologists proposed guidelines for biopsy to diagnose stage and grading of gastric Precancerous conditions, including the management guidelines. It is suggested four biopsies should be done from the lesser, greater curvature, the antrum and the corpus each.[162] Even pepsinogen levels may help in atrophic gastritis which is decreased in early gastric Cancer and gastric dysplasia. Preventive measures may involve treating the Helicobactor Pylori infection and decreasing the high-risk factors like high salt intake which is an irritant. A few hereditary gastric Cancer syndromes have been recognized which accounts for 5-10% and have increased risk of gastric Cancer. Molecular gene testing will help in identification of these syndromes.[161]

Colorectal: GLOBOCON 2020 statistics showed colorectal Cancer (CRC) ranks third in incidence and second in terms of mortality. CRC are the one of the potentially preventable Cancer by adopting the preventive measures to detect and remove Precancerous lesions i.e., adenomas. Though there is very well documented genetic predisposition, majority of these lesions are sporadic. The sequences of adenoma progressing to carcinoma is very well documented.

Colorectal adenomas are usually exophytic or polypoidal growth pattern and a few may be flat lesions. These neoplastic polyps are precursors of majority of colorectal adenocarcinomas and are characterized by the presence of epithelial dysplasia. Based on the architecture, adenomas are three types-tubular, tubulovillous, or villous. Villous adenomas are more prone for invasive Cancer compared to tubular adenomas. Flat adenomas will have a concave surface which does not exceed twice the thickness of the adjacent normal mucosa, not visualized on colonoscopy and doubtful precursor lesion.[133,163] High-grade dysplasia and the size of the adenomas are the most important characteristic that correlates with risk of malignancy. Added to this the sessile serrated lesions which lack the dysplasia are also precursors of CRC. High degree of inter observer variability and non-reproducibility is documented in reporting the grade of dysplasia and villous component of adenoma among pathologists, including gastrointestinal (GI) pathologists.

Inflammatory bowel diseases of colon like Ulcerative colitis and Crohn disease with epithelial dysplasia are the other precursor of CRC. In sporadic cases of CRC, which constitutes 70%-80%, there is sequential mutation and inactivation of APC suppressor gene in addition to KRAS gene, in about 10%-15% DNA mismatch repair MSH2, MLH1 pathway and Hypermethylation MLH1, BRAF in 5%-10% cases in an adenoma which causes progression of adenoma to carcinoma.[133,164] As such there is no definitive diagnostic criteria say which adenomas will progress to malignant transformation. Common screening tests for colorectal Cancer include colonoscopy and fecal immunochemical testing (FIT). Follow up with Surveillance colonoscopy is used to detect and remove Precancerous lesions. Because of cost effectiveness of the colonoscopy in mass screening, implementation of diagnostic and treatment services is not feasible in high risk regions especially in low middle income countries.[146]

Pancreas: Pancreatic Cancer carries poor prognosis and is the seventh leading cause of Cancer death in both sexes. Pancreatic Cancers are known to develop from the precursor lesion through transformation of the pancreatic cell and not 'de novo'. Intraductal papillary mucinous neoplasms and mucinous cystic neoplasms, are Precancerous. Precursor lesions including pancreatic intraepithelial neoplasia, intraductal papillary mucinous neoplasms and mucinous cystic Histopathology 186 WHO classification of digestive system tumors neoplasms. Intraductal oncocytic papillary neoplasm and intraductal tubulopapillary neoplasms. Precursors may be divided into solid and cystic, mucinous and nonmucinous, benign lesions, and with a malignant potential of different degrees. At present, the following precursors are distinguished: serous microcystic adenoma (SMCA), intraductal papillary mucinous neoplasm (IPMN), intraductal tubulopapillary neoplasm (ITPN), mucinous cystic neoplasm (MCN), pancreatic intraepithelial neoplasm (PanIN), and solid pseudopapillary neoplasm (SPN).[164-165] Precursors participate in a recently suggested model of pancreatic carcinogenesis. It starts from the centro- acinar–acinar compartment and develops into PanIN and pancreatic ductal adenocarcinoma (PDAC) through the metaplasia–dysplasia sequence.

The prerequisite for early findings of precursors is the repeated indication of high-resolution imaging methods and **Liver**, Hepatocellular Carcinoma (HCC) is the sixth most commonly diagnosed Cancer and the third leading cause of Cancer death recorded worldwide. The known risk factors for HCC are chronic infection with hepatitis B virus (HBV) or hepatitis C virus (HCV), aflatoxin-contaminated foods, heavy alcohol intake, excess body weight, type 2 diabetes, and smoking.2020). Earlier HCC were clinically diagnosed at a terminal stage, and the average survival after diagnosis was only 3 to 6 months. Precancerous lesion was not concentrated by the clinicians and pathologists, but after the progress in the imaging techniques and careful follow up of the high rick individuals, helps in the early-stage diagnosis of HCC. Hence the histopathological studies of these resected early lesions, biopsy study of small cirrhotic nodular lesions and radiologically suspicious lesions with surveillance and the management strategies like liver transplant has directed the thought of Precancerous lesions in the liver. So, studies have revealed that in noncirrhotic liver, hepatocellular adenoma with β catenin activating mutation and in cirrhotic liver, the large and small cell dysplastic changes, a dysplastic nodule with specifically small cell change are the precursors of HCC. A dysplastic nodule has got the risk of 9% - 31% malignant transformation. Histopathologic examination will help to differentiate dysplastic nodule and well differentiated HCC in most of the cases. Serum Alfa fetoprotein it is not sensitive test for early tumors. Ultrasonography can be used as screening test in high-risk patients like cirrhosis. Computed tomography imaging with contrast studies are diagnostic of HCC by enhancement characters like early arterial phase enhancement, followed by rapid venous washout. Image based Surveillance is very important in high risk individuals and Hepatitis B vaccine may also contribute to the primary prevention of the liver Cancer.[133,164,166]

The Lower Urinary Tract and Male Genital System

Bladder Cancer is the 10th most commonly diagnosed Cancer worldwide, ranks higher among men, for whom it is the 6th most common Cancer and the 9th leading cause of Cancer death. Tobacco smoking and infection with Schistosoma haematobium are the major risk factors and occupational exposures to aromatic amines and others are chemicals affecting workers in the painting, rubber, or aluminum industries and arsenic contamination in drinking water.[133,146]

The two very well documented precursor lesions which progress to invasive urothelial carcinoma are non-invasive papillary tumors and flat non-invasive urothelial carcinoma in situ (CIS). Two relatively different distinct molecular pathways of tumor progression are identified in precursor lesions and invasive bladder Cancer. The non-invasive papillary tumors are the most common which are known to originate from the papillary hyperplasia. In CIS the cytologic features of malignancy are confined to the epithelium, showing no evidence of basement membrane invasion. Not all cases have marked. To differentiate from the reactive Atypia the most reliable criteria are the nuclear enlargement and irregular nuclear chromatin condensation (i.e. nuclear hyperchromasia) because all cases may not show nuclear pleomorphism, full thickness involvement or even a high NC ratio. These "flat" lesions are considered to be high grade and the majority of muscle-invasive bladder Cancers are progression from these precursor "flat" CIS lesions. Very rarely keratinizing squamous metaplasia and dysplasia as well as intestinal mataplasia with high grade dysplasia in cystitis gladularis are considered in view of these lesion can progressed to carcinoma.[133,167]

Cystoscopy is the gold standard test, but Urine cytology is the gold standard non-invasive test for screening the bladder neoplasms in-spite of low sensitivity and subjective diagnostic criteria, it has an excellent specificity.[138]

Prostate: Prostate Cancer (PCA) is the second most frequent Cancer and the fifth leading cause of Cancer death among men. The known factors are limited to advancing age, family history of this malignancy, and certain genetic mutations (e.g, BRCA1 and BRCA2) and conditions like Lynch syndrome.[146] High-grade PIN is the recognized precursor of the majority of prostatic adenocarcinomas. It is also documented in the literature that atypical adenomatous hyperplasia (AAH), Post Inflammatory Atrophy (PIA) and Atypical Small Acinar Proliferation (ASAP) may progress to PIN. Studies have shown that both PIN and PCA are multicentric and majority of PIN occurs in the peripheral zone like the occurrence of PCA. Diagnosis of PIN is characterized by acinar epithelial cellular proliferation in the form of tufting, micropapillary, cribriform, and flat, with cytologic changes of neoplasia with nuclear and nucleolar enlargement. Immunohistochemistry may help in problematic cases like the study of by keratin 34bE12 m (high molecular weight keratin) which distinguishes high-grade PIN (intact or fragmented basal cell layer) from adenocarcinoma. Suggested management is the active surveillance.[152,168-170] Screening for prostate Cancer often involves a prostate-specific antigen (PSA) test.

Penis precursor lesions encompass the umbrella term penile intraepithelial neoplasia (PeIN). All are squamous lesions confined to the epidermis by an intact basement membrane. PeIN may be HPV-related (undifferentiated PeIN) or non–HPV-related (differentiated). Undifferentiated PeIN - Bowen disease, In 10% of patients, Bowen disease gives rise to infiltrating squamous cell carcinoma.

Testis: Germ cell neoplasia in situ is a precursor lesion associated with most GCTs. Seventy percent of patients with documented germ cell neoplasia in situ will develop invasive GCTs. This precursor lesion is found in about 90% of testes involved by germ cell neoplasms and is associated with all types of GCTs except spermatocytic tumor and unusual types that arise in infancy. Germ cell neoplasia in situ also is frequently found in testes at high risk for developing GCTs, such as cryptorchid testes. Germ cell neoplasia in situ is believed to arise in utero and stay dormant until puberty, when hormonal influences may stimulate germ cell growth.

There are a few genetic tumor syndromes which are inherited disorder, in which there is a higher-than-normal risk of certain types of Cancer and caused by mutations in genes passed from parents to children. Some of the lesions seen in these syndromes are not only the precursors, but the mutated gene itself is the factor pathogenic for increased risk for malignancy involving multisystems. The list is very big, mainly involving the digestive system and only their names will be enumerated in this section with the mention of the gene involved in the braces. They are **Familial Adenomatous Polyposis syndrome (APC),**Cowden syndrome (PTEN), MYH-associated polyposis(MYH), Juvenile polyposis (SMAD4,BMPR1A), Peutz-Jeghers Syndrome(STK11), serrated polyposis (Gardner syndrome (APC), Turcot syndrome (APC), **Gastric Adenocarcinoma & proximal polyposis Syndrome (APC),Lynch Syndrome (MLH1, MSH2, MSH6, PMS2,** and **EPCAM** genes),**MUTYH-Associated Polyposis (MAP) syndrome.**(**MUTYH),** Familial pancreatic Cancer (BRCA1 & BRCA2), Li-Fraumeni syndrome(**TP53**), Hereditary Breast and Ovarian Cancer (HBOC) syndrome, Hereditary Diffuse Gastric Cancer (HDGC) syndrome(**CDH1)** and others.[133]

Precursors to Cancers are increasingly recognized as universal, relevant to carcinogenesis, and providing a unique potential for primary and secondary prevention. As the molecular, imaging, and genomic tools to investigate them evolve.

Conclusion

In conclusion, pathology and pathologists play a critical role in Cancer prevention by examining tissue samples and diagnosing Precancerous or Cancerous changes. By identifying early warning signs, pathologists can work with clinicians to develop personalized prevention and treatment plans for patients. In addition, pathologists contribute to Cancer research by studying the molecular and cellular changes that lead to Cancer development and progression. Through their efforts, pathologists help to advance our understanding of Cancer and improve patient outcomes. While the field of Cancer prevention continues to evolve, pathologists remain integral to the ongoing efforts to reduce the incidence and impact of this devastating disease.

10

ROLE OF PUBLIC AWARENESS AND HYGIENE IN CANCER PREVENTION

Dr. Sumita Shankar, Dr. Limalemla Jamir

Background

As per the global Cancer trends in 204 countries and territories over ten years (2010 to 2019), an estimated 23.6 million new Cancer cases and 10.0 million Cancer deaths were reported.[171] Additionally, Cancer burden differed across sociodemographic index (SDI) groups, with the highest increase in Cancer burden among those in the low and low-middle SDI groups.[171] In India, the north-eastern region reportedly has the highest Cancer burden, and across the country, the most common Cancer sites are breast, lung, mouth, cervix uteri and tongue.[172]

Overall, 30-50% of all Cancers are preventable, and the most cost-effective long-term strategy for Cancer control is prevention. While non-modifiable inherited genetic defects contribute to 5–10% of all Cancer cases, environmental factors, which are mainly modifiable, contribute to the remaining 90–95%. The various environmental factors that increase the risk of Cancer include tobacco, alcohol, carcinogens in diet, infectious agents, environmental pollutants and radiation. However, the significant challenges in preventive programs range from deep-rooted cultural practices to unhealthy lifestyles, with the compelling demands of modern living. Therefore, repeated and prolonged exposure to Cancer-causing agents has been known to activate inflammatory pathways, trigger genetic mutations and result in Cancerous tissue in the body.

Hygiene and Cancer

Another important causal pathway in Cancer pathogenesis is poor hygiene, which predisposes to infections and chronic inflammation. Hygiene derived from the word *'Hygiea'*, the name of the goddess of health in Greek mythology, also finds mention in the ancient Indian texts of Ayurveda (*Svastha-vṛtta*), which specify measures for practicing hygiene. In general, maintenance of hygiene at the individual level includes oral hygiene, clean nails and feet, bathing, washing hands after toilet use, clean clothing, and cough and sneeze hygiene; at the domestic level, it includes a clean home, proper storage of food and water, proper waste disposal, a home without insects and rodents etc. At the community level, hygienic practices include sanitary housing, safe drinking water, well-laid drainage, proper excreta and waste disposal, vector control, and market and food outlet hygiene. As per the latest National Family Health Survey (NFHS-5) of India, 19.4 % of the total population does not have access to a toilet, although sanitation facilities have increased from 49 % (NFHS-4) to 70 % (NFHS-5). The vicious cycle of poor hygiene and Cancer remains to be broken in the country in the prevailing circumstances of low awareness and resource constraints.

Several Cancers are associated with poor hygiene. Starting with oral hygiene, poor dental hygiene (tooth brushing once or less per day) is an established risk factor and a possible prognostic factor of head and neck Cancer.[173] Poor oral hygiene alone or tobacco intake, a significant risk factor for multiple Cancers, causes chronic mucosal inflammation and periodontitis, impairs mucosal defense barriers and predisposes to oral, lung, pancreatic, and gastrointestinal Cancers, etc. Alcohol intake has been attributed to an increased risk of oral squamous cell carcinoma through the release of carcinogenic metabolite, acetaldehyde and disruption of the oral microbiome.[174] Carcinogenic infectious agents *(Epstein Barr virus, Helicobacter pylori, Schistosoma haematobium, Opisthorchis viverrine etc.)* and chemicals (pesticides, heavy metals, nitrates, etc.) in unhygienic food and water have been attributed to gastrointestinal Cancers.

As per the International Agency for Research on Cancer, there is a strong causal association between human papillomavirus (HPV) and Cancer cervix uteri, penis, vulva, vagina, anus and oropharynx, including the base of the tongue and the tonsils. Poor genito-oral and sexual hygiene predispose to infections with HPV, trichomonas etc., leading to genital Cancers in both males and females. Additionally, poor hygiene in females disrupts the protective vaginal microbiome increasing the risk of carcinogenesis in the cervix uteri. In males, myiasis in the genitalia is more common among those with poor hygiene and low socio-economic level.[175] At the same time, circumcision and early phimosis treatment are known to prevent penile Cancer.

Cultural practices and personal habits such as unprotected sun exposure, warming the body with hot charcoal-containing vessels and repeated wound trauma have been attributed to skin Cancers such as melanomas, Kangri Cancer in Kashmir and Marjolin's ulcer, a highly aggressive ulcerating squamous cell carcinoma, respectively.

Prevention of Cancer through Public Awareness

Public awareness is essential for Cancer prevention. Following the extensive mass media coverage of the United States Surgeon General's report on the health effects of smoking in 1964, smoking cessation rates rose among middle-aged US adults. Such awareness generation can be made at the individual level through the interactive facility or home-based communication; at the group level through role plays, workshops, lectures, demonstrations, seminars, panel discussions etc. and mass awareness through television, radio, print media, audio-visuals in public places, folk media, public events etc. Social media platforms are increasingly being used to generate awareness at all levels. Online modes of public awareness strategies are also convenient, cost-saving and easily accessible once connectivity is available. Role models (change champions, Cancer survivors, celebrities, and public leaders) also play a key role in various awareness campaigns. Public awareness interventions should be relevant to the target population, culturally appropriate and scientifically sound, behavior change-centered, and aimed at removing social stigma and moving progressively from awareness to motivation and action.

However, prevention efforts through public awareness comprise multi-level strategic approaches based on the disease process. The levels of Cancer prevention through public awareness can be broadly classified into primordial, primary, secondary and tertiary groups (Figure 1). The benefits of hygiene should be emphasized at all levels of prevention so that it is ingrained from the beginning and progresses from awareness to practice.

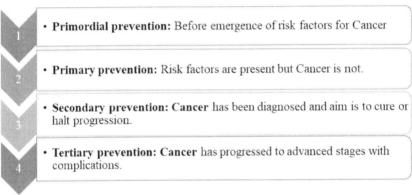

Figure 1

Levels of prevention in the context of Cancer for public awareness strategies.

The strategy for public awareness programs at the primordial prevention stage should be to catch the public attention and get them interested (Figure 2) Well-planned awareness programs must prevent the emergence of risk factors such as alcohol intake due to stress, irrespective of socio-economic and environmental pressures. From educational institutions to workplaces, context-specific awareness sessions should be conducted. For example, a school-based football game program integrated with health education improved knowledge of general and personal hygiene.[175] One can even organize events where people hang out, such as parks, clubs, marketplaces, malls etc. Successful campaigns include mass awareness events in Japan against viral hepatitis and liver Cancer, with proactive advocacy by celebrities to administrators and the involvement of hepatologists in awareness programs at workplaces and educational institutions.[176] Public awareness of the regulations imposed in the public interest by the Food and Drug Administration (FDA) upon the tobacco industry also induced positive sentiments towards FDA and a hostile stance towards the tobacco industry.[177]

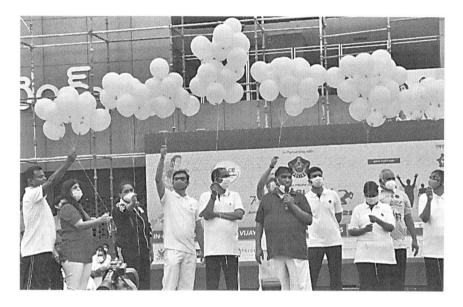

Figure 2

Marathon organized on World Cancer Day [Image courtesy: Dr. S. Shankar]

Once risk factors are present, primary prevention efforts should include risk factor mapping with awareness campaigns at the population level and targeted high-risk group interventions with basic hygiene etiquette. For example, in India, there are pictorial health warnings (PHWs) on cigarette packets to raise awareness of tobacco as a risk factor for oral Cancer, as per The Cigarettes and other Tobacco Products (Packaging and Labelling) Amendment Rules, 2020 (Figure 3). These PHWs have also been reported to motivate smokers to quit smoking or reduce consumption of cigarettes and prevent relapse in ex-smokers.[178] Public awareness intervention trials on alcohol labels, drinking guidelines and warning messages about Cancer also resulted in a significant increase in knowledge gain and retention of the information compared to no such targeted interventions. [179]

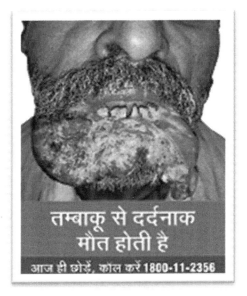

Figure 3

Health warning on cigarette packet [Source: PIB, MoHFW, GoI]

Breast Cancer is one of the most devastating public health problems affecting women worldwide. Willingness (54.3%) to perform breast self-examination, although low awareness (11.5%) indicates the unmet need among women.[180] Awareness programs are yet to penetrate all sections of society. Another important aspect is designing health education material. The content (textual and images) should be culturally sensitive yet scientifically sound.[181] Also, pre-event motivation for encouraging participation in awareness programs is equally important. These can be done through outreach visits to the community stakeholders supplemented with video clips encouraging enrolment.

High cervical Cancer mortality persists in low- and middle-income countries. Early detection and treatment of cervical Precancer through screening programs is a cost-effective measure in preventing deaths due to cervical Cancer. Although screening with a pap smear is considered the most economical and efficient method, associated stigma and fear are significant barriers to screening uptake. However, one-to-one health education and printed educational materials have been reported to increase participation by women.[182,183] Therefore, opportunistic communication, integration with maternal-child services and HPV vaccination programs should be explored for increasing uptake, and these could be more cost-effective as well. Another resourceful human capital for public awareness is laid community volunteers, found to increase knowledge and willingness by women to get screened, clear misconceptions and reduce the stigma associated with cervical Cancer.[184] Although HPV vaccination, and screening with pap smear are the primary modalities for cervical Cancer prevention, personal hygiene education and practice remain more suitable approaches in countries struggling to meet the costs of HPV vaccination and mass screening programs.[185] Starting awareness early among young girls, whether in or out of school, that includes education on menstrual hygiene, would go a long way in healthy behavior behavior throughout the life course.

Colorectal Cancer (CRC) is one of the most common Cancers in Asia. The increasing incidence of CRC among younger age groups reflects the influence of changing environmental and lifestyle factors. Several barriers to CRC health-seeking behavior behavior include lack of knowledge, fear of procedure and result, anticipated costs, and lack of symptoms. Moreover, information leaflets and videos on CRC reportedly have less impact on screening uptake than audio-visual aids and physician recommendations.[186,187] It is, therefore, essential to understand Cancer-specific community facilitators and barriers before designing generic mass awareness campaigns.

Another critical challenge in Cancer prevention is occupational exposure to carcinogens. Asbestos exposure, a commonly used building construction material, has been found to cause malignant mesothelioma and Cancers of the lung, ovary, larynx, and peritoneum.[188] Apart from ensuring that organizations and industries follow government regulations on occupational safety, awareness programs on personal hygiene should be conducted routinely. The use of personal protective equipment, including gloves, hand hygiene, changing clothes, and being mindful of eating or smoking away from the source of contamination are essential preventive measures.

Once carcinogenesis has begun, secondary-level prevention efforts should aim at early diagnosis and prompt treatment. However, low awareness, lack of resources and the concomitant fear of testing and the outcome of the results often prevent people from coming forward. For instance, cervical Cancer screening with a pap smear is often met with such challenges. Therefore, prior sensitization in layperson language, addressing queries, and allaying fears should be done well before institutional opportunistic screening or mass screening camps. Once the diagnosis is made and treatment initiated, a common problem that Cancer patients and their caregivers face basic amenities, including accommodation and transport. To quote, *"My family and village managed to raise resources for transportation and starting treatment at the hospital, but I hardly have any money left for food and accommodation."-* *(Cancer patient).* Therefore, it is also essential to provide information related to these needs by the hospital social services department to enable treatment adherence and prevent progression to advanced stages of Cancer. Additionally, involving patients in the management process by supporting them with information resources, including digital health tools, has improved well-being and treatment adherence.[189] Cancer survivors can also volunteer to experience sharing and motivation of new Cancer patients in treatment initiation and adherence.

Once Cancer progresses to advanced stages, tertiary prevention efforts include awareness of patients and caregivers on disability limitation and rehabilitation modalities, including reconstructive surgeries (Figure 4). Motivation and reminders on daily self-care activities such as oro-genital hygiene are crucial aspects that must continue, as patients are immunocompromised and susceptible to secondary infections. Emphasis should also be made on maintaining the hand hygiene of caregivers and healthcare providers with periodic audit mechanisms.[190]

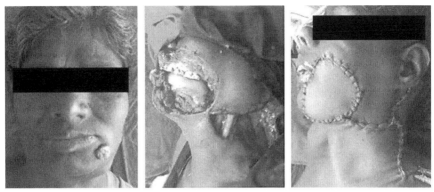

Figure 4

Reconstructive surgery for oral Cancer [Image courtesy: Dr. S. Shankar]

Conclusion

The need to improve public awareness and facilitate community participation is only increasing with the rising trends of multi-modal risk factors for Cancer. Intensified health education and public awareness campaigns are required to remove the social stigma attached to risk factors and Cancer. Awareness of basic hygiene in Cancer prevention must translate to behavior behavior change and adoption as a lifestyle across all sections of society. The motivation of health personnel, involvement and training of lay volunteers, and encouraging participation of the general public in planning and advocacy activities are crucial strategies in Cancer prevention through public awareness.

Audio-visual and print mass media must be used per the target audience's cultural context. Monitoring systems must be established to sustain behavior behavior change with inter-sectoral and inter-disciplinary collaborations. Relevant research must be conducted to inform policy, such as the duration and content of a public awareness campaign to sustain positive Cancer prevention practices. It is also time to go beyond public awareness by recognizing and integrating community-led best practices in Cancer prevention.

11

HABITS & CANCER

Dr. Mythri Shankar

Habits can be good or bad for the body. One can delve into psychological and neurobiological studies to understand it better. Brain networks of habitual behaviors and new decisions we make are molded over time. This can be changed on how we respond to a stimulus or develop new habits through multiple simultaneous signaling processes in the brain.

New emerging basic neuroscience research on habits has broadened our understanding of how habits arise from changes in neural activity in the brain. [192]

Two different behavioral control systems contribute to the reward circuit and influence our decisions - Cognitive (a goal-directed mechanism which weighs the balance between action and consequence) and Habitual (an automated process with no decision-making involved).[193]

Some studies show that new Neural circuits in the brain cortex play a role in influencing and supporting goal-directed and habit behavior via Cellular signaling. In the striatal subregion of the brain, the spiny projection neurons (SPNs) are of two types - GABAergic inhibitory cells that directly (dSPNs) or indirectly (iSPNs) which have Dopamine D1 and D2 receptors which in turn communicate to the project to basal ganglia output nuclei. Which, in turn, have both been implicated in habit-forming behavior. [194]

Establishing long-term changes in habit-related plasticity is related to long-lasting neuroplasticity, changes in the strength of the synapse, alteration in the structure of the dendrites in striatal SPNs have been reported to influence habit learning. There is also evidence to suggest certain changes in the expression of genes can alter neuronal function. Epigenetic mechanisms, therefore, are fundamental regulators of the transcriptional processes mediating the changes in neuronal function and memory. [195]

For example, the histone deacetylases (HDACs) remove acetyl groups from histone tails, creating a repressive chromatin state that prevents active gene transcription. [196]

Multiple variables like Habit strength, Goal-congruent behavior performance, and self-control capacity can make researching this difficult. For example, Habit strength can be assessed by bi-weekly with the Self-Report Habit Index (Verplanken and Orbell, 2003), Goal-congruent behavior performance on a daily basis in their self-chosen context, Self-control capacity was assessed bi-weekly with the Brief Self-Control Scale (Tangney et al., 2004).

But what is crucial is to identify goals and control our actions by building good habits. [197] Many healthy habits can help prevent Cancer. Here are some of them, one on each pillar of Lifestyle Medicine:

a) Quit smoking

Tobacco use is the leading cause of Cancer, and quitting smoking is one of the best things you can do to reduce your risk of Cancer. There are about 4,000 chemicals in a cigarette, 60 of which are Cancer-causing (carcinogens) agents, but the primary culprit is the addictive nicotine. Cigarettes also cause bronchitis, pneumonia, chronic coughs, ear infections, reduced lung function, an increase in severity and episodes of asthma, impotence/ infertility, heart disease and Cancer on various sites. [201]

b) Limit alcohol consumption

154

Drinking too much alcohol can increase the risk of certain types of Cancer, so it is important to limit your intake. It causes an increased risk of mouth Cancer, pharyngeal Cancer (upper throat), oesophageal Cancer (food pipe), laryngeal Cancer (voice box), breast Cancer, bowel Cancer, and liver Cancer. It also increases the levels of estrogen and, therefore, hormone-sensitive Cancers (breast, etc.). [202]

c) Protect your skin

Excessive exposure to the sun's harmful UV rays can increase the risk of skin Cancer, so be sure to protect your skin by using sunscreen and wearing protective clothing. [203]

d) Get vaccinated

Certain viruses, such as HPV and hepatitis B, can increase the risk of Cancer, so it is important to get vaccinated if you are at risk. [204]

e) Regular screenings

Regular Cancer screenings can help detect Cancer early when it is most treatable. Be sure to discuss with your healthcare provider which screenings are recommended based on age, gender, and medical history. Cancer screening can catch Cancer early before symptoms occur to be treated successfully.

Breast, cervical, and oral Cancers are India's most common Cancers. All these Cancers are amenable to easy screening and early detection. Mammography for breast Cancer among women ages 40 to 74, especially those over 50, and regular breast self-examination is advised. [205] Pap test and human papillomavirus (HPV) testing help in the early detection and prevention of cervical Cancer; generally, testing is recommended beginning at age 21 and ending at age 65 in women.

Breast MRI and trans-vaginal ultrasound are often used for women who carry a harmful mutation in the BRCA1 gene or the BRCA2 gene; women with these mutations have a high risk of breast Cancer. The CA-125 test is often done together with a transvaginal ultrasound and may be used to try to detect ovarian Cancer.

155

Visual examination for oral Cancer in high-risk populations is advised for early detection of oral Cancer or premalignant lesions. Clinical examination of the skin should be done routinely, especially in the presence of any suspicious moles or other lesions on the skin.

Colonoscopy, sigmoidoscopy, and stool tests (high-sensitivity fecal occult blood tests and stool DNA tests) detect colorectal Cancer early and help prevent the disease in the first place by finding abnormal colon growths (polyps) that can be removed even before they turn into Cancer. Expert groups generally recommend that people at average risk for colorectal Cancer have screening with one of these tests at ages 50 through 75. Low-dose computed tomography is recommended to screen for lung Cancer in smokers aged 55 to 74.

Alpha-fetoprotein blood test helps to detect liver Cancer early in people at high risk of the disease. Prostate Specific Antigen test is also advised in elderly males to detect prostate Cancer.

f) Food & Nutrition

Eat a healthy and balanced diet: Consuming a variety of whole foods such as fruits, vegetables, whole grains, lean protein, and healthy fats can provide the necessary nutrients and antioxidants that your body needs to prevent Cancer. Say no to red meat and processed foods. Red meat and processed meat are considered carcinogens. They increase colon Cancer risk and breast Cancer recurrence. Fiber-rich foods reduce the risk of Cancer. Poor diet and consuming of fatty foods, processed sugars, and red meat are associated with increased Cancer incidence. Foods rich in phytonutrients, vitamin B12, lycopene, and ellagic acid can help fight Cancer. The more colorful fruits and vegetables are, the more nutrients they have. These foods also help you maintain a healthy body weight, which is vital in preventing Cancer. Greens, herbs, and leaves are rich in green phytonutrients and thylakoids. More than 25,000 phytonutrients are found in plant foods. These foods are rich in Cancer-blocking chemicals, such as sulforaphane, isocyanate, and indoles which inhibit the action of carcinogens.

Reduce or avoid processed meats, smoked meat, meat cooked over an open flame, and red meat. BHA and BHT (petroleum-derived antioxidants used to preserve fat) can cause Cancer. BPA is a chemical used in plastics, which imitates the sex hormone estrogen (endocrine disruptor) and has been linked to Cancer.

Folate and vitamin B protect against colon, rectum, and breast Cancers. Lycopene (tomatoes and tomato products such as juice, sauce, or paste) reduces the risk of several types of Cancer, particularly prostate Cancer. Berries have a phytochemical called ellagic acid, an antioxidant that deactivates certain Cancer-causing substances and slows the growth of Cancer cells. Green tea slows colon, liver, breast, prostate cells, lung tissue, and skin Cancer. Water protects against bladder Cancer by diluting concentrations of potential Cancer-causing agents in the bladder. Beans have potent phytochemicals that may protect the body's cells against damage that can lead to Cancer. Curcumin (the main ingredient in the Indian spice turmeric) can suppress the transformation, proliferation, and spread of Cancerous cells of many Cancers. Much research is still ongoing. [198]

g) Maintain a healthy weight

Being overweight or obese can increase the risk of certain types of Cancer. Therefore, it is important to maintain a healthy weight through regular exercise and a balanced diet. [199]

h) Exercise regularly

Exercise can help reduce Cancer risk by promoting weight loss, reducing inflammation, and regulating hormones. Physical activity reduces mortality and the risk of recurrent breast Cancer by approximately 50%. It can lower the risk of colon Cancer by over 60%. [200]

Read labels and avoid Toxins

These are listed on the label and can be checked off the items before buying. Chemicals to ban from your home.

Sl. No.	Chemicals
1.	Phthalates

2.	BPA
3.	Chlorine
4.	Radon
5.	PFCs
6.	Lead
7.	Pesticides and Fertilisers
8.	Formaldehyde
9.	Parabens
10.	PBDEs and PBBs

Of the 113 agents listed by IARC as known human carcinogens (Group 1), at least 11 have been or are currently used in personal care products: formaldehyde, phenacetin, coal tar, benzene, untreated or mildly treated mineral oils, methylene glycol, ethylene oxide, chromium, cadmium and its compounds, arsenic, and crystalline silica or quartz. Many beauty alternatives are available. Home-made coffee tans, sugar wax, banana peel or cucumber for eye bags and dark circles, and ladyfinger gel hair de-tanglers, aloe vera for skin and hair, flax gel face masks, lemon for de-tanning and nail color, coconut oil and shea butter foot cream. Shampoos made with bio enzymes may be stretching it a bit. Hopefully, soon, someone will come up with a better option. [206]

Minimize exposure to radiation

In 2011, the American Cancer Society (ACS) stated that the IARC classification (a system to evaluate the carcinogenicity of an agent to humans) indicates that there could be some Cancer risk associated with radiofrequency radiation. IARC currently categorizes RFR as a possible human carcinogen (2B). The evidence is not strong enough to be considered causal and must be investigated further. The American Academy of Pediatrics website states that radio frequency electromagnetic radiation emitted from cell phones and phone station antennae can cause headaches, memory problems, dizziness, depression, and sleep problems. It may be associated with Cancer, neurodegeneration, and infertility.

Radiofrequency radiation (RFR) is now recognized as a new type of environmental pollution. Individuals concerned about radiation exposure can limit their exposure to radiofrequency, including using an earpiece and limiting cell phone use, particularly among children.

Some tips to reduce radiation from wireless devices:

a)   Turn them off when not in use.

b)   Use plugged or corded versions (i.e., internet cable, mouse, headsets, or keyboards).

c)   Maximize distance, keeping away from these devices.

d)   Minimize usage of streaming, WIFI, or Bluetooth.

e)   Avoid phone/device usage while sitting in vehicles.

f)   Avoid cell phone usage when the battery power or signal is low.

g)   Use laptops or tablets on hard surfaces (not laps or beds).

h)   Use speaker phones or text messages.

i)   Do not sleep with your phone close to you.

In 2011, the American Cancer Society (ACS) stated that the IARC classification means that there could be some Cancer risk associated with radiofrequency radiation. Still, the evidence is not strong enough to be considered causal and must be investigated further. Individuals concerned about radiofrequency radiation exposure can limit their exposure to it, including using an earpiece and limiting cell phone use, particularly among children. [207]

Adopting these healthy habits can reduce your risk of Cancer and lead a healthier life. The brain and body are designed to give you results. It will happen gradually. Neurogenesis and Neuro Plasticity take time. The Basal Ganglia in the brain learns slowly and inherits functions from the prefrontal cortex and makes it automated. The goal is to make it "Basal," building a culture around this so that it drips down to the subconscious and sticks better.

It takes time to form new habits. Success is influenced by multiple factors - frequency, consistency, and difficulty level. 21/90 rule; it takes about 21 days to form a habit and 90 days to break one. Meaning it takes a few days to form a habit partially and more days to form a habit ultimately. Repetition over time (weeks and months) is what makes it stick hard. And it becomes second nature and automated as long as you keep at it. Challenging habits take a longer time. The higher the frequency, the sooner it becomes a habit. The magic number seems to be at least four times a week.

Habits prevent decision fatigue by reducing time and energy spent making choices and keeping things simple. Keeping options simple also helps - this or that (peanuts/ apple versus chips/chocolate). One can also introduce an element of time limits; it's easier -- "out of it," "by this weekend," or "the end of the month."

Good Habits to Prevent Cancer

a) Eat healthy (Plant-based, low-fat whole food diet), rich in fiber.

b) Weigh less maintain a normal BMI.

c) Move and exercise regularly.

d) Quit smoking and quit chewing tobacco.

e) Reduce alcohol intake.

f) Breastfeed your baby.

g) Get screened or tested early. Don't neglect this.

12

FAMILY HISTORY OF CANCERS. IS IT SIGNIFICANT?

Dr. K. Govind Babu

Introduction

The family is the basic unit of society and is an intimate group of people related to one another by bonds of blood, marriage, emotion, and legal ties. We inherit genes from our ancestors and risk inheriting genes causing Cancer. We have various genomic tools to investigate hereditary Cancer predisposition, but family history remains an essential and often neglected part of patient evaluation. Knowing one's family history not only ascertains the risk of developing Cancer but also opens new treatment options for such hereditary Cancers and provides opportunities for screening tests for early detection for unaffected family members.

Cancer: A Genetic disease

Globally, Cancer is the second most common cause of non - communicable diseases rating next to heart diseases. There has been an exceptional improvement in the understanding of Cancer in the last two decades. The Human Genome Project has clarified that Cancer is a genetic disease. Genes are the functional unit of heredity and are made up of DNA. We inherit genes from our ancestors. A mutation is a change in the gene that may alter its function of the gene. Such modifications can be acquired from our ancestors (Germline mutations) or may develop due to exposures later in life (Somatic mutations). Genes causing Cancers are of two types, Oncogenes (Cancer promoting genes) and Tumor suppressor genes (which prevent the formation of Cancer) (Figure 1). The imbalance between oncogenes and tumor suppressor genes leads to Cancer formation. Such oncogenes can be inherited from our ancestors, or we may have inherited a defective version of the tumor suppressor gene, which might lead to Cancer predisposition.

Does Everyone Who Inherits Cancer-Causing Genes Develop Cancer?

A complex interplay exists between genes and environmental exposures (Figure 2). The expression of inherited genes may be modified by diet, lifestyle factors like smoking and alcohol, and occupational/ environmental exposure to chemicals/ radiation. It is observed that family members share the genes and food habits, lifestyle, and environmental exposures. Cancer affecting multiple family members in many families is due to obesity or infective agents like Helicobacter pylori. Not everyone who inherits Cancer-causing genes develops Cancer. Various risk reduction strategies help individuals change their lifestyles or use surgery or pharmacologic agents for risk reduction.

Correlation To Cancer

Factors that point to a hereditary Cancer predisposition are multiple affected family members with the same or related Cancers and younger age of onset compared to sporadic Cancers. Family history's significance can be easily understood with two hereditary Cancer predisposition syndromes-Hereditary breast-ovarian Cancer syndrome and Lynch syndrome.

Hereditary breast-ovarian Cancer syndrome (HBOC)

Family history of breast and ovarian Cancer is common, but HBOC accounts for less than 10 % of breast Cancers and less than 15 % of ovarian Cancers. HBOC is associated with germline (inherited) genetic mutations in Tumor suppressor genes BRCA 1(located on chromosome 17q21) and BRCA2 gene (located on chromosome 13q). BRCA 1 and 2 play several roles in maintaining genome integrity, like DNA repair, regulation of cell cycle checkpoints, and homologous recombination. The characteristics of HBOC are multiple cases within the same family, early onset, bilateral breast Cancer, synchronous Cancers, associated malignancies in patient/family members, and male breast Cancer. As outlined in Table, the Cancer risk varies in BRCA 1 and 2. Other Cancers associated with BRCA 1 are Cancers of the cervix, uterus, fallopian tube, primary peritoneum, pancreas, esophageal, stomach, and prostate Cancer. BRCA2 is associated with the stomach, gallbladder, bile duct, esophagus, stomach, fallopian tube, primary peritoneum, and skin Cancers. Indications for testing for BRCA 1 and 2 are outlined in Table 2.

Therapeutic Implications for Patients with BRCA Mutation

Assessment of BRCA mutations is no longer a tool for planning secondary prevention and genetic counseling for the family but is also crucial for treatment planning (Figure 3).

Choice of chemotherapy: DNA-damaging drugs like Platinum agents cause DNA double-strand breaks, and the absence of *BRCA1* expression leads to hypersensitivity of cells to DNA damage-based chemotherapy. Patients with BRCA mutation have shown very high pCR and ORR with platinum compounds compared to sporadic BC.

Targeted therapy: PARP inhibitors

Poly (ADP-ribose) polymerase (PARP) is a family of nuclear enzymes with a critical role in recognizing and repairing DNA single-strand breaks. In *BRCA*-mutated cells, homologous recombination is defective, and these damages cannot be efficiently repaired, resulting in cell deaths. Based on the results of phase III randomized controlled trial (RCT) OlympiAD,single-agent PARPi olaparib is approved as the first targeted therapy for patients with *BRCA*-mutated HER2-negative metastatic breast Cancer.

For high-risk patients with BRCA mutations, following surgery (High-risk factors- Tumor size more than 5cm and positive lymph nodes), Adjuvant Olaparib for one-year improved iDFS (Olympia). Neoadjuvant Talazoparib for 24 weeks in BRCA-mutated patients resulted in exceptional response rates (pCR 48%) in the NEOTALA study.

Role of Immunotherapy

Patients with BRCA 1 mutation have an aggressive subtype of breast Cancer, triple-negative breast Cancer (TNBC), which tests negative for estrogen receptor, progesterone receptor, and HER2 neu. Expression of PD-L1 in the tumor microenvironment, on both tumor cells and tumor-infiltrating immune cells, can inhibit antitumor responses.PD-L1 expression has been observed in more than 50% of advanced TNBC tumors. Therapies targeting the PD-L1 / PD-1 pathway enhances the immune response. Pembrolizumab and Atezolizumab (PD L1 +) have provided clinically meaningful progression-free survival and median Overall Survival in patients with metastatic disease. (Keynote 355, Impassion 130)

Preventive Strategies

Family members of affected individuals undergo genetic counseling before and after genetic testing. Depending on their risk, individuals who test positive for BRCA-1 mutation can opt for risk reduction surgeries like bilateral mastectomy with or without bilateral salpingo-oophorectomy.

Surveillance is a must for unaffected BRCA mutation carriers. Breast self-examination, annual clinical breast examination by the clinician, and yearly breast MRI examination are required for early detection of breast Cancer. Maintaining a healthy lifestyle with regular daily exercise to maintain healthy body weight and abstaining from smoking and alcohol are emphasized.

Lynch Syndrome (Hereditary non-polyposis colorectal Cancer)

Approximately 5% of Colorectal Cancers are hereditary. Lynch Syndrome (LS) is the most common inherited colon Cancer susceptibility syndrome. LS is associated with an increased risk of malignancies like colorectal Cancer, Endometrial Cancer, gastric, ovarian, pancreas, urinary tract, biliary tract, brain, small intestine, and skin. LS is caused by Inheriting a germline mutation in one of several DNA mismatch repair (MMR) genes. MMR genes proofread DNA for mismatches generated during DNA replication. Inactivation of MMR leads to an increased mutation rate in dividing cells, increasing tumorigenesis risk. Microsatellites are short repetitive DNA sequences. Defective MMR genes cause abnormalities in microsatellite length, leading to microsatellite instability (MSI). Cancers with more than 40% microsatellite variations are said to be high-frequency MSI (MSI High). MSI High is the molecular signature of Lynch-associated Cancers.

Patients with LS inherit one abnormal allele of MLH1, MSH2, MSH6, or PMS2. 70% of MLH1 and MSH2 are associated with EPCAM Epigenetic silencing of MSH2. Defective MMR is due to the inactivation of both alleles MMR gene. The second allele is lost through mutation, loss of heterozygosity, or epigenetic silencing by promoter hypermethylation.

LS is suspected if Colorectal or uterine Cancer is diagnosed in a patient who is less than 50 years of age, if the Presence of synchronous, metachronous colorectal, or other HNPCC-associated tumors, regardless of age, if Colorectal Cancer with MSI-H histology is diagnosed in a patient who is less than 60 years of age, if Colorectal Cancer diagnosed in one or more first-degree relatives with an HNPCC-related tumor, with one of the Cancers being diagnosed under age 50 years or if Colorectal Cancer is diagnosed in two or more first- or second-degree relatives with HNPCC-related tumors, regardless of age. (Revised Bethesda Guidelines for testing colorectal tumors for microsatellite instability (MSI).

Screening recommendations for LS

For colorectal Cancers:

a) Colonoscopy, starting at age 20, is repeated every 1 to 2 years until age 40. Colonoscopy every year after age 40.

b) Acolectomy (removing the entire colon) should be considered if cancer is found. Continue annual screening for rectal Cancer.

c) Prophylactic (preventative) colon removal is sometimes considered when a colonoscopy cannot be performed.

d) Regular colonoscopy, every 1 to 2 years, for individuals with Lynch syndrome has been proven to decrease the colorectal Cancer risk by more than 50 percent.

For endometrial and ovarian Cancers:

1. Transvaginal ultrasound and a CA-125 blood test every year beginning at age 30. Unfortunately, screening for ovarian Cancer is not adequate. Therefore, some women with Lynch syndrome are advised a total hysterectomy (removal of the uterus) with salpingo-oophorectomy (removal of both fallopian tubes and ovaries) to eliminate their risk for developing endometrial Cancer and to reduce the risk for ovarian Cancer. This should be considered after age 35 after childbearing is complete, whichever is later.

2. **Stomach Cancer:** Upper endoscopy starts at age 30, with follow-up no less than every three years.

3. **Skin Cancer:** Annual exam beginning the year after diagnosis.

4. **Urothelial Cancer (bladder, ureters, urethra) Cancer or a mutation in the MSH2 gene:** Ultrasound is repeated every five years after diagnosis.

5. **Small bowel Cancer:** Capsule endoscopy starts at age 30, with follow-up every three years.

6. **Urine testing:** All patients diagnosed with Lynch syndrome should have a urinalysis every year beginning at age 35.

Conclusion

Even in the era of genomic medicine, documentation of complete family history is essential. It helps in making an accurate diagnosis of familial Cancer syndrome. It has important therapeutic implications for the index case, including prophylactic therapies and agents like chemotherapy, targeted therapy, or immunotherapy for treatment. The unaffected family members need to be counseled and should undergo genetic testing. Depending on the results, they should be advised of screening methods for early detection and preventive strategies. In the era of nuclear families, it is unfortunate that family ties are loosening at a fast pace, and patients hardly know anything about the health condition of the family members! Documenting family history remains a neglected aspect of daily practice but can through light regarding diagnosis, treatment options, and prevention.

13

INFLUENCE OF CIRCADIAN RHYTHM AND SLEEP ON CANCER

Dr. Sharan B Singh M

Biological clock

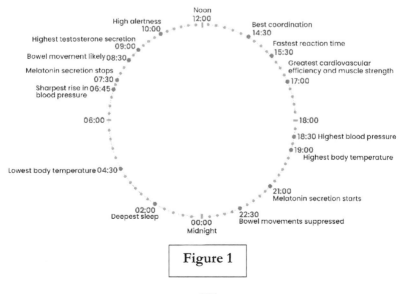

Figure 1

Pineal gland

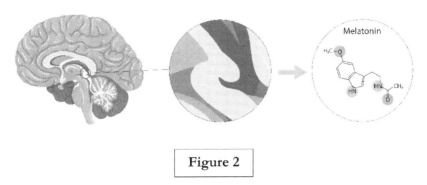

$$\boxed{\textbf{Figure 2}}$$

Melatonin appears to play a role in both physiological and pathophysiological processes, including the control of sleep, circadian rhythms, retinal physiology, seasonal reproductive cycles, Cancer development and growth, immune activity, antioxidation, and free radical scavenging, mitochondrial respiration, cardiovascular function, bone metabolism, intermediary metabolism, and gastrointestinal physiology.

Melatonin suppresses the initiation phase of tumorigenesis by suppressing the accumulation of DNA adducts formed by carcinogens that cause damage to and permanent alterations in DNA, which lead to neoplastic transformation. This may be accomplished directly via melatonin's ability to act as a potent free radical scavenger and/or through its indirect actions to detoxify carcinogens via activation of the glutathione and related antioxidative pathways.

Melatonin has a well-known enhancement of many immune functions, including the production of various cytokines. There is a tight correlation between the nocturnal production of melatonin and the nocturnal rise in circulating T lymphocytes. The synthesis and release of melatonin from human immunocompetent cells- Endogenous melatonin interacts with the immune system in an endocrine, intracrine, autocrine, and/ or paracrine manner to physiologically regulate the IL-2 and IL-2 receptor system in these cells, i.e., oncostatin action of melatonin on Cancer cells.

In modern 24-h a day society, the overall prevalence of sleep disturbances and daytime sleepiness has increased. In contrast, sleep duration during each night has decreased by several accounts. Furthermore, exposure to artificial light at night, particularly during night shift work and television, has been responsible for altering our lifestyles and sleep habits. The increase in breast Cancer associated with living in modern-day societies cannot be accounted for by the usual risk factors.

Exposure to artificial light at night in the built environment in, the causation of circadian disruption, particularly the suppression of nocturnal melatonin production and circadian phase shifts, is emerging as a potential new etiologic agent in the genesis of a variety of human Cancers.

Roles of circadian clock components in Cancer

At the molecular and cellular levels, there is close crosstalk between the circadian clock machinery and the cell cycle, DNA repair, apoptosis, senescence, autophagy, and other oncogenic and immune pathways. Circadian perturbations dysregulate these processes, leading to uncontrolled proliferation, escape from apoptosis, metastatic spread, immune evasion, enhanced angiogenesis, and anti-cancer drug resistance, all hallmarks of Cancer.

In this regard, multiple loss- and gain-of-function studies with cellular and animal models have demonstrated the direct involvement of clock genes in Cancer predisposition and development. Epigenetic or genetic inactivation of Bmal1 and Clock genes has been shown to increase tumor proliferation or growth rates in several types of Cancer, such as hematologic Cancer, colon Cancer, pancreatic Cancer, tongue squamous cell carcinoma (TSCC), breast Cancer, lung adenocarcinoma, hepatocellular carcinoma (HCC), nasopharyngeal carcinoma (NPC), and glioblastoma (GBM).

Conversely, overexpression of these circadian activators suppresses proliferative and malignant phenotypes in tumor cells via mechanisms involving cell cycle arrest and p53-dependent apoptosis.

Similarly, downregulation or upregulation of Per1, Per2, and Cry1, the principal target genes of BMAL1/CLOCK, has been shown to promote or suppress tumor incidence and proliferation, respectively, in multiple Cancer cell types, including Lewis lung carcinoma and mammary carcinoma cells, pancreatic Cancer, lung carcinoma, leukemia, glioma, ovarian Cancer, and oral squamous cell carcinoma.

The potential anti-cancer mechanism exerted by PER1/2 has been suggested to involve the inhibition of PI3K/AKT/mTOR-mediated glycolysis and cell cycle arrest and apoptosis induction.

Also, some studies show that the core clock genes exert tumor-promotive functions, depending on the Cancer cell status or type. For example, BMAL1 silencing led to a substantial increase in apoptosis with mitotic and morphological abnormalities in malignant pleural mesothelioma (MPM) cells44. Similarly, knockdown of either BMAL1 or CLOCK has been observed to induce cell cycle arrest and apoptosis in Cancer Circadian clock systems.

The SCN central clock in the brain, primarily entrained by light, orchestrates circadian phases not only in nonSCN subordinate brain clocks via rhythmic release of neurotransmitters and neuropeptides but also in peripheral organ clocks via systemic hormonal secretion and neural innervations.

Nonphotic external cues (e.g., temperature changes, food intake, exercise, and pathogens) can reset circadian rhythms in peripheral clock tissues, thereby influencing rhythmic output physiology and behaviors. Furthermore, a recent study showed that BMAL1 overexpression promotes breast Cancer cell invasion and metastasis by upregulating the expression of matrix metalloproteinase 9 (MMP9), a mediating factor for local invasion and distant metastasis of tumors. More recently, CRY1 has been suggested to be a critical factor for efficient DNA repair in tumors, acting as a protumorigenic factor.

Knockout of Cry1/2-/- in mice enhances apoptosis pathways in genotoxic responses to UV or cisplatin, a DNA-damaging agent, by causing increased expression of the proapoptotic Factor p7349. The tumor-promoting function of CRY1 has been further suggested in a recent study showing that CRY1 enhances p53 tumor suppressor degradation via p53 binding to its ubiquitin E3 ligase MDM2 proto-oncogene in bladder Cancer cells, thereby increasing anticancer drug sensitivity. Altogether, these results suggest divergent roles of circadian clock genes in tumor pathogenesis depending on the cell type and/or state.

Consistent with these results, a recent large-scale systems analysis of 32 human Cancer types revealed that PERs and CRYs, among several other clock genes, are downregulated in multiple Cancers. These findings highlight the tumor suppressor function of canonical clock components in most Cancer types.

Targeting circadian rhythms in Cancer Treatment

Further insights into circadian rhythms and their related diseases have ignited growing interest in how these processes can be utilized to improve Cancer prevention and treatment.

Chronotherapeutic approaches can be categorized into three types:

(1) Training the clock: Interventions to enhance or maintain a robust circadian rhythm in feeding-fasting, sleep-wake, or light-dark cycles;

(2) Drugging the clock: Using small-molecule agents that directly target a circadian clock; and

(3) Clocking the drugs: Optimizing the timing of drugs to improve efficacy and reduce adverse side effects.

14

GERIATRIC ONCOLOGY

CAN WE PREVENT CANCER AMONG THE ELDERLY?

Dr. Meena Kumari B.T

What is the definition of the Old Age?

Though there is a chronologic definition of old age as people above 65, it is ideally defined based on functional status.

Why should we focus on older adults?

We are currently in the midst of a demographic revolution due to the aging of populations worldwide, particularly in Western countries. Notably that people 85 and older are the most rapidly growing segment of the population.[210] Cancer incidence is increasing in older people as a logical consequence of a longer life span that promotes prolonged exposure to carcinogens and accumulation of genetic alterations. Cancer represents a significant cause of mortality in this population, and Cancer-specific mortality increases as a function of age, despite recent progress in managing Cancer in the general population.[211] Given the dramatic demographic shift observed in developed countries, the medical community, especially the oncologists, geriatricians, and primary care providers, are confronted with the expanding challenges of managing the elderly with Cancer. Aging is associated with accumulating multiple and various medical and social problems. With a prevalence comparable to that of other chronic conditions in this age group, such as diabetes or dementia, Cancer is prominent among diseases of the elderly.[212]

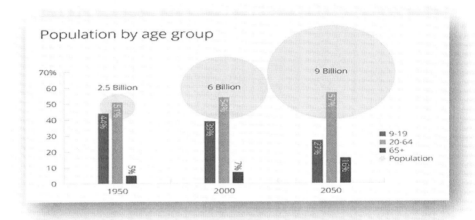

Figure 1

Increasing life expectancy-worldwide phenomenon [213]#

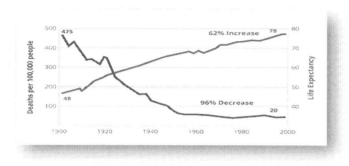

Invasive Cancer incidence, by Age, U.S., 2009

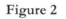

Figure 2

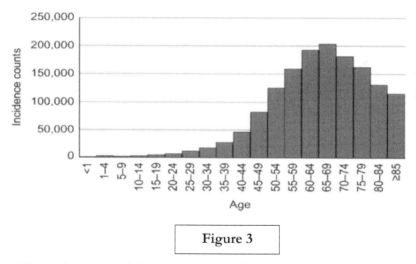

Figure 3

The total number of Cancers is projected to increase by 45% from 2010 to 2030. 70% of all Cancers will occur among adults aged ≥65 years. Lifetime risk (%) of receiving a diagnosis or dying of Cancer by Age, U.S.[214]

One of the main characteristics of elderly patients is the simultaneous presence of more than one morbid condition.[220]

Current age (years)	Risk of receiving a cancer diagnosis				Risk of dying of cancer
	≥10 years	≥20 years	≥30 years	Ever	
0	0.17	0.35	0.79	41.24	21.00
10	0.18	0.63	1.67	41.62	21.25
20	0.45	1.5	4.13	41.65	21.31
30	1.06	3.73	9.85	41.74	21.45
40	2.72	8.98	20.14	41.55	21.57
50	6.57	18.29	31.00	40.77	21.55
60	13.09	27.28	35.94	38.20	20.86
70	17.85	28.74	—	31.59	18.56
80	16.83	—	—	21.23	14.15

Figure 4

Cancer in older people – Pathophysiology [215] United Nations and WHO declaration.. Adding life to years.

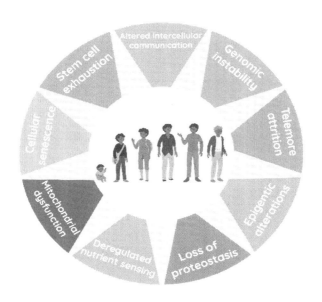

Figure 5

Hallmarks Of Ageing [216]

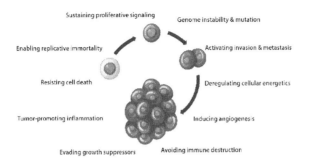

Sustaining proliferative signaling

Genome instability & mutation

Enabling replicative immortality

Activating invasion & metastasis

Resisting cell death

Deregulating cellular energetics

Tumor-promoting inflammation

Inducing angiogenesis

Evading growth suppressors

Avoiding immune destruction

Figure 6

Hallmarks Of Cancer [216]

United Nations and WHO declaration......

Adding Life to years

In 2020 first time in history, people aged >60 years outnumbered children younger than five years.

The proportion of elderly---

In 2017 the ratio of people aged >60 to children younger than five years was 1:8; in 2030, it is expected to be 1:6, and in 2050, 1:5.

Personal characteristics

Genetic inheritance

Health characteristics
- Underlying age-related trends
- Health-related behaviours, traits and skills
- Physiological changes and risk factors
- Diseases and injuries
- Changes to homeostasis
- Broader geriatric syndromes

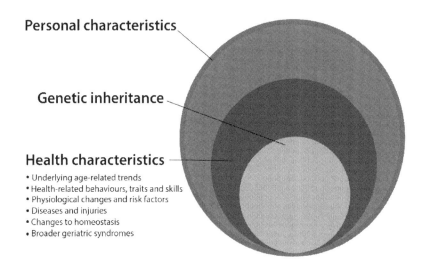

Figure 7

Strategies to reduce Cancer incidence

Screening Strategies- To catch them early and Cure. Our aim should be to Prevent Cancers or Prevent Advanced Cancers.

1) Reduce social isolation and loneliness.

Meditation, Mindfulness-based-stress-reduction, cognitive-behavioral therapy, Relaxation techniques, Biofeedback. Poor health behavior's influence Cancer risk and inadequate physical activity.

Pro-inflammatory gene expression pathway. Psychosocial and behavior interventions (e.g.) increase meaningful activity & social connection, which have been claimed to have the potential to slow cell aging & Cancer development.

Optimism and social engagement – "2 PILLS" that may increase healthy life span by ten years.

2) **To reduce environmental exposure (Cancer Initiators, Cancer Promoters).**

a) Reduce exposure to ionizing radiation (e.g., ultraviolet radiation from the sun).

b) Radiation from medical imaging procedures.

c) Drinking water contaminants (arsenic &Trichloroethylene).

d) Air pollutants such as ozone, sulfur oxides, and nitrous oxides.

e) Pesticides and chemicals.

3) **Place as a determinant of health.**

4) **Better access to preventive services, better social conditions.**

5) **Improve access to health literature - Better/understandable health messaging.**

6) **Quit smoking.**

I. Within 12 hrs, the carbon monoxide level in the blood drops down.

II. Within three months, lung circulation and function improve.

III. After 15 years, the risk of coronary heart disease is the same as that of a non-smoker.

Areas of Need- Cancer prevention in elderly

I. More Research.

II. Build healthy communities - Eg- Access, Environmental exposure.

III. Eliminate health disparities -Eg- Rural-urban divide, Health literacy.

IV. Evidence-Based Clinical &Community Preventive services - Eg:

Cancer screening, Tobacco cessation.

V. Empower people to make healthy choices -Eg: Ageism, Care-giver concerns.

Cancer Screening

Screening is available for breast, prostate, cervical, colon, and lung Cancer.

a) Breast Cancer - Screening starts at age>40 years, yearly Mammogram, and until Age 84 years.

b) Prostate Cancer - Age 55-75 years, PSA and DRE annually, stop beyond 75/Stop if PSA <3 Years even at 75years.

c) Cervical Cancer ----- Age > 24 years. PAP smear and HPV test -3 yearly, Stop at 60 years of age.

d) Colorectal Cancer - Age>50 years, Colonoscopy at least every ten years, Continue till 75 years.

e) Lung Cancer --- Age ≥50 years and ≥20 pack-year histories of smoking, Low dose CT yearly. Stop at 77 years/Continue if fit.

How does screening help?

a) Prevent Cancer deaths by Better Treatment.

b) Reduce Cancer deaths and provide better supportive care.

Polypharmacy and interactions

Financial toxicity

1. The population of older people will boom in times to come.

2. Cancer in the elderly is and will be a significant public health problem in times to come.

3. There is a renewed focus on preventive oncology older people.

4. Prevention efforts include:

a) Strategies to reduce social isolation.

b) Reduction in environmental exposure to carcinogens.

c) Better access, better social conditions.

d) Efforts to improve health literacy.

e) Avoid Ageism.

5. Continue to screen for Cancers in elderly.

Cancers remain frightening, and the geriatrician/primary care provider can recognize the aspects of depression related to the Cancer diagnosis. Besides the technical tools focused on specific elements of Cancer management, other domains like social, familial, spiritual, and psychological support should also be explored to improve the care and health of elderly patients with Cancer. Rehabilitation with appropriate nutritional intervention, physiotherapy, and occupational therapy should also be encouraged through specifically organized programs. Last but not least, the social environment may determine access to care and the exact position of the elderly Cancer patient within his family group. Therefore, personal and cultural aspects must be integrated into the comprehensive management of elderly patients with Cancer.[217]

Palliative care is a domain shared by both geriatric medicine and oncology.[218] Pain, anxiety, fatigue, and dyspnea are among the problematic symptoms experienced not only by elderly dying people but also by all metastatic Cancer patients, regardless of age. However, elderly patients are at higher risk of poor treatment because their sensitivity and tolerance to pain may be underrated.[219]

15

BARIATRIC SURGERY- ITS IMPACT ON REDUCING CANCER RISK

Dr. Pradeep Chowbey

Introduction

Obesity is an established global pandemic showing no signs of abating. The global prevalence of overweight and obesity has increased by 27% in adults and 47% in children.[221] By 2025, global obesity prevalence will reach 18% in men and surpass 21% in women; severe obesity will exceed 9% in women and 6% in men.[222] From 1975 to 2016, the prevalence of obesity in children and adolescents increased from 0·7% to 5·6% in girls and 0·9% to 7·8% in boys.[223] The link between obesity and Cancer is well established. In 2012, 3.6% of all new Cancers were linked to obesity. Population attributable fraction PAFs were more significant in women than men (5·4% versus 1·9%).[224] A study in 2003 found that a BMI of at least 40 Kg/m2 was associated with death rates from all Cancers combined that were 52 percent higher (for men) and 62 percent higher (for women) than the rates in men and women of normal weight.[225]

The association between obesity and Cancer is related to an increased incidence and a poorer prognosis. Esophageal, pancreatic, gastric, hepatocellular, gallbladder, thyroid, colorectal, multiple myeloma, meningioma, ovarian, postmenopausal breast, and endometrial and renal Cancers have all been found to have an increasing incidence with increasing body mass index (BMI).[226-228] Cancer is the second most typical cause of mortality following cardiovascular diseases in the world.[229] An increase in these life-shortening non-communicable diseases NCDs is likely to neutralize any benefit of longevity and improved quality of life after a decrease in infectious diseases and progress in medicine in addition to increasing the overall healthcare costs. The International Agency for Research on Cancer (IARC) working group states that the absence of excess body fat lowers the risk of Cancer. A review of experimental animals and mechanistic data studies suggested a causal Cancer-preventive effect of intentional weight loss.[214] Bariatric surgery has proved to be the best treatment option for significant and sustained weight loss, reversal/ improvement in comorbid conditions, and decreased associated mortality. There is increasing evidence of the positive effect of bariatric surgery on obesity-related Cancers.

Obesity and Risk of Cancer

Obesity is associated with a greater incidence of Cancer; additionally, being overweight and obese increases the risk of death for patients with obesity-associated Cancers and non-obesity-related Cancers like premenopausal breast Cancer and squamous cell oral tongue Cancer.[231-232] An umbrella review of 204 systematic reviews and meta-analysis on adiposity and Cancer showed that out of 36 primary Cancers studied, associations for nine Cancers with obesity were supported by solid evidence, predominantly comprising Cancers of digestive organs and hormone-related malignancies in women. The increase in the risk of developing Cancer for every 5 kg/m² increase in body mass index ranged from 9% for rectal Cancer to 56% for biliary Cancer in men. The risk of postmenopausal breast Cancer among women who have never used Hormone Replacement Therapy increased by 11% for each 5 kg of weight gain in adulthood, and the risk of endometrial Cancer increased by 21% for each 0.1 increase in waist-to-hip ratio,[233] according to the IARC working group. Obesity is linked to Cancers of at least 13 different anatomical locations. It is endometrial, esophageal, renal, and pancreatic adenocarcinomas, hepatocellular carcinoma, gastric cardia Cancer, meningioma, multiple myeloma, colorectal, postmenopausal breast, ovarian, gallbladder and thyroid Cancers.[230] A review of 203 studies[234] comprising more than 6.3 million patients studying the overall survival OS, Cancer-specific survival CSS, disease-free survival DFS, and tumor progression-free survival PFS showed obesity to be an independent prognostic factor in determining the outcome in these patients. It was associated with a worse product for all four parameters (viz. OS, CSS, DFS, PFS) compared to patients with the reference range BMI except in patients with lung Cancer and melanoma, a phenomenon called the "obesity paradox".[235] This is likely due to the use of BMI, which is a crude measure of obesity and does differentiate adipose tissue from lean body mass; selection bias and confounding factors have been suggested as the reason for this phenomenon. This assumes importance in the face of being misinterpreted as obesity being protective against some Cancers.

Pathophysiology linking obesity to Cancer

Obesity is a state of excess adipose tissue that creates an environment of cellular proliferation by activating growth factor signaling pathways and potentiates the risk for neoplastic transformation. The mechanism by which obesity creates an oncogenic environment involves:

1. Hyperinsulinemia, Insulin resistance resulting in high levels of circulating insulin and changes in insulin-like growth factors IGF signaling. These changes act by promoting cellular proliferation and inhibiting apoptosis. This rapid proliferation may result in DNA damage and induce mutations that are tumorigenic.[236]

2. The high visceral fat volume in hormonal pathways forms a source for increased oestrogen production. The increased levels of circulating estrogen are responsible for hormone-dependent Cancers like post-menopausal breast and endometrial Cancers.[237-239]

3. Excess adipose tissue causes altered adipocytokines levels such as high leptin levels pro-inflammatory and low adiponectin levels known as anti-inflammatory, insulin sensitizer, and anti-tumorigenic, have growth, immune, and tumor-regulatory functions.[240]

4. A chronic inflammatory environment and oxidative stress resulting from ectopic fat deposition, a pathological expansion of white adipose tissue into areas it should not be in (e.g., intrahepatic, intra-abdominally, intramyocellular, etc.). This ectopic fat causes metabolic, inflammatory, and immunologic alterations that affect deoxyribonucleic acid (DNA) repair, gene function, cell mutation rate, epigenetic changes permitting malignant transformation, and progression.[241-243]

5. The gut microbiome is a complex symbiosis system between the host and the microbiota. The gut microbiome is known to get altered in obesity and exert its tumor-inducing effect by promoting inflammation and producing Cancer-promoting substances.[244-247]

6. Mechanical trauma - The incidence of esophageal adenocarcinoma EAC has risen in parallel with the rising incidence of obesity. The association of EAC with obesity is multifactorial, and one contributing factor is the high incidence of gastroesophageal reflux disease GERD seen in the obese population.[248-249] GERD causes recurrent trauma due to acid reflux and is associated with Barrett's esophagus and EAC.

Cellular growth and proliferation are controlled by a delicate balance of several factors, including internal and external signaling for cellular growth and division and sufficient nutrients to provide the energy for the process. Obesity provides excess nutrition and altered growth factors, which can disturb this critical balance resulting in cellular neoplastic transformation.

Broadly the changes in the pathways mentioned above promote neoplastic transformation by creating a pro-inflammatory state. Conversely, does weight loss counter these mechanisms and reduce the risk of obesity-induced tumorigenesis? Weight loss is associated with a decrease in all-cause mortality due to obesity.[250] Weight loss decreases the risk of postmenopausal breast Cancer recurrence [251]and endometrial Cancer.[236] Intensive lifestyle intervention to improve the patient's overall health can reduce obesity-related Cancer risk by 16%.[253]

Bariatric surgery - Cancer risk-reducing mechanisms

Bariatric surgery (BS) is a treatment option for weight loss in morbidly obese patients. It is safe and has been documented to help achieve well-sustained weight loss.[254] The benefits of bariatric surgery in improving obesity-related comorbid conditions and increasing life expectancy are well documented.[255-256] The use in reducing Cancer incidence is linked to the sustained weight loss and weight loss-independent mechanisms following BS.

Mechanisms associated with weight loss are predominantly decreased circulating estrogen levels and improved insulin sensitivity.[257-258] The suggested weight loss-independent tools linked to Cancer reduction suppress the inflammatory markers and correct the pro-inflammatory state caused by obesity. Apart from a substantial decrease in pro-inflammatory molecule secretion, alteration of gut microbiota, changes in glucose and fat metabolism, improvement of insulin sensitivity, and modification of gastrointestinal peptides are proposed mechanisms of the antineoplastic effect of BS.[259-263] Knowing how these mechanisms function offers the potential to find better and safer Cancer control strategies and are active research areas.

Bariatric surgery - impact on obesity-related Cancers

The association of obesity with Cancer is well established. [231,264] Despite epidemiological evidence suggesting weight loss and increased physical activity contribute to decreasing Cancer burden, [250-253] the evidence is insufficient for weight loss methods to be recommended as part of Cancer treatment protocols.

The risk and incidence of hormone-related Cancers in female patients have been shown to decrease following BS.[271] A recent meta-analysis involving 1,50,537 BS patients versus 1,461,938 non-surgical women in the control arm showed the risk of breast Cancer being reduced by 49%, the risk of ovarian Cancer decreased by 53% and the risk of endometrial Cancer reduced by 67%.[265] Similar results have been demonstrated in an observational study by Schauer DP et al.,[266]where the hazard ratio HR for postmenopausal breast Cancer, endometrial Cancer, and pancreatic Cancer decreased significantly post-bariatric surgery. A cohort-matched study comparing 8794 operated patients with 8794 matched non-operated patients found a five-fold reduction in the incidence of hormone-related Cancers following bariatric surgery.[267] This benefit was seen maximally in post roux en y gastric bypass patients. Similar results have also been demonstrated in the Swedish obesity subject study, which showed that the overall incidence of Cancer decreases following bariatric surgery in patients with obesity and diabetes. There was also a positive correlation between prolonged diabetes remission and decreased Cancer incidence.[264] The effect of bariatric surgery on prostate Cancer in men is controversial, with the study by Mackenzie et al. showing a lower rate of ca prostate following BS (OR 0.37). However, a meta-analysis by Wiggin et al. did not show a significant impact of BS on prostate Cancer.[268]

The reduction in hormone-dependent obesity-related Cancer incidence following bariatric surgery is better seen in women [266,269,270] than men. This variation in response and outcomes in the surgical group based on gender has been shown in several studies, and a fall in blood estrogen levels is hypothesized as the underlying cause.[257]

Bariatric surgery and its effect on non-hormone, obesity-related Cancers

The effect of BS on certain Cancers like esophageal adenocarcinoma (EAC), gastric Cancer, and colorectal Cancer remains controversial. Procedures like sleeve gastrectomy (SG) have increased the incidence of GERD and Barrett's esophagus.[271,272] The incidence of EAC has risen in the surgical cohort of patients. However, this increase is likely due to the rise in bariatric procedures rather than an actual increase in EAC following bariatric surgery.[273] Epidemiological studies have also shown no increase in the risk of EAC and gastric malignancies following BS.[274] However, it is advisable for patients undergoing SG to have regular endoscopic surveillance on follow-up.[275]

The risk of colorectal Cancer (CRC) following BS doubled in a case-matched study of 8794 surgical patients with non-surgical obese patients following the gastric bypass procedure.[267] However, other studies have shown the risk of CRC in surgical patients to be reduced to the risk of CRC in the general population versus the non-surgical obese, where the risk is higher by 34%.[276] Several extensive patient database studies and meta-analyses have also concluded that BS has little or no impact on CRC.[277,278,279] The reasons for the controversial link between BS and CRC are the confounding factors, including a decrease in statin intake following BS, which are known to have Cancer-preventive effects. Also, the alteration in the gut microbiota, changes in food habits, reduction in circulating bile acids, and the phenomenon of colonic epithelial proliferation following BS have all been hypothesized to contribute to this effect.[280]

Bariatric Surgery and its Impact on Cancer Outcomes

Bariatric surgery reduces Cancer risk and mortality in formerly obese patients. On stratification by gender, the effect of bariatric surgery on oncologic outcomes is protective in women but not in men[61]. The frequency of Cancer found in the surgical group compared to non-operated controls, with Cancer-specific mortality, decreased by 46% in the former group. However, Cancer incidence declines only for obesity-related malignancies (i.e., esophagus, colorectal, pancreas, postmenopausal breast, uterus, kidney, liver, gallbladder), and mortality drops for all Cancer type.[280]

Conclusion

Obesity increases the risk of Cancer and is associated with a poor prognosis. Bariatric surgery, by weight loss dependent and independent mechanisms, decreases the risk of obesity-related Cancers and is also associated with improved treatment and survival outcomes in patients who develop Cancer following BS.

16

AUTOIMMUNITY AND CANCER

Dr. Veena Viswanath, Dr. BG Dharmanand

The relationship between rheumatic diseases and malignancies is bidirectional, complex, dynamic, and poorly understood. According to recent epidemiological studies, there is an increased risk of cancer in adults younger than 50. This increase is concurrent with an increasing trend of autoimmune diseases, suggesting a causal link between the two. Malignancy can affect the quality of life, prognosis, and survival rates and influence treatment decisions in a patient with an autoimmune disease.

Systemic autoimmune rheumatic diseases have been associated with an increased risk of malignancy. The reasons for an increased risk of malignancy in the context of autoimmune diseases are not well defined. The various reasons that may result in an elevated risk include chronic inflammation and repetitive cycles of antigen-specific cell damage, tissue regeneration, and wound healing, contributing to cancer initiation and propagation. Diverse immune and inflammatory pathways activate tumorigenesis and trigger malignancy. In certain instances, autoimmune diseases may result from cancer-induced autoimmunity, which is a by-product of naturally occurring anti-tumor immune responses.[282] Immune responses that limit tumor growth may become cross-reactive with self-tissue resulting in autoimmunity. In addition, treatments for rheumatic diseases may also increase malignancy risk.

Some malignancies are associated with or even present with joint, bone, muscle, and soft tissue manifestations or systemic autoimmune phenomena due to the generation of autoantibodies. These manifestations can be either a part of paraneoplastic syndromes or a more direct consequence of cancers. Additionally, various musculoskeletal diseases or connective tissue disorders may arise due to treatment of malignant diseases. Also, further studies may help explore the possibility of a shared genetic susceptibility to develop cancer and autoimmune diseases. Exposures to a common inciting environmental factor that can trigger both diseases' development should also be considered.

Pathophysiology

Epidemiological studies suggest that the rise in the incidence of autoimmune diseases parallels the increase in their respective cancers, as evident in autoimmune gastritis, gastric cancer, inflammatory bowel diseases, and colon cancer. Further associations between autoimmunity and cancer have become more apparent in studies of patients with CTLA4 haploinsufficiency. These patients present with a complex syndrome, including autoimmunity and an increased risk for gastric cancer and lymphoma.

Professional antigen-presenting cells (APC) activate T cells by providing co-stimulation through antigen-loaded MHC and CD80/CD86. CTLA4 is a crucial checkpoint for regulating T cell activation and thus maintaining immune tolerance. CTLA4 negatively regulates T cell activity through at least three mechanisms.

a) CTLA4 can bind to CD80/CD86 with high affinity and block co-stimulation.

b) CTLA4 can bind to CD80/CD86 and actively elicit an intrinsic inhibitory signal.

c) CTLA4 binds to CD80/CD86 and removes them from the APC by trans endocytosis.

Thus, CTLA4 insufficiency can lead to impaired regulation of T cells, which can further result in dysregulated immune responses.

Autoimmunity initiates organ-specific cell damage and triggers a reparative response mediated by type 2 immunity. Type 2 inflammation further induces epigenetic changes, genetic modifications, and reactive oxygen species. production These mechanisms may underlie autoimmune tumorigenesis. It is not known how autoimmunity triggers type 2 inflammation and tumorigenesis. But IL33 could be a significant player which binds to ST2R and upregulates type 2 inflammation by skewing naïve $CD4^+$ T cells toward Th2 or $CD4^+$ T helper cell differentiation.[283]

Tumor initiation is due to a dysregulated IL4/IL13-driven type 2 immunity. In secondary lymphoid organs, dysregulated Th2 cell-B cell interaction may lead to the development of lymphoma, while in mucosal epithelia, Th2 cell-epithelial cell crosstalk leads to epithelial cell transformation. Type 2 inflammation through IL4 IL13 may contribute to tumorigenesis in several ways, including:

a) Epigenetic-driven mechanism of cellular reprogramming.

b) Influencing the expression of genes related to proliferation, survival, metaplasia, and ultimately malignant transformation, which works in tandem with epigenetic changes.

c) Inducing expression of the specific NADPH oxidase homologs, dual oxidase, DUOX2, and NADPH oxidase 1 (NOX1), and the subsequent production of reactive oxygen species (ROS).

Is cancer more common in autoimmune diseases?

Certain systemic autoimmune rheumatic diseases, including dermatomyositis, rheumatoid arthritis (RA), systemic lupus erythematosus (SLE), Sjogren's syndrome, and systemic sclerosis (SSc), are associated with an increased risk of malignancy.[284] Different types of cancers are observed in these disorders, increasing the risk of solid organ and hematologic malignancies. Multiple mechanisms drive the relationship between autoimmune diseases and malignancy. Chronic inflammation and damage can stimulate cytokines and chemokines that further the development of malignancies through various pathways (Table 1). Other potential mechanisms contributing to cancer development in autoimmune diseases include cytotoxic or biological therapies and the inability to clear oncogenic infections.[285]

Table1: Mechanisms through which cytokines stimulate tumorigenesis.

1.	Induce DNA damage.
2.	Inactivate tumor suppressor gene.
3.	Stimulate enhanced cell growth and survival.
4.	Trigger angiogenesis.
5.	Enhance invasion.

Rheumatoid arthritis

Whether the development of malignancies in RA patients results from the inflammatory process, the immunological imbalances, or the use of cytotoxic and immunosuppressive agents remains controversial. The overall risk for malignancy is about 10% higher than the general population and is primarily driven by increased risks of lymphoproliferative cancers. There is an increased risk of Hodgkin's and non-Hodgkin's lymphoma, large granular lymphocyte (LGL) leukemia, lung cancer, liver and oesophageal cancer, and melanoma. In contrast, the risk of colorectal malignancy, breast cancer, and prostate cancer is reduced.[286] Incidence and mortality rates due to leukaemia or lymphoma are approximately twofold higher than expected.

Cancer risk appears to be greater in patients with persistently high disease activity, high cumulative disease activity, and more severe disease and in those with positive rheumatoid factor and elevated inflammatory markers.[287] The extra-articular disease of rheumatoid arthritis, particularly Felty's and Sjogren's syndrome, confers a further increased risk of non-Hodgkin's lymphoma.[288] Drugs used to treat the disease, including cyclophosphamide, azathioprine, and methotrexate were thought to increase the risk of malignancy. However, not all patients with RA who develop malignancies have been treated with these agents. But Cyclophosphamide and Azathioprine are not regularly used to treat RA. Methotrexate has been studied extensively, and no suggestion of an increase in malignant potential has been found.

The most common type of lymphoma is diffuse large B cell lymphoma (DLBCL). Large granular lymphocyte (LGL) leukemia is a clonal lymphoproliferative characterized by increased large granular lymphocytes. Almost all individuals with RA who develop LGL leukemia have the T cell type (T-LGL), and nearly one-third of people with T-LGL have RA.

Systemic Lupus Erythematosus

The risk of certain malignancies appears to be increased in patients with SLE. Overall, a small increased risk was estimated across all cancers. But there is a substantially increased risk of lymphoid malignancy, primarily non-Hodgkin lymphoma, and leukemia, among patients with SLE. Non-Hodgkin lymphoma in patients with SLE is often an aggressive histologic subtype, predominantly diffuse large B-cell lymphoma.[289]

Risk factors for developing hematologic malignancies may relate to inflammatory burden and disease activity, immunologic defects and overexpression of *Bcl*-2 oncogenes, and viruses, especially Epstein-Barr virus (EBV) while leukopenia, independent of immunosuppressive treatment, was a risk factor for developing leukemias. Disease characteristics predisposing to non-Hodgkin's lymphoma include longer disease duration and increased disease activity with moderately severe end-organ damage. There also appears to be an increased risk of cancers of the vulva, cervix, lung, thyroid, buccal mucosa, and possibly liver.[290] Smoking is a predictor of a higher risk of lung cancer.

Disease-induced immune dysregulation or treatment with immunosuppressants may reduce the ability to clear oncogenic infections.

The risk of virus-associated cancers is elevated and notably human papillomavirus (HPV) associated malignancies, including anal cancer, vaginal/vulvar cancer, cervical dysplasia, and non-melanoma skin cancers.[291] The risk is also high for other potential virus-associated cancers, including liver cancer (hepatitis B and C viruses), bladder cancer (polyomavirus), and non-Hodgkin's lymphoma (Epstein-Barr virus, EBV).[291] Various longitudinal epidemiologic studies have also identified a reduced risk of breast and prostate cancers and possibly ovarian and uterine cancer.[292] Race, ethnicity, and antimalarial use do not affect the relative risk of developing malignancy. Although the overall risk of death due to malignancy does not appear to be increased in SLE patients, the risk of death due to specific malignancies, particularly non-Hodgkin lymphoma, is significantly increased among SLE patients compared with the general population.

Sjogren's Syndrome

Patients with Sjogren's Syndrome have an increased risk of non-Hodgkin lymphomas, which is evident for both primary and secondary forms of SS. Clinical, histopathologic, and laboratory features that identify patients with SS who are at increased risk for developing lymphoma, including persistent salivary gland enlargement, cutaneous vasculitis, lymphadenopathy, splenomegaly, cryoglobulinemia, low serum complement C3 or C4, an IgM kappa monoclonal protein, neutropenia, high focus score and possibly germinal center-like structures on labial salivary gland biopsies.[293]

Marginal zone lymphomas, especially extra nodal marginal zone lymphoma of mucosa-associated lymphoid tissue (MALT lymphoma), involving the parotid gland, the orbital adnexa, nasopharynx, thyroid, stomach, and lung is the most common histopathological subtype. It is followed by DLBL and nodal marginal zone lymphoma. Monoclonal gammopathies occur in patients with SS and are associated with an increased risk of myeloma and lymphoma. B cell activation characteristic of Sjogren's syndrome is a predisposing risk factor, and infectious agents, including Hepatitis C, EBV, and H. Pylori, have been implicated in the pathogenesis of malignancy.

Systemic Sclerosis

Chronic inflammation and fibrosis of affected organs may lead to an increased risk of malignancy in patients with systemic sclerosis. The link to smoking is controversial. The risk is higher early in the disease, and patients who are older at the time of diagnosis are also at higher risk.[294] Systemic sclerosis is associated with an increased risk of lung, liver, hematologic, skin, bladder, oropharyngeal, and oesophageal cancer. The most significant association appears to be with lung cancer, which accounts for approximately one-third of the cancers seen in SSc patients.

Data from the Prostate, Lung, Colorectal, and Ovarian Cancer Screening Trial, which had more than 65,000 participants, demonstrated that baseline pulmonary scar is associated with an increased incidence of future ipsilateral lung cancer. This mechanism may also apply to patients with SSc, in whom an increased risk of lung cancer is seen in patients with interstitial lung disease.[295] Similarly, oesophageal disease in systemic sclerosis is the likely reason for the increased incidence of Barrett's esophagus and cancer. Reports of patients with concurrent cancer and SSc also suggest that cancer therapy may be a rheumatic disease. Localized scleroderma has not been associated with an increased risk of cancer.

Inflammatory Myopathies

Inflammatory myopathies are associated with malignancies in a significant minority of cases. The association of malignancy and autoimmune rheumatic disease is strongest with inflammatory myositis. Cancer can be diagnosed simultaneously with, before or after the diagnosis of myositis, but it is commonly reported in the first few years of onset of myositis. Hence all patients newly diagnosed with PM or DM should be evaluated for the possibility of an underlying malignancy. There is an increased risk of ovarian, pancreatic, gastric, colorectal, breast, lung, and cervical adenocarcinoma. The link to malignancy in newly diagnosed patients with dermatomyositis is strongest, while the association between malignancy and polymyositis and inclusion body myositis is less intense.

Clinical factors associated with an increased risk of malignancy include older age of disease onset, pharyngeal and diaphragmatic weakness, distal extremity weakness, capillary damage on muscle biopsy, cutaneous necrosis, and leukocytoclastic vasculitis.[280] Some serum autoantibodies in DM and PM (anti-TIF-1 gamma or anti-p155/1anti-NXP2ti NXP2 or anti-p140) confer a positive risk of malignancy. In contrast, myositis-specific antibodies (anti-synthetase antibodies, anti-Mi-2, anti-SRP) and myositis-associated antibodies (anti-RNP, anti-PM-Scl, anti-Ku) are associated with a decrease in the incidence of malignancy.

Myositis, associated with cancer, responds more poorly to treatment than myositis in the absence of cancer. The presence of a tumor does not appear to affect the severity or distribution of weakness, the duration of liability prior to diagnosis, or the height of creatine kinase elevation. In dermatomyositis, the course of the disease also parallels the course of cancer, with remission of dermatomyositis following effective cancer therapy and relapse of dermatomyositis heralding cancer relapse.

Others

There is insufficient data to support an increased risk of malignancy in patients with vasculitis. The overall risk of cancer does not appear to be increased in the seronegative spondyloarthropathies except for one study in which an increased rate of cancer in Asians with ankylosing spondylitis was reported, with the risk highest for hematologic malignancy and higher in the first three years following diagnosis of ankylosing spondylitis.[297]

Can cancer cause autoimmunity?

Autoimmunity can be induced by malignancy, with a diagnosis of cancer shortly preceding or following the first presentation of a rheumatic illness. is explained by the concept of tumor defense-induced autoimmunity, where an immune response that is initiated against cancer targets host cells. The two best examples of this are dermatomyositis and SSc. In both diseases, patients significantly increase the risk of cancer. There is a special temporal relationship between cancer diagnosis and the onset of rheumatic diseases. A particular immunological profile of autoantibody subsets is associated with an increased risk of cancer development in both disorders (e.g., anti-RNA polymerase III in SSc and anti-NXP2 and anti-TIF1 gamma in dermatomyositis.[282] The autoimmunity concept also applies in the context of the thyroid, where thyroid autoimmunity and cancer are highly associated.

More than a two-fold increased risk for the development of malignancies is seen among patients with SSc. The most common scleroderma-associated cancers are breast and lung cancers. Most cases of breast cancer are diagnosed shortly after or before the diagnosis of scleroderma, commonly within two years. This temporal relation between the diagnosis of breast cancer and SSc may suggest a common genetic background, a possible shared etiology/risk factor, or a paraneoplastic process. Multiple studies have observed a close temporal relationship between the onset of cancer and SSc among patients with autoantibodies to RNA polymerase I/III,[42,43] particularly in patients with breast cancer, although it might be seen in other tumor types too. Patients with RNA polymerase III autoantibodies were found to have a striking clustering of cancer within 2 to 5 years of onset of systemic sclerosis, and these patients had unique nucleolar RNA polymerase III expressions in their cancerous tissues, suggesting that tumor autoantigen expression and SSc-specific immune responses were associated.[299]

The prevalence of malignancy is about 25% inflammatory myositis. Cancers are reported more frequently in dermatomyositis than polymyositis. The most common cancers occurring among patients with inflammatory myopathies are breast and gynecological cancers among women, lung cancer among men, and gastrointestinal malignancies among both sexes. Cancer can be diagnosed before, simultaneously with, or after the diagnosis of inflammatory myopathy, with the peak incidence of a cancer diagnosis co-occurring with and during the first two years after the diagnosis of the muscle disease and falling off gradually over the subsequent five years of follow-up Cancer-associated myositis (CAM) in adults has been associated with antibodies to intermediary transcription factor (TIF)-1gamma (anti-p155, anti-p155/140) and with antibodies to nuclear matrix protein (NXP)-2 (anti-MJ or anti-p140). Inflammatory myopathies may initially manifest with the recurrence of a previously diagnosed cancer, and a previously diagnosed but inactive inflammatory myopathy may reactivate with the occurrence of cancer.

Autoantibodies in Cancer patients

Cancers, including hematologic malignancies and solid tumor, may lead to the induction of autoimmunity. Antibodies are also produced against numerous self-antigens expressed in tumor cells—a large group of autoantigens designated as tumor-associated autoantigens.[300] More than 400 such autoantigens have been identified to which tumor-associated autoantibodies bind. The autoantibodies in patients with malignancies include anti-oncoprotein antibodies (Anti-HER-2/neu and anti-c-myc, c-my, and l-myc Antibodies), anti-tumor suppressor gene antibodies (Anti- P53 antibodies), anti-proliferation associated antigens (anti- CENP-F antibodies), autoantibodies against onconeural antigens (anti-Hu and anti-Ki) amongst many others. Though these autoantibodies can be seen in various cancers, including breast, ovarian, colon, and lung cancers, the exact significance of their detection in sera is unclear. Some of these autoantibodies have been detected in healthy volunteers (anti- c-myc and anti-c-myb) a few in autoimmune diseases (anti-P53 in miners with SLE), and some may result in paraneoplastic neurologic syndromes (Anti-Hu and Anti-Ri). Studies are needed to determine whether those autoantibodies have a diagnostic or diagnostic value or if they can be used to monitor response to specific anti-cancer therapy.

Can malignancy mimic rheumatologic disorders?

Autoimmune thrombocytopenia, Sjogren's syndrome, autoimmune hemolytic anemia, rheumatoid arthritis, SLE, and autoimmune thyroid diseases have all been reported among patients with hematological malignancies. Antinuclear autoantibodies, DNA, histones, anti-Ro, anti-La, anti-Sm, and anti-RNP antibodies have been detected in sera patients with various malignancies. Patients with multiple myeloma, Waldenstrom's macroglobulinemia, and chronic lymphocytic leukemia have rheumatoid factor activity. Antiphospholipid autoantibodies (aPL) were also found in the sera of patients with malignant diseases with varying frequency and can confer a two-fold increased risk of thrombosis. Myeloma-associated amyloid arthropathy can present with polyarthritis, often symmetrical, and should be considered in the differential diagnosis of especially seronegative rheumatoid arthritis and seronegative spondyloarthropathies.

Lymphomas may have clinical feat characterized by vascular and granulomatous inflammation that can cause diagnostic confusion with systemic inflammatory and autoimmune rheumatic disorders. Patients with lymphoma, especially angioimmunoblastic T cell lymphoma, may have arthritis, Coombs-positive hemolytic anemia, skin rash, fever, and weight loss that suggest SLE or Still's a disease. Angiocentric and angioinvasive lesions of various organs due to large B cell lymphomas may be confused with granulomatosis with polyangiitis, especially when there is a predominant extranodal disease, T-cell-rich tissue infiltrates extensive necrosis and inflammation. Multiple cancers can cause paraneoplastic manifestations categorized as vasculitis secondary to underlying malignancy. Certain malignancies, especially leukemia and lymphomas, are vasculitic mimics that should be considered while evaluating patients with suspected vasculitis. Intravascular large-cell lymphoma can resemble CNS vasculitis, while atrial myxoma can cause vascular manifestations mimicking medium and large vasculitis and result in cutaneous manifestations.[301] Conversely, autoimmune diseases like SLE can mimic lymphoma when patients present with lymphadenopathy and hepatosplenomegaly with or without constitutional symptoms (pseudo-lymphoma-like presentation).

Paraneoplastic rheumatic and autoimmune manifestations

About 7–10% of patients with cancer develop one of the many paraneoplastic syndromes. Paraneoplastic manifestations may result from the tumor cells' secretion of various hormones and hormone-like peptides. These can also be secondary to the activation of autoimmune phenomena. The presence of malignancy can be associated with diverse musculoskeletal, immunological, and vasculitic manifestations that can remit with the treatment of underlying cancer and thus can be considered paraneoplastic.

Malignancy-associated vasculitis, though uncommon, has been reported more often with hematologic malignancies (typically lymphoproliferative) than solid malignancies. Vasculitis may occur a few years before the diagnosis of a malignancy concurrent with or following the diagnosis of malignancy. The most common presentation is an small isolated vessel cutaneous leukocytoclastic vasculitis, typically presenting with palpable purpura preferentially located in dependent areas. Small vessel vasculitis affecting the blood vessels of the peripheral nerves and muscles, vasculitis isolated to a single internal organ, or a systemic form of vasculitis have also been described in patients with malignancies. Solid tumors are associated with various types of vasculitis, including polyarteritis nodosa, IgA vasculitis (Henoch-Schoenlein purpura), and small-vessel vasculitis.[302] Hairy cell leukemia and lung cancer are the most common malignancies associated with vasculitis.

Hypertrophic osteoarthropathy, characterized by digital clubbing, periostosis of tubular bones, and synovial effusions, which are most prominent in the large joints, can be associated with lung cancer and, to a lesser extent, Hodgkin's lymphoma. Improvement in hypertrophic pulmonary osteoarthropathy has been noted after treatment of the underlying malignancy. The RS3PE syndrome refers to remitting seronegative symmetrical synovitis with pitting edema, usually characterized by acute onset distal extremity symptoms and signs. Synovitis has been associated with a wide array of hematologic and solid tumors.

Multicentric reticulohistiocytosis (MRH) is a rare multisystem disease consisting of a cutaneous histiocytosis, xanthelasma and destructive polyarthritis that can rapidly progress to arthritis mutilans. MRH is associated with underlying malignancy in one-quarter of patients; breast, hematologic, and gastric cancers are the most common.

Paraneoplastic inflammatory arthritis is described with a variety of tumor types. Though these can cause symmetrical polyarthritis involving small joints of the hands resembling rheumatoid arthritis, asymmetric presentation can also occur. Palmar fasciitis, accompanied sometimes by polyarthritis, is most frequently reported with ovarian cancer and, to a lesser extent, with stomach, pancreas, lung, colon, and prostate tumors. Eosinophilic fascia, characterized by woody induration of the skin of the extremities and trunk with sparing of face and digits, a mimic of scleroderma, is associated with hematologic disorders in 10% of cases, which includes lymphoproliferative malignancies, myeloproliferative diseases and multiple myeloma.[303]

Malignant Diseases with Musculoskeletal Manifestations

In addition to the various paraneoplastic rheumatologic syndromes, articular and systemic autoimmune phenomena can also be a more direct consequence of some malignancies, especially lymphoproliferative and myelodysplastic disorders, and in some cases, can be the presenting feature of the disease. Joint involvement is unusual in lymphoma, is primarily seen with T cell types and may result from secondary gout, as a reaction to adjacent lymphomatous involvement, or due to direct lymphomatous infiltration of the synovium. Hodgkin lymphoma can have bone pain, which may be worse at night and pathologic fractures, particularly involving the vertebrae. Articular manifestations due to leukemia are more common in children compared in adults. These may include bone pains, arthralgias, and symmetric or migratory polyarthritis. Leukemic arthritis is characterized by severe pain and frequently unresponsive antirheumatic medication and often reveals more osteopenia and earlier lytic lesions.[304]

Autoimmune abnormalities may be present in up to one-quarter of patients of MDS and include polyarthritis or monoarthritis resembling rheumatoid or undifferentiated polyarthritis, polymyalgia rheumatica, RS3PE, relapsing polychondritis, Raynaud phenomenon, Sjogren's syndrome, and vasculitis.

Can treatment of autoimmune diseases cause cancer?

Pharmacologic therapy of rheumatic diseases may increase the risk of malignant disease. Assessing the risk of cancer associated with various biological and nonbiological DMARDs is often tricky for the following reasons:

a) Variable cancer risk associated with different autoimmune diseases.

b) There is a potential risk of malignancy associated with various immunosuppressants.

c) Concurrent and sequential use of various agents makes it difficult to assess the risks with individual agents.

There is no increased risk of malignancy with NSAIDs, glucocorticoids, hydroxychloroquine or sulfasalazine. The risk of cancer is increased with chemotherapeutic DMARDs, particularly cyclophosphamide, and the risk of certain cancers, particularly lymphoproliferative disorders, may be increased with drugs such as azathioprine, methotrexate and cyclosporine. Data is sparse for many drugs because of the lack of long-term follow-up. No increase in cancer occurrence has been reported with leflunomide. Cyclosporine has been associated with developing EBV-associated lymphomas in a few patients with rheumatoid arthritis.

Though the overall malignancy risk is not increased with methotrexate, some studies suggest that the risk of lymphoproliferative disease may be increased, most of which is B cell lymphoma.[305] Some studies have reported an increased risk of lymphoma with azathioprine, with the highest risk in patients on higher daily doses of azathioprine of up to 300 mg per day.[306]

Cyclophosphamide is an alkylating agent associated with an increased risk of bladder cancer, leukemia, lymphoma, and skin and solid malignancies, with the highest risk for bladder malignancy. Acrolein, a metabolite of cyclophosphamide, is excreted by the kidneys and concentrated in the urine and causes bladder toxicity, including cystitis and cancer. Bladder cancer may occur within one year of initiation of therapy and up to 15 years or longer after discontinuation of cyclophosphamide treatment and higher cumulative doses, an oral route of administration, and current or former smoking are all associated with a higher risk of subsequent cancer.[307] At the same time, concurrent mesna, which inactivates acrolein in the urine, can reduce the risk.

Data on cancer risk with mycophenolate mofetil is less clear. Certain studies show an increased risk of non-melanoma skin cancers and lymphomas, whereas others do not. Data suggest that primary CNS lymphoma risk may be increased, in particular with mycophenolate use.[308]

No unusual increase in malignancy has been observed with Rituximab and Abatacept. Anakinra has been associated with an increased risk of lymphoma, and many solid tumors have also been reported in various case series. Janus kinase inhibitors, including Tofacitinib, are suspected to increase the risk of malignancy. But data so far has failed to establish a statistically significant increase in the incidence of malignancies except for non-melanoma skin cancer.

In the 2000s, anti-tumor necrosis factor therapy for rheumatoid arthritis was linked to an increased risk for infection and malignancy, especially non-melanoma skin cancer. However, evidence from recent studies suggests that using anti-tumor necrosis factor therapy after an initial cancer diagnosis does not influence the risk of recurrence or result in the development of new cancer. Patients with inflammatory bowel disease treated with this therapy have lower rates of colorectal cancer.

Can treatment of malignancies cause autoimmune diseases?

Various musculoskeletal or other connective tissue disorders may arise from treating malignant disease. These phenomena are referred to as post-chemotherapy rheumatism or chemotherapy-related arthropathy.

Bleomycin and gemcitabine are potential triggers of sclerosis of the skin and may lead to the development or worsening of Raynaud's phenomenon and digital ischemia. This reaction is secondary to vascular toxicity and neurotoxicity, resulting in endothelial dysfunction and aberrant sympathetic arterial vasoconstriction.[309] Nonspecific manifestations like myalgias and arthralgias, rheumatoid-like polyarthritis and reactive arthritis may also develop with various anti-cancer therapies. Taxanes, such as paclitaxel and docetaxel, can cause severe musculoskeletal manifestations, photo distributed skin rashes clinically and histologically similar to subacute cutaneous lupus and SSc-like disease.

Aromatase inhibitors are often associated with significant joint and muscular symptoms commonly referred to as aromatase inhibitor-associated musculoskeletal syndrome (AIMSS), adversely affecting the quality of life and reducing compliance. AIMSS can be classified into two major groups: AI-induced bone loss and AI-induced arthralgias (AIA). High-dose glucocorticoids are associated with an increased risk of osteonecrosis and osteoporosis, which increases the fracture risk. Severe musculoskeletal pain and osteonecrosis of the jaw can rarely be associated with the use of bisphosphonates.

Many immunotherapies, such as IL-2 therapy, anti-tumor T cell infusions, cancer vaccines, and immune checkpoint inhibitors, are increasingly used to treat cancer. These agents stimulate the host immune response to destroy neoplastic cells, which can result in autoimmunity— [LC36–41]. Cancer immunotherapy upregulates anti-tumor immunity through immune checkpoint blockade targeting cytotoxic T lymphocyte-associated protein 4 (CTLA4), programmed cell death protein 1 (PD-1), or the programmed cell death one ligand 1 (PD-L1). But these new therapies can induce autoimmunity in patients without pre-existing autoimmune conditions or cause exacerbations in patients with pre-existing and previously quiescent rheumatic and autoimmune diseases. Among those with pre-existing autoimmune diseases, flares of illness or the development of symptoms of another autoimmune disease may occur.

Immune checkpoint inhibitors cause nonspecific specific activation of T cells, leading to a spectrum of immune-related adverse events (irAEs) with different rheumatologic phenotypes. The manifestations include inflammatory arthritis, myositis, sicca syndrome, vasculitis, polymyalgia rheumatica, eosinophilic fasciitis, sarcoidosis and scleroderma. Inflammatory arthritis is the most common clinical presentation, can develop at any time during therapy and vary in severity and pattern of expression. Treatment includes NSAIDs, glucocorticoids and DMARDs in refractory cases.[310]

Radiation and autoimmune diseases

Radiation therapy and chemoradiotherapy for head and neck cancer can cause xerostomia, which may mimic Sjogren's syndrome. Radiation therapy may trigger severe skin thickening in patients with pre-existing systemic sclerosis or new developmental or localized scleroderma. However, whether it can start de novo systemic sclerosis remains unknown.[311] Some small studies have suggested that patients with systemic rheumatic diseases, especially those with systemic sclerosis and possibly those with SLE, are at greater risk for toxic effects from radiotherapy used to treat malignant conditions. But based on the currently available data, the presence of connective tissue disorders is not a contraindication to radiotherapy. Radiation therapy has also been implicated as a potential trigger for developing eosinophilic fasciitis, though the data is sparse.

Screening for malignancies in autoimmune diseases and preventive strategies

Though there are reviews that provide guidance based on expert opinion, there is a lack of evidence-based recommendations for screening and monitoring cancer in rheumatic diseases. As with all cancer screening, care is needed to ensure that proposed interventions result in meaningful risk reduction minimizing harm. All patients should receive cancer screening based on age, sex, family history of malignancy and conventional cancer risk factors, such as smoking. Age and sex-appropriate cancer screening for colorectal cancer, prostate cancer, breast cancer, and cervical cancer are indicated in all. More aggressive cancer screening may be warranted in patients with systemic sclerosis and dermatomyositis, which are associated with cancer at the time of disease onset. For patients with high-risk characteristics in these categories of diseases, a more rigorous initial screening and serial follow-up are indicated. Because cancers can develop at an accelerated rate in the first few months to the first year or so of treatment, patients should be seen at frequent intervals and examined closely for signs and symptoms of malignancy, especially during the initial treatment period throughout their disease.

Malignancy risk is significantly elevated in patients with scleroderma with RNA polymerase III or those who did not show centromere or topoisomerase antibodies. In dermatomyositis, over 80% of patients with malignancy have anti-NXP-2 or anti-TIF 1γ antibodies, which confers an a27-fold increased risk for cancer. Certain factors in patients with scleroderma or dermatomyositis may alert them to the possibility of underlying malignancy in systemic sclerosis and dermatomyositis (Table 2).

Table 2: Red flags that signal the presence of underlying Cancer.

1.	New onset disease above 60 years of age.
2.	Aggressive nature of the disease.
3.	Atypical features.
4.	Poor response to treatment.
5.	Unexplained weight loss or constitutional symptoms.
6.	Personal history of previous malignancy.
7.	Family history of malignancy.

Mammography, PSA and CT of the chest, pelvis, and abdomen may be considered, as indicated, in patients with scleroderma in the high-risk subgroup. In patients with dermatomyositis, assessment for tumor markers such as CA-125 and radiographic imaging of the chest, abdomen, and pelvis may be appropriate when clinically indicated. Whole-body positron emission tomography (PET)/CT can also be considered as needed instead of conventional screening involving multiple tests, particularly for patients with refractory disease.

Regular monitoring of hemograms, including differential counts and LDH levels with peripheral smear examination when new symptoms develop, can aid in the early detection of hematological malignancy. Due to an increased incidence of lung cancer in many rheumatic diseases, low-dose CT screening for lung cancer can be considered in high-risk individuals. Increased prevalence of human papillomavirus infection and increased incidence of cervical dysplasia and malignancy have been noted in patients with SLE and thus necessitate a regular Pap smear monitoring immunization with the HPV vaccine. Patients taking alkylating agents such as cyclophosphamide may be at a particularly high risk of cancer. These patients should undergo routine cancer screening, Pap smears, and urinalyses for at least 15 years from cyclophosphamide therapy. Drugs like cyclophosphamide should be used when absolutely indicated. Exposure to medications with possible malignant potential, including azathioprine, should be minimized. Lifestyle modification, including a healthy diet and regular exercise, should be encouraged with an emphasis on smoking cessation since smoking increases the risk of the development of malignancy in certain rheumatic disorders.

17

SCOPE OF RESEARCH AND CHALLENGES IN PREVENTION OF CANCERS

Dr. Sandhya Ravi

Introduction

Cancer prevention is a mission that needs to be prioritized. The Global burden of the disease continues to rise because of the increase in population and longevity and also the increase in cancer-promoting lifestyle and environment, especially in low and middle-income countries (Stewart & Kleihues, 2003; Boyle & Levin, 2008; Stewart & Wild, 2014).

Screening for cancer and early detection aimed at active prevention are practical approaches to reducing the burden of cancer. Broadly defined, prevention is "actions aimed at eradicating, eliminating, or minimizing the impact of disease and disability, or if none of these is feasible, retarding the progress of disease and disability" (Porta, 2014).

Prevention can be:

a) <u>Primary Prevention</u>: Avoidance of exposure to carcinogens, lifestyles that decrease risk (e.g., never smoke), or vaccinations. So, actions that can be taken to lower the risk of developing cancer.

b) <u>Secondary Prevention</u>: Slowing, blocking, or reversing the progression of carcinogenesis to invasive cancer (e.g., consider the importance of molecular endpoint biomarkers and their validation). So, it entails methods that can find and alleviate precancerous conditions or find cancers in the early stages, when they can be treated more successfully.

c) <u>Tertiary Prevention:</u> application of measures aimed at reducing the impact of long-term disease and disability caused by cancer or its treatment.

Why is cancer prevention research important?

Cancer incidence is rising globally and in India. An estimated one in nine people are likely to develop cancer in their lifetime. It is a public health imperative to do what we can to decrease the incidence through prevention and control using existing and emerging knowledge of ways to reduce cancer risk.

Cancer prevention, using the knowledge from epidemiology and molecular biology, has achieved many successes. However, the accessibility of effective and affordable screening is not always available for the people who need it.

Tobacco control efforts help reduce the cancer burden. HPV vaccines protect against several kinds of cancer. Screening with colonoscopies can find precancerous growths and have them removed.

Cancer shares common risk factors with cardiovascular diseases, diabetes, chronic respiratory diseases, and alcohol dependence, so any preventive measures will bring down the risk overall.

I - Scope of Research in Cancer Prevention

As early as 1964, based on a report from the WHO, it was known that lifestyle and other environmental factors, including environmental carcinogens, hormonal factors, and dietary deficiencies could be implicated in the cause of fatal cancers, many of which could be potentially preventable.

In 1981, the landmark study of Doll and Peto refined and clarified the evidence of such preventable factors, particularly to reduce the burden of cancers in USA and England. This study was the starting point for subsequent studies of cancer causes and strategies for cancer prevention.

Risk Identification

Research in Cancer prevention is inextricably associated with risk identification and assessment. Long -term prospective studies are needed to follow people over time to relate the exposure to the risk factors. These have some inherent difficulties in conduct. Data from multiple studies are analyzed to conclude the etiology of cancers. These studies are subject to bias as compared to prospective studies.

The most commonly used scheme to identify this risk is through:

A) Structured data summaries-

    a)   Meta-analyses.

    b)   Pooled analyses.

Observational epidemiologic studies show associations between modifiable lifestyle factors or environmental exposures and specific cancers. Therefore, lifestyle modification (i.e., changing one's risk profile from bad to good) would actually reduce cancer risk, at least partially. This expectation can be fulfilled if the association is due to a causal (and ideally, reversible) relationship. Observational studies rarely provide conclusive evidence of such relationships.

Randomized controlled trials are additionally required to test whether interventions suggested by epidemiologic studies and leads based on laboratory research result in reduced cancer incidence and mortality.

Major known risk factors that have a significant impact on cancer burden are

1) Tobacco use.

2) Alcohol use.

3) Physical inactivity, dietary factors, obesity, and being overweight.

4) Physical carcinogens, such as ultraviolet (UV) and ionizing radiation.

5) Chemical carcinogens, such as benzo(a)pyrene, formaldehyde, and aflatoxins (food contaminants), and fibers such as asbestos.

6) Biological carcinogens, such as infections by viruses, bacteria, and parasites.

Interventions aimed at reducing the above risk factors in the population will reduce cancer risk and other conditions that share these risks. Among the most important modifiable risk factors for cancer (Ezzati et al., 2004, Danaei et al., 2005, Driscoll et al., 2005) are:

Tobacco use – (1.5 million cancer deaths per year)

Being Overweight, obesity, and physical inactivity – together responsible for 274,000 cancer deaths per year

Harmful alcohol use – responsible for 351000 cancer deaths per year

Sexually transmitted HPV infection -responsible for 71,000 cancer deaths per year.

Occupational carcinogens – responsible for at least 15200 cancer deaths per year.

Prevention measures, including the scope of research in these areas, must be cost -effective and inexpensive to be widely implemented and adopted.

B) <u>Understanding etiologic pathways in cancer.</u>

Cancers are complex and demonstrate genetic heterogeneity, so it is rational to intervene early and prioritize prevention.

Novel early -detection preventive strategies can be based on:

- Molecular mechanisms of cancer– gene expression profiling, proteomics, methylation analysis, and high throughput genotyping.

- Angiogenesis and lymphangiogenesis occur early in the disease and are important markers.

- A Growing catalog of mutational events, altered cellular protein concentrations.

Epidemiological studies can help translate biomarkers from the lab to the field to determine risk and help diagnosis. Self-sampling with HPV DNA testing for cervical cancer screening is an example.

C) <u>Precision Cancer Prevention.</u>

The present scenario is promising for developing a 'precision cancer prevention' (NCI Dr Philip Castle). Knowledge of genetics, risk factors, and lifestyle can help tailor prevention strategies for an individual.

Chemoprevention uses synthetic agents to block, retard or reverse the carcinogenic process.

Classification of carcinogens as per the IARC system

1) Definite carcinogen – association established between exposure and outcome and chance, bias, and confounding can be ruled out with reasonable confidence.

2) Probable carcinogen – association established but chance, bias and

confounding cannot be ruled out with reasonable confidence.

3) Possible carcinogen – no definite association between exposure and outcome because of insufficient quality, consistency and statistical power of available studies.

Preventive research must establish this categorization before targeting specific biochemical pathways (enzyme, specific protein, or other molecular targets) in order to reduce risk.

The process of carcinogenesis is not a biological continuum but a series of steps, an agent that works on one step may not work on another and may produce unexpected adverse effects.

D) Advances in the scope of research in the prevention of cancers.

The National Cancer Institute's Early Detection Research Network (EDRN) is working to discover, develop and validate biomarkers and imaging methods to detect early-stage cancers and assess the risk for developing cancer, and translate these biomarkers and imaging methods into clinical tests. A consortium of more than 300 investigators at academic institutions and the private sector are working collaboratively to bring biomarkers and imaging methods to clinical use.

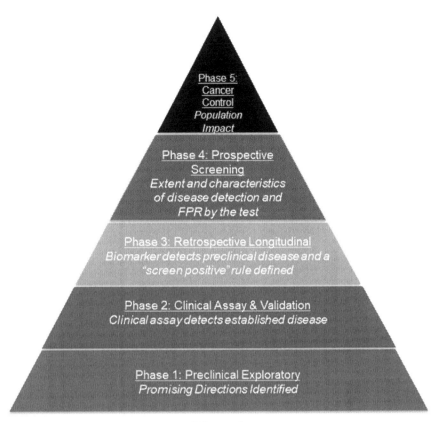

Figure 1

This systematic approach to discovery, development, and validation is used to help identify "winners" or "losers" among biomarkers. The multi-step approach includes Phase 1 – Discovery; Phase 2 – Clinical Assay and Validation; Phase 3 – Retrospective Longitudinal; Phase 4 – Prospective Screening; and Phase 5 – Cancer Control.

EDRN has also developed and adopted the Prospective specimen collection, Retrospective Blinded Evaluation study design, an approach to reduce bias during all biomarker discovery and validation phases. The Prospective specimen collection, Retrospective Blinded Evaluation study design has four key elements:

1. Clinical context and outcomes.

2. Criteria for measuring biomarker performance.

3. The test itself.

4. The size of the study.

Critical features of this design are:

A. All patients are enrolled prior to diagnosis.

B. Cases and controls are enrolled under the same conditions.

C. All samples are collected and processed identically.

D. Other areas of expanded scope of research in cancer prevention are:

1. Immuno prevention studies.

2. Using AI for screening and early detection.

3. The use of spatial proteomics technology that captures protein positioning within cells to characterize tumor microenvironment – especially useful in understanding what drives DCIS to transition to invasive cancer - a critical unmet need and opportunity for prevention.

4. The Discovery and development of natural products for cancer interception and prevention which are safe, non-toxic, and productive.

5. Advances in robust high-throughput screening (HTS) strategies and medicinal chemistry could alter the pharmaceutical landscape for developing many new cancer interception-prevention strategies .

6. Multi-cancer detection assays (MCD), a new advancing technology, is a promising screening tool for early cancer, although overdiagnosis of indolent disease and potential harm from unnecessary and invasive procedures in individuals with no known malignancies is a concern.

7. Studies on compounds from foods and their effect on cancer risk.

Research in the area of prevention should focus on improving understanding of the cancer process and work towards developing effective measures to intervene. Interventions can include biomarkers for early detection and new screening methods and technologies, as well as drugs, vaccines, surgery, or behavioral modifications that interrupt the molecular and biological pathways involved in cancer risk and development. Simultaneously, screening strategies especially for breast, cervical, oral, and lung cancer must improve.

Health education programs must improve awareness about identifying risks, risk-reducing behavior, and lifestyle changes. Only then will this form the foundation of all interventions and strategies. Health education programs focusing on improving awareness about identifying risks, risk reducing behavior and lifestyle changes form the foundation of all interventions and strategies.

Cancer prevention research programs focus on the population that does not have cancer yet. Essentially, the benefit of the intervention must far outweigh the risk to the individual. Research must look at ways to identify cancer risk, and to map the molecular and genetic pathways that lead to cancer. Intervention must interrupt the path to prevent the disease without harming the person at risk.

F) Prevention and Cancer Survivorship

The number of cancer survivors is rising, and it is important to consider prevention intervention in them to prevent second malignancies. However, such an intervention is challenging as each cancer has its own factors related to the tumor biology, treatments undertaken, co-morbidities, average patient age and gender, among many others.

II Challenges in cancer prevention research

The complexity and inter-relatedness of many of the interventions in preventive health research pose a significant challenge. Cancer prevention management should focus on individuals at high risk and primary localized disease in which screening and detection also play a major role. The timing and dose of (chemo-)preventive intervention also affect response. The intervention may be ineffective if the target population is very high risk or already has premalignant lesions with cellular changes that cannot be reversed. The field needs to move beyond general concepts of carcinogenesis to targeted organ site prevention approaches in patients at high risk, as is currently being done for breast and colorectal cancers. Establishing the benefit of new cancer preventive interventions will take years and possibly decades, depending on the outcome being evaluated.

Design Challenges

The design of trials in prevention is confounded by:

1) Difficulty in validating population -based epidemiological data in clinical trials – issues of bias, sample size, false subgroup interpretations, differentiating host (genetic) from environmental (lifestyle factors).

2) Issues that affect the assessment of risk.

A risk assessment tool can be highly predictive but still be poorly calibrated. Calibration determines the extent to which the predicted risk corresponds to the actual risk observed in a given population. Prevention research must focus on high -risk individuals for the following reasons:

-Improves the benefit-risk ratio and is an important factor in achieving good adherence to treatment, which tends to be required for a long period.

-Some preventive agents are expensive, so they need to be used only on those likely to benefit.

-Risk assessment can also identify those at low risk of specific diseases, where preventive activities, including routine screening, are much less important and efforts are best focused on other aspects of health.

Cancer risk assessment challenges concerning

Physical activity

Risk assessment is of less value as benefits are sufficiently widespread and side effects are less. Almost all individuals stand to benefit from the intervention or lifestyle change, with greater benefit seen in higher-risk individuals like the obese.

Dietary factors

Food and eating patterns are complex and multifaceted, so testing exposures or assessing risks related to dietary factors is particularly challenging. Focus on specific foods can be misleading because foods are consumed as part of an overall dietary pattern with other characteristics, with a variable mix of healthy and less healthy dietary factors. Even a highly plant-based diet may have numerous potentially beneficial components, so focusing on a specific nutrient or bioactive food component may not be effective.

Additional challenges

a) Since many variables such as diet quality, physical activity, weight management, and smoking status are clustered, it is challenging to tease out a single behavioral pattern.

b) Gut microbiome variability in health and disease adds another dimension of complexity between identified exposures in observational studies and the response of individuals to interventions.

c) Difficulty in analyzing the response to one component in the diet, which has multiple components, makes predicting outcomes un-reliable .

d) Cancer outcome-focused trials require a large sample size and are time and resource intense. The results may not be generalizable to the broader population as they are done on high-risk individuals.

e) Identifying the effects of modification of lifestyle factors on markers of cellular activities instead of cancer outcomes require shorter-term intervention studies, which are less expensive and involve a smaller sample size. However, limitations are:

    i) The observed short-term effects on biomarkers or proposed mechanistic factors do not necessarily translate into effects on cancer or other clinical outcomes.

    ii) In any clinical trial of a lifestyle intervention, the trial is actually testing the intervention itself in addition to testing the effect of a specific diet or level of physical activity.

iii) Adherence to the prescribed behavior or dietary change is challenging.

iv) Testing the effect of foods or dietary constituents in feeding studies or supervised exercise activities on cancer biomarkers produces only very short-term changes that may not be sustained and, thus, may not necessarily affect cancer outcomes.

v) Treatment duration in diet intervention trials is limited, usually not exceeding an average of five years. Given the long latency of most cancers, this brief timeframe is not a true test of the diet-cancer connection.

vi) The intervention may be too late in the cancer continuum; this issue is particularly important in the design and interpretation of diet intervention trials because nutritional effects on physiological factors are known to be particularly critical during developmental periods.

In summary, one strategy proposed to better test the relationship between dietary factors and other lifestyle factors and cancer is to target a group likely to benefit from behavioral modification. Realistic, convenient, and achievable goals are necessary, and strategies to support the maintenance of behavior change are crucial. Finally, focusing on foods and dietary patterns may produce findings transferable to public policy and recommendations.

Effect of demographics and co-morbidities

The development and impact of age, sex, ethnicity, culture, and comorbidities on preventive intervention need to be recognized in the design and interpretation of all trials. The presence of comorbidities is another confounding factor in cancer prevention trials. The impact of comorbidities on intervention and outcomes needs to be routinely assessed, particularly in older individuals, as comorbidities accumulate with age and affect both the intervention and health and mortality outcomes.

Limitations of preclinical studies

It is difficult to reproduce the complexities of human tumors in preclinical animal models as many of the animal models available to date have limited physiological relevance to human disease. Patient-derived xenografts are more promising tools to identify therapeutic targets and may be useful in cancer prevention studies in the future.

Studies in mouse models are done under strictly controlled laboratory conditions and protocol- driven nutritional regimen. This is not possible in conducting human intervention trials. Humans enrolled in clinical trials usually have diverse genetic backgrounds and have engaged in wide-ranging dietary habits and other lifestyle factors such as smoking, alcohol consumption, and food preparation methods that may affect biologically active constituents and thus exposures. In vitro studies can only provide mechanistic guidance.

Challenges in screening

Screening interventions are for the early detection of precancerous conditions. Although guidelines exist for screening oral, breast and cervical cancers in low and middle income countries, there are many challenges. Unlike organized screening, opportunistic screening poses unique challenges related to cost, training, access and follow up treatment. Educational programs to improve health literacy and awareness among the general public, leading to an earlier diagnosis, can improve preventive care outcomes.

The National Cancer Grid (NCG), a consortium of more than 180 cancer institutions in India, the largest cancer network in the world, aims to provide evidence-based resource-stratified strategies and approaches for a sustainable implementation of population-based cancer screening and early detection program in India.

Developing meaningful practice guidelines from cancer prevention research should take into consideration the following:

1. The clinical risk-benefit and not a singular molecular target. should be the driver for human clinical trials.

2. Developing more accurate models for risk assessment using both genetic and environmental /lifestyle factors to improve the cancer prevention strategy.

3. New, more effective (enhanced benefit and diminished risk) chemoprevention agents need to be developed with a major emphasis on Phase 0 and I pharmacodynamics studies before moving forward to correlative Phase II studies.

4. For primary prevention, a moderate increase in physical exercise, weight loss, decreased caloric consumption, and an improved vegetable-based diet should be integrated into practice and lead to a "healthy lifestyle."

5. Chemoprevention is not ready for routine adoption in cancer survivors. Emphasis should be on primary prevention and managing long-term side effects.

6. Assessing the impact of and improving the success and implementation rates of lifestyle, dietary and pharmacological interventions.

7. Effective prevention research must lead to discoveries that improve the quality and quantity of life. Screening and prevention must be part of primary health care as screening can provide a teachable opportunity for cancer prevention advice.

18

BREAST CANCER PREVENTION

Dr. Nanda Rajaneesh, Dr Samhitha Venkatesh

Introduction

Breast cancer is one of the most lethal and commonly diagnosed malignancies worldwide, with around 2.3 million new cases in 2020. In women, it has the highest incidence (24.5%) and is the leading cause of cancer death. [319]

Women's breasts undergo constant changes throughout their lifetime under the influence of various hormones in the form of proliferation, differentiation, and involution, a balance between which is crucial to their health and life.

Abnormal cells are continuously formed in the breast tissue during these processes, influenced by inherent mutations (15%) and external environmental factors (85%). These abnormal or "initiated" cells are the first step in cancer formation and are usually repaired/removed by the immune system. But, when there is a high proliferation in the breast tissue due to factors like late childbirth, vitamin-D deficiency, improper diet, exogenous hormones, and obesity, there is little time for these cells to undergo DNA repair. Moreover, the over-burdened immune system cannot remove them, thereby promoting them to form benign tumors such as fibroadenoma/fibrocystic disease.

Over time, they accumulate more and more mutations and progress to breast cancer. Therefore, the larger the number of such "initiated" cells in the body, the greater the risk of developing breast cancer.

Breast cancer thus arises due to the interaction between normal breast development and the process of carcinogenesis by initiation, promotion and progression (Figure 1).

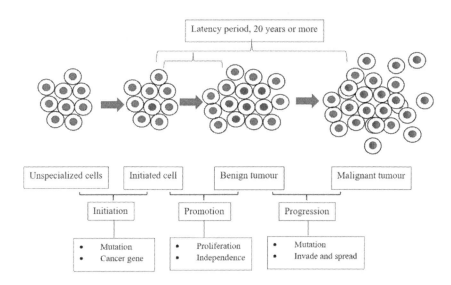

Figure 1- The process of breast cancer formation.

The two-hit model for breast cancer provides a valuable basis for assessing the interplay of factors contributing to oncogenesis. It suggests that a genetic or environmental "first hit" disrupts some elements of breast development, making it vulnerable to a subsequent "second hit" later via improper lifestyle/diet or increased exposure to exogenous hormones, eventually disrupting the compensatory mechanisms and resulting in tumorigenesis.

Risk factors

Reproductive factors: Women's breasts constantly change under the influence of estrogen and progesterone. Reproductive factors that increase the duration/levels of exposure to these hormones, such as the early onset of menstruation (<12 years), late onset of menopause (> 55 years), later age at first pregnancy, and nulliparity have been associated with an increase in breast cancer risk. Menarcheal age is a well-established risk factor, with an estimated 10% reduction in risk for every two-year increase in menarcheal age. [320]

Conversely, pregnancy and breastfeeding, which reduce a woman's lifetime number of menstrual cycles and cumulative exposure to endogenous hormones, are associated with decreased breast cancer risk. [321] Additionally, they cause breast cells to differentiate to produce milk. Some researchers hypothesize that these differentiated cells are more resistant to transforming into cancer cells than undifferentiated ones. [322,323]

The age at first pregnancy and the number of pregnancies affect the risk significantly. Women aged ≥ 35 years at their first childbirth are 40% more likely to get cancer than those aged < 20. Each subsequent birth lowers the risk. [324]

Age: Advancing age is another crucial risk factor. Most breast cancers are diagnosed after age 50. [325] This is attributed to the time and number of premalignant steps required between mutagenic initiation and complete tumor promotion to generate a clinically evident cancer.

Overweight/Obesity: Women being overweight or obese, especially after menopause, have an increased risk of breast cancer. This is attributed to the associated increased levels of oestrogens derived by peripheral conversion of adrenal androgens in fat tissue after menopause. [326]

Dense breasts: High breast density is shown to be a vital, independent risk factor. The relative breast cancer risk associated with breast density is ~1.2 for women with heterogeneously dense and 2.1 for women with extremely dense breasts. [327]

Personal history of breast cancer: A personal history of prior breast cancer is associated with a higher risk of acquiring subsequent new breast cancers and recurrence. This risk increases over time; 3-5% and 14% more women are diagnosed after 7-8 years and 25 years, respectively. [328,329] Several factors influence the risk –

a) Primary tumor features - tumor size, nodal status, pathological grade, molecular sub-type, presence of skin invasion.

b) Type and efficacy of the treatment given.

The lobular component in the initial tumor is associated with an increased risk of second breast cancer. [330] Furthermore, a history of ductal carcinoma in situ (DCIS) is known to confer an additional risk for ensuing second cancer. Women had a 3% and 6% chance of acquiring DCIS/invasive breast cancer after five and ten years post-treatment, respectively. [331] Multiple studies have also shown that women with hormone receptor-negative (HR-negative) breast cancers, especially those diagnosed at an earlier age (20s-30s), have a higher propensity to develop second contralateral breast cancer later in their lifetime. [329,332] In HR-positive cancers, endocrine therapy using aromatase inhibitors reduces the risk by approximately 33%. [333]

Second breast cancers usually had high histologic/nuclear grades, high Ki67 and HER-2-positive/triple-negative subtypes and were detected at stage III/IV. [334] Such aggressive phenotypes may be due to the selective prevention of other phenotypes by prior systemic adjuvant therapy.

Genetic factors: Most breast cancers are associated with acquired mutations, but about 5-10% of breast cancers are hereditary.[335] Breast Cancer gene (BRCA-1 and 2) mutations account for most cases. Hereditary breast cancers are seen to cluster in families and develop at an earlier age than sporadic cases. Relative to women without a family history, those with one and two pre-menopausal first-degree relatives with breast cancer are at 3.3-fold and 3.6-fold more significant risk, respectively. [336]

BRCA1 and BRCA2 are tumor suppressor genes, and mutations in them can impair DNA repair and increase DNA breakage and genomic instability, thereby promoting carcinogenesis.[337]

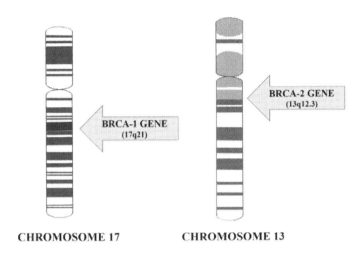

CHROMOSOME 17   CHROMOSOME 13

Figure 2- Location of Breast Cancer genes

Breast cancers associated with these mutations were usually found to be triple-negative (bad prognosis) and develop in younger women, often in both breasts.[338] BRCA1-associated cancers exhibit more pleomorphism, increased mitoses, and less tubule formation, all pointing toward high-grade tumors. [339]

These mutations account only for 16-20% of the general population's familial risk of breast cancer. A significantly increased risk is found in several rare genetic syndromes such as Cowden syndrome (PTEN), Li-Fraumeni syndrome (TP53), Hereditary diffuse gastric cancer (CDH1), and Peutz-Jeghers syndrome (STK11). [340]

Another major epidemiologic characteristic of familial breast cancer is its strong association with ovarian cancer. Several studies have found these cancers to occur in the same woman, especially with a strong family history, suggesting the presence of common risk factors between them. [341]

Diet: Incorrect nutrition plays a significant role in breast cancer. The hormones in meat or plants (exogenous hormones) are thermally stable, function agonistically to endogenous hormones, and cannot be wholly degraded during downstream processing. Small concentrations of the hormones escape the liver's digestive actions and enter the circulation. Their presence in circulation, along with endogenous hormones, increases the overall concentrations of the hormones near the hormone-sensitive breast tissues. They activate the downstream signaling pathway and disturb the Hypothalamic-Pituitary-Gonadal (HPG) axis causing changes in breast histology.[342] Plant products like soy, nuts, cereals, seeds, and grains contain phytoestrogens (isoflavones, lignans, phytoalexins), which can bind to estrogen receptors and influence transcription factors, thereby exerting estrogen/antiestrogen–properties.[343] Similarly, growth hormones used for improving feed efficiency/nutritional quality and increasing milk production can influence human tissue. Accumulating these hormones act as a carcinogenic tool and aggravates breast disease risk.

Fruits and vegetables such as legumes, allium vegetables, carrots, melons, tomatoes, dark-green vegetables, and citrus fruits provide a rich supply of dietary fiber, minerals, vitamins, and bioactive compounds. [344] They prevent carcinogenesis by regulating interleukins (IL-6), inhibiting the activities of lipoxygenase, cyclooxygenase, and transcription factor NF-$\varkappa$B. A study by Farvid et al. in 2016 showed that a higher intake of fruits and vegetables rich in α-carotene, vitamin C, fiber ,and isothiocyanates (apples, bananas, kale, and cruciferous vegetables) during adolescence was associated with a lower risk of breast cancer, due to their antioxidant and anti-proliferative properties. [329] An antioxidant diet rich in vitamin E, β-carotene, zinc, iron, copper, and selenium can neutralize free radicals that cause oxidative damage, protect the immune system and prevent cancer.

The role of red meat was studied by Guo et al., which showed that higher red and processed meat intake is associated with an increased risk of breast cancer. Pro-oxidant property of iron (heme-iron), the presence of carcinogenic compounds like heterocyclic amines (HCAs)/polycyclic aromatic hydrocarbons (PAHs), and hormone residues in the meat are the probable explanations for the association.[346] Moreover, a study by Brinkman et al. showed that red meat consumption was inversely associated with circulating concentrations of sex hormone-binding globulin (SHBG). [347] Lower SHBG concentrations indicate higher circulating total estrogen/estradiol levels, which explains the higher risk. Conversely, consuming fish, poultry, and egg show heterogeneous effects on breast cancer risk.

Dairy products are found to have both pro- and anti-carcinogenic effects. Components such as conjugated linoleic acid, branched-chain fatty acids, calcium, and vitamin D can affect cell proliferation/differentiation and inhibit tumorigenesis, thereby protecting against breast cancer.[348] Conversely, full-fat dairy products contain a high amount of lipophilic steroid hormones and xenobiotics like harmful pesticides and recombinant bovine somatotrophin (rBST) that can disturb hormonal homeostasis, increasing the risk. [349]

Intermittent fasting: It plays a significant role in ameliorating obesity, insulin resistance, dyslipidemia, hypertension, chronic inflammation and cancer via- [350]

a) Metabolic switch from glucose to ketone bodies as the primary energy fuel- Mutations found in cancer cells reduce their ability to adapt to such metabolic changes. The ketotic state exacerbates the metabolic oxidative stress in cancer cells and inhibits their growth.

b) Increasing stress resistance and antioxidant defenses- Fasting induces protection in normal cells by prioritizing maintenance pathways and inactivating growth factor signaling, but not in oncogene-driven cancer cells (differential stress resistance), making them vulnerable to cytotoxic treatment. [351]

c) Stimulating autophagy helps eliminate damaged and mutated cells, improving immunity and preventing cancer. [352]

Physical activity: Several epidemiological studies have shown an inverse relationship between breast cancer risk and physical activity levels in pre-and post-menopausal women. [353,354] Multiple mechanisms are proposed to explain this influence via its effects on-

1. Sex hormones (estrogens, androgens).

2. Insulin levels and resistance.

3. Metabolic hormones (leptins, adipokines).

4. Growth factors (IGF-1).

5. Inflammatory markers (prostaglandins, C-reactive protein).

6. Immunological parameters (NK-cells, WBCs, T-helper cells).

7. Free radicals.

Physical activity during the reproductive years reduces the exposure to estrogen by delaying the onset of menses, reducing the luteal phase of the menstrual cycle, lowering the follicle-stimulating hormone (FSH) levels, and causing secondary amenorrhea, particularly in adolescence. [355] Women who maintain an activity level of 1-3 hours/week and ≥4 hours/week can reduce their pre-menopausal breast cancer risk by about 30% and 50%, respectively, relative to inactive women.[353] Women in their post-menopausal years who exercise regularly have lower circulating estrone levels and higher levels of SHBG. Exercise enhances insulin sensitivity and reduces plasma insulin levels, thereby minimizing its mitogenic potential.

Oral contraceptive pills (OCP): Data from ≥ 54 epidemiological studies showed that women who ever used OCPs had a minimal increase (7%) in the relative risk of developing breast cancer when compared to "never-users". [356]

Current users of OCPs, especially combined OCPs, had a 24% increase in risk. The risk declined with the termination of use, and no increased risk was evident after ten years of cessation. [357] Moreover, women exposed to OCPs before their first full-term pregnancy experienced an increased risk of pre-menopausal breast cancer with increasing duration of use.

Smoking: Tobacco smoke contains potential human breast carcinogens, including PAHs, aromatic amines, and N-nitrosamines. They pass through the lung alveolar membrane, enter the bloodstream and are transported to the breast through plasma lipoproteins. They can have estrogenic and anti-estrogenic effects. Studies have shown that smoking is associated with an increased risk of ER+ and luminal breast cancers, which is attributed partly to the estrogenic properties of these carcinogens.[358] Conversely, antiestrogenic smoking effects are suggested to be more dominant only among post-menopausal women. Therefore, smoking is associated with an overall increased risk of breast cancer, especially luminal-A. [359]

Alcohol intake: Moderate consumption causes increased breast cancer risk. The overall estimated association is an approximate 30-50% increase in risk for 15-30 grams/day of alcohol consumption (~1-2 drinks/day). [360] Acetaldehyde, the primary ethanol metabolite, is suggested to have a role in breast cancer pathogenesis by binding to DNA and inducing damage. [361] A higher intake of alcohol is also shown to increase circulating estrogen levels among pre-and post-menopausal women. [362] It is associated with luminal-A–like breast cancer (ER+, PR+/-, HER2-), and no significant association was seen with HER2-positive or triple-negative breast cancer. [363]

Vitamin-D deficiency: The immunogenic and anti-carcinogenic properties of Vitamin D include- inhibition of cancer cell proliferation, invasion, metastasis, angiogenesis, induction of apoptosis, and differentiation in normal cells. [364] Breast cells contain all the components of a vitamin-D signaling axis that coordinates the local synthesis and metabolism of 1, $25(OH)_2D$ and its signal transduction via Vitamin D receptors (VDRs). Therefore, impaired activity of such genes due to deficiency can increase breast cancer risk. [365] Low serum levels of vitamin D are common at breast cancer diagnosis and associated with a poorer prognosis in terms of overall and distant disease-free survival, particularly in post-menopausal females. [366] It was found that 94% of women with serum vitamin D levels < 20 ng/ml were likely to develop metastases, and 73% were likely to die of advanced disease. [367]

Vitamin-B$_{12}$ levels: Prospective studies investigating the relationship between vitamin-B$_{12}$ and breast cancer risk show mixed results. Although, according to some studies, no association between vitamin-B$_{12}$ levels and risk of breast cancer was found in the overall population, an inverse association was reported independently among either post- or pre-menopausal women. [368,369] Other studies have shown a positive association between plasma/dietary vitamin B12 and breast cancer risk. [370] These inconsistent findings could be attributed to the varying functions of vitamin B12 and confounding factors such as differences in nutrient interactions in one-carbon metabolism, genetic polymorphisms, and alcohol intake.

Hormone Replacement Therapy (HRT): Although the benefits of HRT in post-menopausal women are widely accepted, it is associated with certain risks such as stroke, heart disorder, and breast cancer. This depends on the treatment's composition and duration and the women's health risks. The Million Women study showed that the breast cancer risk was substantially greater for combined (estrogen-progestogen) than for estrogen-only HRT. [355]

Breast biopsy: It is vital to establish a breast lesion's true nature by providing a pathological assessment of a palpable/radiologic breast abnormality. The histologic features, age at biopsy, and degree of family history are significant determinants of breast cancer risk after diagnosing benign breast disease. The risk associated with different findings on biopsy reports is summarised below. [372]

Biopsy report	Risk
Non proliferative breast disease a) Adenosis. b) Fibroadenoma. c) Apocrine metaplasia. d) Duct ectasia.	No increased risk.
Proliferative breast disease without atypia: 1. Florid hyperplasia without atypia. 2. Intraductal papilloma. 3. Sclerosing adenosis.	1.5-2 times increased risk.
Proliferative breast disease with atypia: I. Atypical ductal hyperplasia. II. Atypical lobular hyperplasia.	4-5 times increased risk.

Radiation exposure: The breast is sensitive to radiation-associated carcinogenesis, especially after exposures at young ages. Women aged < 20 years at the time of exposure are at higher risk of radiation-associated breast cancer than those exposed at older ages. [373] There is a concern that ionizing radiation from mammography might disproportionately increase the breast cancer risk for women with specific BRCA1/BRCA2 mutations, which affect DNA repair. [374] But the benefits of screening mammogram far outweigh the risks and is thus safe.

Bacterial infections: The microbiota plays a significant role in human health, and any imbalance in it (dysbiosis) can influence the immune system and subsequently promote breast cancer.[375] External infection, inflammation, and extensive use of antibiotics can lead to dysbiosis. The increased risk of breast cancer due to prior puerperal mastitis also relates to establishing a pro-malignant environment through immune system activation and inflammatory process via phagocytes and proinflammatory cytokines (IL-6, TNF- α, leptin). [376]

Race and ethnicity: Disparities in breast cancer incidence, stage, and mortality due to race and ethnicity are well-known. Breast cancer incidence rates are highest in non-Hispanic white women, followed by African American women, and are lowest among Asian/Pacific Islander women. [377] Compared with non-Hispanic whites, several racial/ethnic groups, including Blacks, Hispanic whites, and American Indians, are more likely to be diagnosed with advanced-stage breast cancer and HR-negative tumors (poor prognosis). [378] This disparity is due to a combination of factors, including differences in lifestyle, socioeconomic status, obesity, comorbidities, stage at diagnosis, tumor characteristics, screening, access, and treatment response.

Further research has shown a high prevalence of infiltrative ductal carcinoma and triple-negative breast cancer subtypes in Indian females, with the highest incidence in pre-menopausal females. [379]

Stress and anxiety: Studies have shown a possible association between stressful events and breast cancer incidence. Persistent activation of the HPA axis and release of stress mediators (catecholamines, corticosteroids) can suppress immune functions. This affects the ability of the body to recognize and remove the neoplastic cells, thereby promoting carcinogenesis.[380] Thus, stress can affect breast cancer directly via the biological stress response or indirectly by affecting the immune system.

Prevention

The primary focus in preventing breast cancer lies in restoring the hormonal balance in the body and boosting immunity. The following simple yet effective methods can achieve this-

Diet modifications:

1. Avoiding food products enriched in exogenous hormones and chemical toxins, such as milk products, red meat, and processed foods, and

switching to more organic alternatives is beneficial.

2. The cells in our body, especially immune cells, depend on cell-cell communication via membrane-bound receptors to transmit signals adequately. The cell membranes are made of phospholipids which, when peroxidized by free radicals, can alter the membrane fluidity and loss of membrane integrity, impairing cellular functions and intracellular signaling. Intake of fruits and vegetables rich in antioxidants such as vitamins E and C, β-carotene, zinc, iron, copper, and selenium can neutralize free radicals that cause oxidative damage and protect the immune system.[381]

3. Intermittent fasting is proven to be highly beneficial in boosting immunity, alleviating obesity and insulin resistance, dyslipidemia, and hypertension, and reducing chronic inflammation and cancer via various mechanisms such as causing a metabolic switch from glucose to ketone bodies as the primary energy fuel, increasing stress resistance and antioxidant defenses and stimulating autophagy, a catabolic process by which intracellular endogenous (damaged organelles, misfolded or mutant proteins, genomic fragments, and macromolecules) and exogenous (viruses or bacteria) components are degraded and recycled. The morphological and molecular mechanisms of autophagy were first elucidated by the Japanese scientist, Professor Yoshinori Ohsumi, for which he was awarded the 2016 Nobel Prize in Physiology or Medicine, which also highlighted the need for cancer prevention. Since then, multiple studies have explored the effects of autophagy in cancers and various other human disorders such as infections, inflammatory diseases, neurodegenerative disorders, obesity and cardiovascular diseases. Commonly practiced intermittent fasting regimens which have proven effective include alternate-day fasting, 5:2 intermittent fasting (fasting two days each week), and daily time-restricted feeding. [382]

Yoga, physical exercise, and meditation:

a) Regular aerobic exercise for 35-45 minutes daily has positive effects in improving the immune system, reducing chronic inflammation, and detoxifying the body, all of which can be beneficial in preventing breast cancer. Moreover, it helps to avoid obesity and maintain a steady weight, reducing the risk even further. [383]

b) Yoga and meditation can improve blood circulation, enhance immune cell distribution, recruitment and better detoxification. They also can relieve stress by reducing stress hormones such as cortisol. The maintenance of the balance between the nervous, immune, and endocrine systems is also mediated by yoga and meditation, which helps improve the hormonal milieu and reduces the risk of breast cancer development. [384]

Vitamin D and B12 supplementation:

a) Vitamin D is known for its immunogenic and anti-carcinogenic properties, inhibiting cancer cell proliferation, invasion, metastasis, and angiogenesis, and induction of cellular differentiation and apoptosis. Vitamin D deficiency is observed in many women with benign and malignant breast pathologies and is associated with a poorer prognosis. Moreover, it is also associated with secondary hyperparathyroidism leading to osteopenia and worsening of osteoporosis, especially in post-menopausal women. This gets aggravated further with chemotherapy and hormonal therapy. Therefore, several benefits lie in supplementing vitamin D, not just in preventing primary breast cancers but also in preventing recurrence in existing breast cancer patients.[385]

b) Vitamin B12 is essential in one-carbon metabolism and DNA synthesis, repair, and methylation. Deficiency of this vitamin may trigger genetic and epigenetic pro-carcinogenic processes; hence, moderate supplementation with multivitamins is protective.[386]

Positive attitude and sound sleep:

I. A positive attitude and happiness significantly influence the immune system by releasing neurotransmitters like serotonin, dopamine, and β-endorphins, receptors for which exist on the immune cells. They are known to increase the CD4+ and CD8+ T cells and the killing capacity of natural killer (NK) cells, thereby enhancing cellular immunity, the primary effector mechanism to prevent carcinogenesis. [387]

II. The circadian rhythm (sleep-wake cycle) is a potent regulator of the immunological process and hormone balance. The different cytokines, hormones and neurotransmitters form the primary basis for this. A good sleep of 6-8 hours helps to maintain this neuro-immuno-endocrinal balance. The effector cells, such as NK cells and CD8+ cells, peak after a good sleep, and plays a massive role in maintaining immunity. During early sleep, there is increased proliferation, differentiation, and migration of T cells along with the formation of immunological memories, all of which can improve and enhance the subsequent immune response. Prolonged sleep curtailment and accompanying stress response lead to the continuous production of pro-inflammatory cytokines and chronic low-grade inflammation, thereby resulting in immunodeficiency and progression of cancer. This highlights the importance of maintaining a good sleep-wake cycle. [388]

Therefore, implementing such relatively simple dietary lifestyle practices, can substantially reduce the risk of acquiring breast cancer. Further awareness is thus needed regarding these aspects, not just among ordinary people and breast cancer patients but also among the treating doctors.

19

INFERTILITY, IVF TREATMENT AND ITS RELATION TO BREAST CANCER

Dr. Kalaivani V

Introduction

Carcinoma of the breast is one of the most common cancers in women and is the cause of death in about 20% of women despite advances in medical sciences.[389] As per WHO's International Agency for Research on Cancer (IARC) predictions, the specific age-standardized incidence rate for female breast cancer worldwide is 46 cases per 100,000 women.[390] Breast cancer is a heterogeneous disease with the incidence, clinical diagnosis, and prognosis varying according to ethnicity and race.

Most breast cancer cases are sporadic; however, 5-10%have a genetic predisposition. BRCA 1 and 2 are the tumor suppressor genes associated with breast cancer in about 40% of cases. These genes are localized on chromosomes 17q21 and 13q12.3, respectively.[391-392] Breast cancer is related to reproductive factors like early menarche below 12 years of age, late menopause above 55 years of age, nulliparity, miscarriages before the first full-term pregnancy, late age at first childbirth(>30y), infertility and, hormone usage.[393-395] The environmental factors associated are high socio-cultural level, obesity, selected dietary habits, alcohol consumption, low physical activity and exposure to ionizing radiation.[396-402]

Infertility is emerging as one of the common diseases affecting young adults, seen in one in several couples trying to conceive.[403] Female causes contribute to more than half of the cases. [404-405] The most common cause found for infertility in women is the hormonal disorder affecting ovulation, including polycystic ovarian syndrome (PCOS), followed by tubal factors. Endometriosis contributes to a smaller number of cases.[404] Several hormonal and reproductive risk factors are related to breast, ovarian, and endometrial cancers. It is found that the causes and consequences of infertility could influence cancer risk, and the relationship is found to be complex.[406]

As per the nationwide population-based study conducted among Swedish women by Frida E. Lundberg et al. in 2018, women born before 1950 and after 1980 were less likely to have a diagnosis of infertility. Infertile women were found to have higher educations, older at first childbirth, and had fewer children at the end of the study follow-up.[406] Among the infertile women, ovulatory disturbances were found in 16.4%(n=19,299) of women, endometriosis in 11.9% (n=14,-030) compared to 1.5% (n=41,617) and 2.0% (n=54,797) women with no infertility. However, in this study, neither infertility nor related diagnosis was associated with a higher incidence of breast cancer in the multi-variate adjusted analysis.

Van der Bolt- Dusebout & colleagues studied a population of 25,018 women, compared the incidence of breast cancer amongst IVF-treated women and women with subfertility who did not receive IVF with a median follow-up of 21 years,[407] and did not report any statistically significant difference in the incidence of breast cancer.

A meta-analysis by Carolyn Cullinane & colleagues published in 2022 analyzed twenty-four studies and concluded that there was significant breast cancer risk associated with fertility treatment with a summary odd ratio of 0.97 (95 percent CI 0.90 to 1.04).[408]

Studies have also shown that women with infertility problems undergoing hormone therapy are more likely to have dense breasts due to controlled ovarian stimulation, a risk factor for breast cancer.[409] Women over 30 are increasingly at risk for breast cancer by initiating IVF cycles.[410] Papps et al. also demonstrated an increase in the incidence of breast cancer in women >/= 40 years of age after controlled ovarian stimulation in their retrospective cohort study.[410]

Ovarian stimulation can affect endogenous estrogen levels, affecting breast cancer risk (G-13,20,40,41). Hormones thus play a role by influencing the proliferation of breast epithelial cells. The part of hormone replacement therapy and assisted reproductive technology (ART) includes - ovarian stimulating agents like clomiphene, human chorionic gonadotropin (hCG) and, gonadotropin analogs.

Mechanisms of Action Estradiol Hormone

Estradiol hormone is an estrogen steroid hormone involved in the reproductive cycle of women.[409] It is synthesized in the breast, ovary, and extra glandular tissue.[411] It stimulates the proliferation of the mammary gland with paracrine, autocrine, and intracrine mechanisms. Estradiol and other estrogenic components accelerate the development of breast cancer by early mutation to the tumor metastasis by increasing cell proliferation or genotoxic effects. [412-413] The breast tissue contains two nuclear receptors and crucial transcriptional regulators: ERα (Estrogen receptor α) and ERβ (Estrogen receptor β). Estradiol attaches to nuclear estrogen receptors α and promotes cancer growth by causing DNA damage, resulting in increased DNA replication. [414-416]

Fertility Stimulating Drugs

Clomiphene citrate is an estrogenic agonist and increases ovulation. It contains a mixture of clomiphene and zuclomiphene isomers. Zuclomiphene is more effective for ovulation induction with both estrogenic and anti-estrogenic attributes. Clomiphene citrate competes with estrogen to bind ERs in cells containing these receptors like the ovary, pituitary and hypothalamus. Stimulating the hypothalamus to release Gonadotrophin releasing hormones which cause the release of luteinizing hormone (LH) and follicle-stimulating hormone (FSH) from the anterior pituitary, causing maturation of follicles, induces ovulation and thus pregnancy.[417-418] Clomiphene citrate binds nuclear ER for a longer time as compared to estrogens.

Women who have received more than six cycles of hCG or hMG in the IVF process are at an estimated 40% risk of developing breast cancer, especially in those with positive family history.

FSH and LH injectables, or a combination of both, might stimulate more than one egg to develop at a time. However, excessive gonadotropins in this procedure can suddenly increase the FSH and LH hormones' levels and stimulate and mature follicles. It can also increase estrogen secretion, gene expression, and possibly the risk of breast cancer.[422]

Studies have shown that increasing the number of menstrual cycles with regular ovulation may increase the risk of breast cancer.[423] Mitotic activity in the breast is low in the follicular phase and peaks during the luteal phase. Therefore, increasing the number of menstrual cycle periods with ovulation will expand mitotic activity in the breast.[424] In a study by Maryam Ghanbari Andarieh et al., women with a history of infertility were found to develop breast cancer much more than those without a history of infertility. It has been suggested that infertility drugs may have a greater malignancy risk as a confounding element than infertility itself and may increase the incidence of breast cancer.[425]

Studies by Oktay, Phillips, and Wang showed low Anti-Mullerian Hormone (AMH) and low ovarian response rates in women with BRCA-1 mutations; this information is more predictive of poor response to ART than true infertility. Data on whether BRCA-1 mutations are an independent predictor of infertility is currently lacking. The study by Reigstad et al. documented an increased risk of breast cancer in infertile patients who had received ART. Analysis done by Brent Hanson et al. showed a link between women who received ART and higher future breast cancer rates.[410] A critical confounding in all these studies has demonstrated an increase in breast cancer risk among nulliparous women, as infertile women are more likely to remain nulliparous.[427]

Association of BRCA with Infertility

Mean oocyte numbers were significantly lower in BRCA1 mutation-positive women.[428] And so had a lower response to ovarian stimulation for fertility preservation via embryo or oocyte cryopreservation according to the COST-LESS protocol.[428] A study conducted on 84 women by Kutluk Oklay et al. in 2010 analyzed the relationship between BRCA mutation and infertility risks. This study demonstrated that BRCA mutations are associated with occult primary ovarian insufficiency. The probable hypothesis is that activated apoptotic pathways may prematurely eliminate the oocyte. DNA repair is deficient in patients with BRCA mutations, so oocytes may be prone to DNA damage. BRCA mutations may contribute to a long-known association between breast and ovarian cancer risks because occult primary ovarian insufficiency is associated with female infertility. In the general population, one in every 1000 women is BRCA mutation-positive, and the incidence could be as high as 2.5% in certain ethnic groups like Jewish-ashkenazi origin.[429,430] Sperm production is altered in BRCA rodent models, which may explain that BRCA mutations may be responsible for male-factor infertility in some oligo-spermic men.[428]

Infertility and Risk of breast cancer in Men

Anthony I. Swerdlow et al. conducted a nationwide case-control study in England & Wales, interviewing 1998 cases between 2005-2017 with 1597 male control.[427] It was found that the risk of breast cancer was statistically significant in males with a diagnosis of infertility (OR = 2.03 - 95% CI 1.18-3.49) for invasive tumors but not if the couples' infertility of origin was from the female partner. The risk was also statistically significant (OR = 1.5-9% CI 1.21-1.86) compared with men who were fathers. The reason is not apparent, explains the author.

20

COLORECTAL CANCER PREVENTION

Dr. K. Lakshman

The word cancer evokes fear and powerful negative emotions. However, science has taken big steps in cancer prevention, diagnosis, and treatment in the past two to three decades. Colorectal cancer is no exception. This article focuses on the science of the prevention of colorectal cancer.

Globally, the burden of cancer is substantial. In 2012, 14.1 million new cancer cases and 8.2 million deaths were recorded. In 2030, the corresponding data will likely be 21.7 million cases and 13 million deaths. [431] In India, all cancers put together, about Eight Hundred Thousand new patients are seen, and 70% of these cases present in an advanced stage.

Colorectal cancer Is the third most common cancer in the world, with a 2012 estimate of 1.4 million. The incidence of this cancer is approximately 50% higher in men than women.[432] It is considered in line with the developed Western countries. However, the developing world has a significant load of colorectal cancer. For example, the figures for India show that each year, one sees 4.4 cases of colon cancer per 100000 population of men and 4.1 cases per 10000 women.[433]

There is also a trend that shows an increase in the incidence of colorectal cancer in developing countries, that too in a younger population. In a study, ten of the 36 countries analyzed showed an increase in the incidence of colon cancer. Among these, India led the most significant increase, followed by Poland. This increased incidence of colorectal cancer in the developing world is attributed to a change in lifestyle mirroring the Western population. The growth seen in a younger people is part of a global trend. [434]

Hence, understanding the disease and looking at practical and feasible steps in reducing the load of colorectal cancer becomes an integral part of preventive healthcare. It is imperative to understand the pathophysiology of the disease before we embark on the preventative steps.

Pathophysiology of Colorectal cancer

Pathophysiology refers to the processes that result in disordered physiology, i.e., normal functioning, leading to disease. In general, various causes like changes in the genetic material, viral diseases, chemical injury, etc., lead to disordered cell proliferation and disturbed cell death, leading to the causation of cancer. In colon cancer, it is well established that the causation of cancer follows stepwise escalation named "adenoma-carcinoma sequence". Figure 1 depicts this sequence diagrammatically.

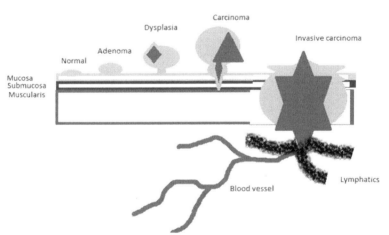

Figure 1 - The Adenoma-Carcinoma Sequence - Diagrammatic representation.

The cells of the innermost layer of the large bowel, called mucosa, start proliferating and give a small lump called an adenoma. In the next stage, the changes in the cells result in uncontrolled proliferation and change in the characteristics of the cell, called dysplasia. However, these changes do not extend beyond the innermost layer. Continued changes lead to further disease expansion and invasion of the deeper layers going beyond the layer next to the mucosa, called the submucosa. At this stage, the condition becomes cancer. Progressing further, it invades the layers of the colon more deeply and starts spreading to other parts of the body through the blood vessels and the lymphatics. This phenomenon of spread is called metastasis.

Polyps follow 1 of 2 methods of development. These include the adenomatous and sessile serrated pathways—the former accounts for most polyps. The adenomatous polyps have a stalk many times and contain filamentous tubular glands. The sessile polyps are flat and have cells with a sawtooth pattern.[435]

Interestingly, polyps have associated genetic changes that accumulate over some time. This phenomenon results in the transformation of a benign polyp into cancer. In the adenomatous polyps, changes are associated with APC, KRAS, and p53 genes. In the sessile polyps, changes are seen in BRAF genes. Common to both is the phenomenon called microsatellite instability seen in the DNA content of the cells. This phenomenon leads to the transformation of normal cells into cancer cells.

It is to be noted that only 10% of adenomas become cancerous, but among all cancers, 70% are from preexisting adenomas, and only 30% are from sessile serrated polyps.[435]

Risk factors and protective factors for Colorectal cancer

The risk factors for colorectal cancer may be modifiable or nonmodifiable. Age, gender, ethnicity, and hereditary and non-hereditary genetic factors are the nonmodifiable risk factors. Hereditary disorders are relatively rare. The two major diseases in the hereditary group are Lynch syndrome and familial adenomatous polyposis syndrome.[435] Genetic counseling may help in reducing the fresh cases of hereditary cancers. Also, screening can be started earlier in the children of patients with hereditary cancer. This enables earlier treatment and can save lives.

Most colorectal cancers belong to the non-hereditary or sporadic group. In this group, interventions through genetic counseling would not be helpful. However, counseling regarding the modifiable factors can be undertaken.

Modifiable factors include the reduction of risk factors and the promotion of protective factors. Further, these interventions may influence general factors or factors specific to colorectal cancer. Figure 2 represents these factors schematically.

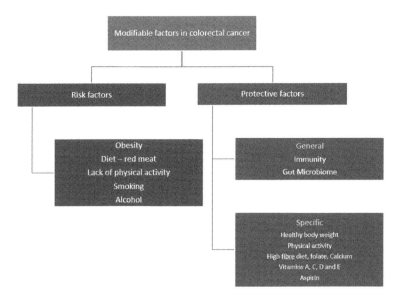

Figure 2 - Modifiable factors in colorectal cancer

Several studies have shown an association between obesity, consumption of large quantities of red meat, lack of physical activity, smoking, and moderate to high intake of alcohol, with the incidence of colorectal cancer.[419] It is estimated that a 50-70 percent reduction in Colorectal Cancer can be achieved by simple changes in Lifestyle.[437-438] The current standard recommendation Is listed in Box 1.

Remain lean within acceptable body weight.	Exercise regularly.
Minimize consumption of alcohol.	Stop smoking.
Reduce consumption of red and processed meat vegetables.	Consume more.
Consume Omega 3 fatty acids.	

Box 1: Standard recommendations about Diet and Exercise [437]

Diet is also shown to have proinflammatory properties, which may lead to cancer. The dietary inflammatory index (DII) measures this property.[439] Foods with high DII include carbohydrates, saturated fats, cholesterol, and Vitamin B12. The anti-inflammatory foods include fiber, Omega 3 and 6 fatty acids, Vitamins A, C, D, and E, Folic acid, carotene, and caffeine.

Prevention of Colorectal Cancer

Prevention of any cancer, including colorectal cancer, can be considered under three headings: primary, secondary, and tertiary prevention.

Primary prevention refers to the manipulation of the modifiable factors that lead to the formation of cancer. Secondary prevention refers to the early detection and treatment of cancer so that the outcomes can be improved. Secondary prevention is carried out primarily by screening. Tertiary prevention refers to the minimization of the after-effects of cancer treatment and an attempt to enhance longevity.

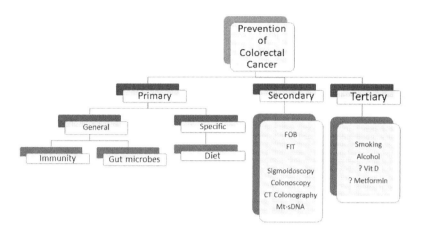

Figure 3 depicts the primary preventive measures that can be carried out in colorectal cancer.

The specific role of diet in colorectal cancer has already been discussed under the risk factors. This section discusses the general role of immunity and gut microbes in preventing colorectal cancer.

Nonspecific Measures

Immune System and Cancer

The immune system plays a vital role in cancer development and prevention. The immune system may be innate or acquired; The innate system is a nonspecific defense we are born with. The acquired system is a specific response to a given immune challenge.

The human tissues are rich in immune cells called macrophages and dendritic cells, which can differentiate between self and non-self (foreign) cells.[440] These are recognized as the non-self through their pattern recognition receptors (PRR). Once the foreign antigen is identified, they affect the release of compounds called cytokines that result in several changes in the metabolism. Interferon-gamma is one such important cytokine.[441] It is produced by a class of T-cells called Natural killer cells (NK) and is responsible for cancer surveillance. NK cells, along with Cytotoxic T Lymphocytes (CTL), kill cancer cells through the release of a compound called Perforin.[440]

Also, good numbers of effector memory cells and CD8+ cells in the tumor suggests a good prognosis. Conversely, some other immune cells can promote cancer cells by increasing their blood supply through angiogenesis and the release of epidermal growth factors:[440]

Gut Microbiota and Cancer

The word microbiota refers to the trillions of bacteria in the human gut. The term microbiome refers to the collective genomes of the microbiota.[441] The microbiota affects local metabolism, immunity, and gene expression.[437] Disruption of the mucus barrier, promoted by the Western diet, is hypothesized to alter how the gut microbiota interacts with the mucosa leading to carcinogenesis.[437] The most studied microbes in this field are Fusibacterium nucleata and Bacteroides fragilis. These induce a proinflammatory state, leading to microsatellite instability and cancer.[438]

Circadian Rhythms and Cancer

Much work has been done on circadian rhythms, melatonin hormone, and its effects on immunity. The hypothalamus sets the circadian rhythm. Nights are when the inflammatory phase peaks; during the day, the anti-inflammatory phase is dominant.[442] Melatonin, the hormone responsible for affecting the circadian rhythm, influences other processes like retinal physiology, cardiac function, immunity, cancer production, etc. Melatonin is also a free radical scavenger and can suppress the DNA product that comes out of the effect of carcinogenic chemicals on DNA. Melatonin is thus a protective agent as far as cancer is concerned. Disturbance of its production due to night-time wakefulness, particularly in brightly lit areas, leads to losing this protective function. Interestingly, night shift workers have been shown to have a higher incidence of malignancies like breast, endometrium, prostate, and colon cancer.[443]

While the nonspecific measures have been studied in detail, the evidence for any clinical intervention that substantially reduces the incidence of colorectal cancer is not robust.

Specific Preventive Measures

The specific measures can be considered under primary, secondary, and tertiary preventive measures.

Primary Preventive Measures

Primary measures consisting of lifestyle changes have been discussed under the risk factors above and listed:

Secondary Preventive Measures

Secondary measures are the mainstay of colorectal cancer prevention. Because of a distinct adenoma-carcinoma sequence, clinicians can detect and treat precancerous lesions and prevent full-blown cancer or detect early stages of cancer and treat them to get good outcomes in terms of longevity and quality of life. Detection of precancerous lesions is done through screening. The five-year survival of early colorectal cancer is 90% compared to 13% in late-stage disease.[435] Screening reduces cancer-related mortality by 30%.[436] Screening can be started early and can be conducted more frequently in individuals known to be at risk for colorectal cancer. These are listed in Box 2.

Age >50

Personal or familial history of CRC

Adenomatous polyps

Inflammatory bowel disease

Hereditary CRC syndromes FAP and Lynch syndrome - HNPCC

Box 2 - Individuals at high risk for colorectal cancer (CRC)

The more intense screening offered to high-risk individuals listed above is called **Targeted Prevention.**

The increased cancer risk in inflammatory bowel disease is thought to be due to the chronic inflammation-induced release of cytokines. This results in changes in cell proliferation and migration enabling transformation into cancer.[444]

CRC falls into the category of a specific disease amenable to screening for the following reasons:

1. The incidence of the disease is significant - even in developing countries.

2. There is a long precancerous stage.

3. There are relatively easy and cost-effective tests to diagnose the disease in the precancerous or early cancerous stage.

4. These tests are reliable.

5. Effective treatment is available to deal with early disease.

Many professional bodies have put forth screening guidelines. There are slight differences in the recommendations among these guidelines. We will list one such approach below.[435] Screening is generally offered to people between 50 and 70 years of age. For patients suspected of having hereditary cancers, the whole family, including first-degree relatives, must be screened. In addition, genetic testing is also carried out. Screening for cancer in inflammatory bowel disease starts after the patient has had the disease for ten years.[438]

Screening starts with the listed examinations in asymptomatic patients. But educating the population about the so-called 'danger symptoms' is essential. These include the following:

a) Rectal Bleeding.

b) Passing altered blood in stool.

c)   Recent alteration of bowel habit.

d)   Persistent lower abdominal pain.

e)   Weight loss, general weakness, and loss of appetite.

Screening Methods

Name	Method	Sensitivity	Frequency
Fecal occult blood	Detection of blood in stool	33-75%	Annual
Fecal immunochemical test	Detection of hemoglobin in stool	60-85%	Annual
Name	Method	Sensitivity	Frequency
Multitarget stool DNA	Detection of DNA aberration and hemoglobin in stool	92%	3 yearly
Sigmoidoscopy	Endoscopy of distal colon	95% - distal colon only	5 yearly
Colonoscopy	Endoscopy of whole	90%	10 yearly

	colon		
CT Colonography	Radiologic visualization of colon	90%	5 yearly

Table 1 - Screening methods in clinical practice [modified from Ref 5]

Fecal occult blood is a simple test to perform. But it has limited sensitivity. The immunochemical test is slightly more sensitive than fecal occult blood but is less specific.[435] The multi-target stool DNA combines tests for abnormal DNA to detect hemoglobin. The patient must have a colonoscopy as the next screening stage if it is positive.

Sigmoidoscopy examines only the distal colon. With the so-called 'rightward' migration of cancers - more and more colon cancers being now detected in the right colon - this test may not be an adequate screening tool. However, it is easier to perform, the preparation is more straightforward, and the cost is relatively less.

Colonoscopy is the most reliable screening tool for CRC. But the preparation is tedious, performance needs considerable training and skill, and expensive.

CT colonography is less invasive and nearly as accurate as a colonoscopy but suffers from the disadvantage that the preparation is akin to a colonoscopy and is tedious.

The clinician must choose an appropriate tool for screening bearing in mind several factors like the prevalence of the disease in the population, comorbidities in the patient, presence of high-risk factors, availability of the test, and the cost of the procedure.

Tertiary Prevention

Tertiary prevention is the limitation of recurrent disease after the first treatment session for CRC. Alcohol and smoking cessation is known to reduce recurrences. Interestingly, unlike in primary prevention, obesity has no effect in tertiary prevention. Administration of Vitamin D and metformin for tertiary prevention is being explored.[432]

Conclusion

Colorectal cancer presents a significant disease burden even in developing countries. An understanding of the pathophysiology of the disease helps in carrying out a logical, scientific screening program. Detection of precancerous or early cancerous lesions significantly improves mortality and morbidity. Several methods of lifestyle modification and screening are available to achieve this. Several guidelines give evidence-based recommendations for screening. The clinician must judiciously choose the screening program to suit the general patient population and the socio-economic status of the community where he/she practices.

21

PREVENTION OF MULTIPLE MYELOMA AND LYMPHOMA

Prof. (Dr.) Vishwanath Sathyanarayanan, Dr. Poonam Maurya and Mr. Bharath A Kashyap

Multiple Myeloma (MM) is a clonal plasma cell malignancy that accounts for around 10% of all hematologic cancers.[445] Multiple Myeloma (MM) is a neoplasm of clonal plasma cells that is characterized by the presence of elevated serum monoclonal protein and end-organ damage, collectively known as CRAB features (hypercalcemia, Renal insufficiency, Anemia, and Bone lesions).[445]

It evolves from a premalignant condition called "monoclonal gammopathy of undetermined significance" (MGUS). MGUS is less prevalent in the younger population (0.34% of 10–49-year-olds) but approximately 3% of the general population over 50 and progresses to MM at 1% per year.[445,446] In certain situations, there may be an entity called "Smoldering Multiple Myeloma" (SMM), which is also a precursor to MM though more advanced than MGUS, with an average of around 10% per year, transforming into MM and invariably most will progress to MM.[447]

Developing treatment and prevention strategies in MM is particularly attractive because MM meets 8 of 10 Wilson and Junger criteria for disease screening and prevention. Two screening blood tests for MGUS and myeloma are unique to myeloma that approach 99% sensitivity and specificity, e.g., serum protein electrophoresis and serum-free light chains. Currently, no interventions are known to halt the progression of MGUS to MM.

There is growing data on treating high-risk SMM to prevent their progression to MM and potentially cure them before they transform to MM. The combination of elotuzumab with lenalidomide and dexamethasone was shown in a phase II trial to prevent progression to MM in this setting. Not all SMM are the same, and hence genomic profiling and NGS can be used to stratify and decide which patients of SMM to treat or observe.

Irene Ghobrial, a medical oncologist at the Dana-Farber Cancer Institute, has been studying the molecular changes that occur as these precursor conditions advance to Multiple Myeloma. This could help researchers identify ways to stop them from progressing. They called the study "Predicting Progression of Developing Myeloma in a High-Risk Screened Population (PROMISE), which aims to enroll 50,000 people who are at high risk for Multiple Myeloma and its precursor conditions, which would probably diagnose 3,000 people who have MGUS or smoldering Myeloma. These patients will be followed up on how their disease progresses.

African Americans are more prone to MGUS, so they have a higher risk of Multiple Myeloma, so aggressive screening strategies should be employed.[448]

In a study, 52 genes were identified and found to be dysregulated in MGUS. Most dysregulated genes (41 of 52) exhibited a progressive expression increase along the transition from MGUS to MM. MGUS gene expression signatures may provide valuable molecular targets for the prevention of the multistep molecular pathogenesis of MM.[449]

The lipid processing disorder Gaucher's disease is associated with MM. Reduction of antigenic stimulation or signaling pathways downstream may be a prevention strategy in Gaucher's and perhaps other patients.

Obesity is additionally linked with an increased risk of MGUS. In a cross-sectional study of women aged 40–79, obese women were significantly more likely to have MGUS (relative risk = 1.8). Studies evaluating the impact of obesity duration suggest that early-life obesity may increase the overall MM risk compared to later-life obesity alone. Reduced lipokine adiponectin expression, as associated with obesity, is related to the progression of MGUS to MM in humans. [450] Hence preventive strategies should be focused on preventing obesity.

Metformin, through its anti-inflammatory function, reduces blood insulin by targeting AMPK or other mechanisms. In a study by Chang et al., 3287 MGUS patients found that four years or longer of metformin use was associated with a decreased risk of MM progression (hazard ratio = 0.47, CI = 0.25–0.87).[451]

Plasma levels of Vitamin D are reduced in patients with MM. In MGUS patients, Vitamin D supplementation improves bone health and metabolism markers. Vitamin D-deficient patients take a supplement because of the low-risk profile of Vitamin D supplements. This is a fantastic potential treatment option.[452-453]

Sleep and obesity-related sleep apnea may be additionally modifiable risk factors in preventing the MGUS to Myeloma transition. Alternatively, sleep duration may impact MM risk independent of obesity. In one of the only studies to directly link sleep quality with MM risk, Gu et al. found an increased risk of MM (Hazard ratio = 2.06, CI = 1.20–3.51) in individuals sleeping less than 5 hours a night compared to those sleeping 7–8 hours a night.[454-455]

Lymphoma is a cancer that affects the lymphocytes and the lymphatic system, the vital cells of the immune system. The lymphatic system includes the lymph nodes, spleen, thymus gland, and bone marrow.

There are two types of lymphoma, Hodgkin and non-Hodgkin.[456] The main difference between the two is the type of lymphocyte it affects. Hodgkin lymphoma affects the lymphocyte known as Reed-Sternberg. Non-Hodgkin lymphoma affects every other lymphocyte. There are more than 100 sub-groups of non-Hodgkin lymphoma.[457] These are divided based on whether B or T lymphocytes are being affected and their speed of growth. Global disease burden (GLOBOCAN 2020).[458] Non-Hodgkin lymphoma: 35828 new cases in 2020; 20390 deaths; 88272 patients in the last five years.[458] The data shows that the number of non-Hodgkin lymphoma cases is rising. Hodgkin lymphoma: 9,221 new cases in 2020; 3513 deaths; 24928 patients in the last five years.[458] The data shows that Hodgkin lymphoma cases are on the rise.

Smoking

Smoking negatively affects the immune system. The innate and adaptive immunity will not perform well, which means the function of the lymphocytes is impaired.[443] This increases the likelihood of infections, leading to a higher risk of lymphoma. If the patient wants to reduce the risk of lymphoma, the patient should quit smoking.[459]

Alcohol

Ethanol, which is present in alcohol, breaks down into acetaldehyde in our body. The acetaldehyde can damage DNA in healthy cells, thus letting cancerous cells grow. The patient should stop drinking to reduce the likelihood of lymphoma.[460]

Chronic Stress

Stress can increase the likelihood of many cancers, including lymphoma. The reason is that when the body is stressed, "neurotransmitters like norepinephrine are released",[461] which will cause cancer cells to be stimulated. To prevent this, one should participate in activities that reduce stress. An example of that would be yoga, that clears the mind, thus reducing the patient's stress levels. Other ways for the patient to reduce stress would be to eat a healthy diet, exercise regularly, meditate, and spend more time with the ones you have good connections with.[461] Walking and exercise can mediate a patient's mood and boost endorphin production.

Obesity

High BMI is an inflammatory state linked to many cancers, including lymphoma.[462] To prevent obesity, the patient should eat a healthy diet and not eat more than needed. Also, exercising is necessary for prevention.

Chemicals

Heavy exposure to industrial chemicals can cause lymphoma to develop.[463] These chemicals most likely contain carcinogens that can damage the cells' DNA and cause cancerous cells to arise.[463] The patient should try to avoid exposure to industrial chemicals. If unable, patients should wear masks and gloves to prevent chemicals from touching the body.

Bacterial Infections

H pylori: H pylori increases the likelihood of receiving a specific type of lymphoma called MALT lymphoma. Although not all people with an H pylori infection get MALT lymphoma, most people with MALT lymphoma have an H pylori infection.[464] To prevent H. Pylori, patients should practice good hygiene. If the patient has H pylori, therapy, including antibiotics, is essential.

Campylobacter jejuni

This is a bacteria that causes food poisoning when infecting humans.[464] This bacteria can increase the likelihood of lymphoma developing in a patient. Safe, hygienic practices are necessary to prevent this bacterial infection and cook meat so it is not undercooked.[464]

Borrelia burgdorferi and Borrelia afzeli

These bacteria cause Lyme disease and can increase the patient's likelihood of lymphoma.[464] Hard-bodied ticks mainly spread these bacterial infections.[464] To prevent this bacterial infection, cover all body parts when entering an area where ticks are prevalent. Also, spraying anti-tick spray on the body can help reduce the chance of a tick infecting the body with Borrelia burgdorferi or Borrelia afzelii.

Chlamydophila psittaci

This is a bacteria that usually infects birds but also infects humans.[464] Humans get infected by this bacteria when they come into close contact with birds already infected by it.[464] When humans are infected with Chlamydophila psittacine, the likelihood of developing lymphoma is increased. To prevent this bacterial infection, be careful when cleaning bird cages.

Hepatitis B

"Hepatitis B (HBV) is a hepatotropic virus accounting for chronic hepatitis and cirrhosis." [465] This does increase the patient to the risk of non-Hodgkin lymphoma. The best way to prevent the infection of hepatitis B is through vaccines. "The vaccine confers protection in more than 90% of healthy adults younger than 40 years who receive the complete vaccine series, and immunity lasts at least three decades." [465] Vaccines provide the best protection from viruses.

HHV-8

This virus can cause lymphoma. HHV-8 is an STD and increases the likelihood of a patient developing lymphoma. The best way to prevent HHV-8 is to perform safe-sex practices such as using contraceptives like condoms.[466] Also, the patient and partner should get tested as an added measure. This will allow the patient to know what precautions to take. Tests like the viral marker test screen the patient's blood samples for HHV-8 and other viral illnesses.[466]

HTLV

This is a virus that can cause lymphoma. It is an STD spread through "infected bodily fluids including blood, breast milk, and semen." [467] The best way to prevent HTLV is to perform safe sex practices. In addition to that, both partners should get tested for safety. The test involves screening the patient's blood samples; this includes the viral marker test, where viruses will be detected.[467]

EBV

The Epstein-Barr virus is a virus under the herpes virus family. This is an STD spread from infected bodily fluids that interfere with the body's immune system and can increase the likelihood of a patient getting lymphoma.[467] The best way to prevent this is through safe sex practices. In addition to that, both partners should get tested for safety. The test involves screening the patient's blood samples; this includes the viral marker test, where viruses will be detected. [468]

HIV

This stands for human immunodeficiency virus and is an STD. HIV causes AIDS, which interferes with the body's immune systems and can increase the patient's likelihood of developing lymphoma.[468] HIV spreads through bodily fluids. The best way to prevent this is through safe sex practices. In addition to that, both partners should get tested for safety. The test involves screening the patient's blood samples; this includes the viral marker test, where viruses will be detected.[468]

Immunosuppressants

Immunosuppressants are drugs that inhibit the immune system. The reason why immunosuppressants are prescribed is to prevent lymphoma since lymphoma is the overproduction of altered lymphocytes. However, immunosuppressants can cause secondary lymphoma since the immune system can't perform at its best.[469] Another reason immunosuppressants are used is so the body does not reject an organ transplant.[469] One should only use immunosuppressants to prevent lymphoma development from immunosuppressants when necessary. Do not take more than what is prescribed by your doctor.

Radiation

Radiation can cause the development of lymphoma.[470] Radiation can cause damage to the DNA in healthy cells, thus leading to a higher likelihood of cancer. [470] However, when treating a patient with cancer, radiation is the best way to kill the cancerous cells, but this radiation can cause second cancers like lymphoma.[470] To be as safe as possible from developing second cancers, safer options for radiation therapy like IMRT, IGRT, INRT, and ISRT are better than IFRT.[470]

Family history

Lymphoma is not genetically inherited. However, the patient is more likely to develop lymphoma if a close relative has lymphoma.[471]

Autoimmune disease

In an autoimmune disease, the immune system's lymphocytes attack the body's healthy cells.[472] Although there is no direct cause and effect of autoimmune diseases and lymphoma, autoimmune diseases can increase the likelihood of developing lymphoma which could be because of the prolonged activation of the immune system.[472]

There is no way to prevent lymphoma development from auto-immune diseases. All that a patient can do is be aware and make sure to get checked by a doctor as soon as any lymphoma symptoms are present. The best way of beating cancer is to get it checked as early as possible.

Chemotherapy

Chemotherapy does increase the likelihood of lymphoma.[473] Chemotherapy can harm healthy cells and the cancer cells intended to kill by the prescriber. The damage to healthy cells can cause cancerous cells to arise.[473]

Age

Age can have a significant effect on the likelihood of developing lymphoma.[474] Non-Hodgkin lymphoma is more frequently developed in older people.[474] This is because there is a better chance of mutations occurring during cell division when you are older.[474]

22

PREMALIGNANT LESIONS OF THE ORAL CAVITY

Dr. Sampath Chandra Prasad Rao, Dr. Nivedita Narayankar, Dr. Ajay Bhandarkar, Dr. Rakshita Kamath

Introduction

A 79-year-old patient came with chief complaints of an ulcer over the left lateral border of the tongue of 3 months duration, which was insidious in onset & non-progressive; the patient did not give history of weight loss or fever. And there was no history of difficulty in breathing or swallowing. Oral examination showed adequate mouth opening, A 2*2 cm ulcer over the anterior two-thirds of the left lateral border of the tongue, as shown in Figure 1. The patient was followed up for one year and was diagnosed with Oral Squamous cell carcinoma.

Premalignant oral cavity lesions (e.g., Leukoplakia and Erythroplakia) encountered during a routine oral examination signify the most important clinical findings in an ENT examination. Oral premalignant lesions are "a morphologically altered tissue where cancer is more liable to occur than in its seemingly normal counterpart". [475–478]

The potentially malignant oral mucosal disease has some ability to give rise to malignancy of the oral epithelium, i.e., Oral squamous cell carcinoma (OSCC). Leukoplakia, Erythroplakia, & Palatal keratosis are categorized as precancerous lesions. [477-478]

Leukoplakia

Historically, leukoplakia is an adherent white patch or a plaque (keratosis).

Oral leukoplakia is the most common disease among precancerous lesions [482] and is found in 65% to 80% of patients.

The age group affected ranges from 30–50 years based on the studies of Indian villagers who chew tobacco and smoke. [493-494]

In some leukoplakia patients, human papillomavirus (HPV) may have a potential role.

Moreover, regarding the site of the lesions, the reports from India or some countries show that oral leukoplakia is significantly dominant in the buccal mucosa and labial commissure, perhaps related to gender and tobacco habits. [482, 486-488, 489-491] Reports from other countries note that oral leukoplakia is dominant in the gingiva/alveolar rim or tongue. [487,489,491] Malignant transformation rates of oral leukoplakia differ from 0.13 to 17.5%.

Among individuals chewing betel quid and smoking, the risks of developing oral cancer after 20 years of follow-up were 42.2%.[499]

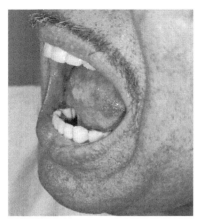

Figure 1: Leukoplakia over the Left lateral border of the tongue

Two major clinical categories of leukoplakia come across in clinical practice, homogeneous and non-homogeneous leukoplakia. The distinction is based on surface color and morphological (thickness and texture) types.

A provisional clinical diagnosis of leukoplakia is made for a white patch after excluding a local traumatic cause & it's confirmed once it cannot be scrapped away and as the color does not disappear after stretching the tissue.

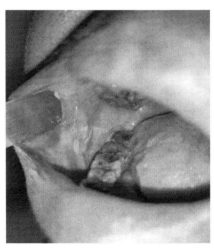

Figure 2: Image showing leukoplakia

On the Right side of the buccal mucosa with nicotine stains over the teeth.

Homogenous Leukoplakia:	Non-Homogenous Leukoplakia:
Flat	Verrucous
Corrugated	Nodular
Wrinkled	Ulcerated
Pumice	Erythroleukoplakia

Table1: The clinical classification of oral leukoplakia (International symposium held in Uppsala, Sweden, in 1994 and supported by the World Health Organization) [477,478]

Type 1	Flat, white patch/plaque without red components.
Type 2	Flat, white patch/plaque with erosion or red components.
Type 3	Slightly raised or elevated white patch/plaque.
Type 4	Markedly raised or elevated white patch/plaque.

Table 2 Clinical classification of oral leukoplakia [493]

Three points which need to be considered while considering the malignant transformation rates of oral leukoplakia are expressed as percentages:

(1) Length of the observation periods.

(2) Type of study population.

(3) Therapeutic approach. [482,487,490]

Proliferative verrucous leukoplakia

A clinical suspicion of proliferative verrucous leukoplakia (PVL)is made when any leukoplakic lesion develops as warty and exophytic. It spreads widely over time and that has recurred after treatment. PVL may involve multiple oral cavity sites such as the gingiva, alveolar mucosa, tongue, and buccal mucosa.

Erythroplakia

Erythroplakia is analogous to leukoplakia and has been defined as a fiery red patch that cannot be characterized clinically or pathologically as any other definable disease'. The lesions of erythroplakia are usually irregular in outline though well-defined and have a bright red velvety surface which is occasionally granular. The soft palate is the most involved subsite.

A diagnostic biopsy is performed & sent for histopathology, which can distinguish specific and nonspecific inflammatory oral lesions because many erythroplakia are dysplastic or may harbor carcinoma *in situ*.[482]

Erythroleukoplakia

Mixed white and red lesions, formerly speckled leukoplakia, are now termed erythroleukoplakia. [475,489] Erythroleukoplakia is a distinct leukoplakia, or erythroplakia might have an irregular margin.[494]

Among individuals chewing betel quid and smoking, the risks of developing oral cancer after 20 years of follow-up were 95.0% for erythroleukoplakia.[499]

Oral Lichen Planus (OLP)

The oral manifestations of lichen planus vary from person to person. The lesions are generally multiple and symmetrically distributed.[490] The clinical presentation of OLP can be divided into several clinical sub-types: linear, reticular, annular, papular, plaque, atrophic, and ulcerative. Bullous lichen planus is unusual in presentation. In dark-skinned people, the affected area shows signs of pigmentation. Patients often exhibit features of more than one subtype concurrently.

A bilateral keratotic lace-like network of white striae on the buccal mucosa and lateral margins of the tongue is usually present in lichen planus. Reticular type is the most frequent type encountered in clinical practice, and most patients are asymptomatic.

Atrophic OLP presenting on the gingivae can be seen as desquamative gingivitis. The bullous type is rare and tends to recur, and it's essential to differentiate this type from pemphigus or mucous membrane pemphigoid.

Some patients may exhibit cutaneous lichen planus, and the medical history may help identify OLP cases. Other extra-oral mucosal sites, such as genitalia, may also be affected.

The differential diagnosis for OLP, when it presents with a reticular/ erythematous appearance, includes lichenoid lesions, lichen sclerosis, lupus erythematosus (DLE), chronic ulcerative stomatitis and when plaque like has oral leukoplakia. Biopsy and histopathological examinations are recommended to make a definitive diagnosis.

Oral Lichenoid Lesions

It is also known as oral lichenoid reaction (OLR). OLL/OLR can be categorized into three varieties:

1) Topographic relationship to a dental restoration 19, often amalgam, also named as oral lichenoid contact lesions (OLCR).

2) Drug-related.

3) It is also found in association with chronic graft versus host disease (cGVHD).

Graft Versus Host Disease (GVHD)

GVHD can be widespread in the mouth. GVHD is a complication in allogeneic hematopoietic stem cells or bone marrow transplantation recipients. The oral cavity is one of the most frequently affected sites.

Discoid Lupus Erythematosus (DLE)

Lupus erythematosus is a chronic autoimmune disease subdivided into three forms: systemic, drug-induced, and discoid. The latter benign variant commonly affects the skin and may involve the mucosal surface of lips and the oral cavity. Oral lesions have been detected in 20% of patients with systemic lupus. The disease is driven by an immune complex deposition in affected sites, which might lead to vasculitis.[482]

DLE has been recognized by the Collaborating Centre of the World Health Organization as a potentially malignant disorder; however, malignant transformation is known to be exceedingly rare.

Oral Submucous Fibrosis

It is a chronic, insidious disease that affects the oral mucosa's lamina propria. When the disorder advances, it involves tissues deeper in the oral cavity's submucosa, resulting in loss of fibroelastic properties, termed Oral submucous fibrosis. Asian patients with a history of betel quid and areca nut chewing with limited mouth opening should arouse suspicion of this condition.[482]

The clinical assessment shows sunken cheeks and inadequacy of opening the mouth may be apparent. In addition, the tongue may be small, exhibit reduced mobility, and show a marked loss of papillae. The palate may appear pale with horizontal bands across the soft palate, and the uvula may be shrunken or deformed. The progressive constraint of mouth opening is a hallmark feature of this disease, and OSF significantly impacts the affected individuals' quality of life.[495]

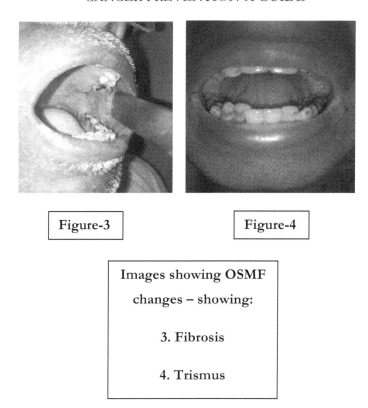

Figure-3   Figure-4

Images showing OSMF

changes – showing:

3. Fibrosis

4. Trismus

Epidermolysis Bullosa

Epidermolysis bullosa (EB) is a skin disease characterized by epithelial fragility that may manifest with blistering and erosions of the oral mucosa. The condition is classified into 32 different subtypes. Intraoral soft tissue manifestations are found in all subtypes and include marked frequency of oral and perioral blistering leading to ulceration, scarring, and obliteration of the oral vestibule and microstomia.[496]

Dyskeratosis Congenita

Dyskeratosis congenita (DC) is a rare inherited bone marrow failure syndrome, and patients with DC have a significantly increased risk of malignancy.[497]Leukoplakic patches of the dorsal tongue and sometimes on the buccal mucosa are features of the classic triad of signs, including lacy reticular hyperpigmentation of the skin and nail dystrophy.

Actinic Cheilitis

Actinic cheilitis (AC) is a chronic inflammatory condition of the lip that results from excessive exposure to solar ultraviolet (UV) radiation and most frequently affects the lower lip. Those with fairer skin are at an enhanced risk,45 may predispose to AC, and men have a stronger propensity than females.

AC has a wide range of clinical presentations comprising white lesions in conjunction with crusting, flaking, dryness or a speckled appearance indicating the simultaneous presence of erythema and white patches.[498]

Conclusion

OPMDs have an expanded risk of developing into oral cancer. Several varieties are recognized. Some of them are solitary lesions, while others are referred to as multifocal or prevalent conditions within the oral cavity. Leukoplakia is the most common OPMD encountered in clinical practice. Clinicians should perform a biopsy or provide an immediate referral to a specialist for patients with a clinically evident oral mucosal lesion considered suspicious of an OPMD.

23

PREVENTION OF GASTRIC CANCER

Dr. Rajesh Pendlimari, Dr. Nagesh N S

Introduction

Gastric cancer is the fourth most common cancer in the world, with 9,89,600 cases in 2008, and the second cause of death among all cancers worldwide. [500-501] Gastric cancer is often silent in the early stages and becomes symptomatic only in the advanced stages. Hence survival rates vary from 10-30%. [502-503] Only in Japan, due to extensive pre-screening, gastric cancer is identified in its early stages; hence, this 5-year survival rate is as high as 90%.

Geographical variation is noted for gastric cancer incidence, with countries such as China, Japan, Eastern Europe, and Central and South America reporting higher cases. In contrast, South Asia, North & East Africa, North America, Australia, and New Zealand report a very low incidence. Over the last few decades, gastric cancer has been declining worldwide.

Risk factors

Gastric cancer occurs due to both environmental factors and certain specific genetic alterations. Primary prevention includes a healthy diet, anti-H Pylori treatment, chemoprevention, and screening for early detection. Dietary factors have an essential role in the carcinogenesis of gastric cancer. Healthy food habits such as fresh fruits, vegetables, low sodium diet, sensible alcohol drinking, and maintaining proper weight are associated with the risk of gastric cancer. [504-506] Established exposure to increased gastric cancer risk includes tobacco use and industrial and chemical pollutants such as those used in wood processing, coal mining, rubber manufacturing, and chromium.

Foods

High salt consumption, especially salt-preserved foods such as fish, vegetables, and meats, has been a probable risk factor since the early studies. A report in 2018 by the world cancer research fund's continuous update program observed a 15% increased risk in patients consuming salted fish and a 9% increased risk per 20 gm of pickled vegetables per day.[507] The exact association of salt dose in food materials still needs to be discovered as reliable quantification of salt intake is challenging. Salt-preserved foods may indicate poor diet quality and low socio-economic status, which also increases the susceptibility to H. pylori infection and hence causes an increased risk of developing gastric cancer. High nitrate and nitrite content in pickled /salted foods promote N-nitroso compounds with carcinogenic properties.[508] Habitual high salt intake can also damage gastric mucosa leading to chronic inflammation and glandular atrophy, increasing DNA damage and cell proliferation and making them susceptible to H. pylori infection.[509]

Obesity

Obesity / increased body fat is associated with multiple cancers, including gastric cancer. The state of obesity paves for low-grade inflammation, hyperinsulinemia, hyperlipidemia, and increased production of endogenous steroids, which can cause tumorigenesis.[510] Increased abdominal fat raises intra-abdominal pressure, leading to GERD, which paves for pre-cancerous lesions. Abdominal obesity, as measured by waist circumference, is positive for gastric cancer risk.

Alcohol

Alcohol consumption of 42 gm/day or more is associated with a 42% increased risk of developing gastric cancer. However, habitual small-quantity consumption did not show any increased risk compared to non-drinkers.[507] A significant linear dose-response association has been reported with alcohol levels greater than 45 gm per day.[507] Alcohol acts as a solvent in the stomach, enabling the penetration of carcinogenic substances into the gastric cells and interfering with prostaglandin production and retinoid metabolism.[511] Also, alcohol increases the production of toxic free radicals, which cause cellular injury, and an alcohol metabolite acetaldehyde has been classified as a class I human carcinogen.

Fruits

High consumption of fruits is associated with decreased gastric cancer risk. The risk reduces by 5% with 100 gm of fruits and 24% with citrus fruits when consumed daily.[513] Citrus fruits have a high concentration of vitamin C, carotenoids, naringenin, and other antioxidants, which protect against oxidative damage.[514] Vitamin C helps regenerate other antioxidant molecules, such as vitamin E, inhibits nitrosamine formation in the stomach, and protects gastric mucosa.[515] Vitamin C, E, carotenoid, and selenium were known to have antioxidant and anti-inflammatory properties and suggested that they may have a preventive or protective effect on gastric cancer.

Smoking

Lifestyle factors such as smoking, lack of physical activity, higher BMI, excessive alcohol, and specific diet patterns have been associated with gastric cancer. Smoking status was a statistically significant factor for overall gastric cancer risk. The other lifestyle factors may act in synergy to increase the risk.

Biomass

Biomass smoke is complex, consisting of pollutants, particulate matter, and volatile organic and inorganic compounds, including polycyclic aromatic hydrocarbons, benzene, and formaldehyde. Biomass fuel increases the risk of developing gastric cancer by 1.8 times.[516] Particulate matter consists of tiny particles and droplets such as dust, soot, or smoke with the size of PM_{10} and $PM_{2.5}$. Particulate matter exposure to $PM_{2.5}$ is associated with the risk of gastric cancer. Exposure over 17 years to $PM_{2.5}$ increases the risk of gastric cancer by 1.8 times. [517]

Occupational exposure

Occupational exposure to rubber production, x-radiation, γ radiation, asbestos, and lead inorganic compounds is associated with gastric cancer. Chemical contamination of water sources with arsenic, fluoride, nitrate, lead, chromium, manganese, cadmium, selenium, and uranium is associated with a higher incidence of gastric cancer. The environmental factors alter epithelial gene expression, which initiates carcinogenesis and irreversible mutations impeding accurate replication and mismatch repair mechanisms. These factors also limit the gastric microbiome and disrupt symbiotic harmony. These factors can also influence the oncogenicity of H. pylori, though this needs further clarification.

Blood group A

The risk of developing gastric cancer was higher in patients with blood group A and lower in blood group AB. The blood group showed no significant effect on the clinicopathological parameters of gastric cancer. The O blood group may be a good prognostic factor for gastric cancer patients. [518]

Helicobacter Pylori

Helicobacter pylori (H. pylori) is a spiral-shaped, flagellated organism positive for urease, catalase and oxidase. H. pylori has been classified as a type I carcinogen by IARC and WHO.[519] The pathogenicity is briefed in Figure 1.[520] H. pylori escape the highly acidic environment due to its shape, flagella, motility, and producing urease enzyme, which converts urea into ammonia and makes a neutral environment around it. Ammonia disrupts the tight cell junctions in gastric mucosa and causes damage to gastric epithelium.[521] The outer membrane proteins of H. pylori interact with receptors of gastric epithelial cells such as blood group antigen, binding adhesin (BabA), outer inflammatory protein (OipA), sialic binding adhesive

(SabA), and H. pylori outer membrane adhesin (HopQ). And this prevents H. pylori from being easily washed out of the stomach.[521] The virulence factors are the CagA protein coded from the CagPAI gene on H. pylori. The other essential proteins, CagT and CagC, potentiate Cag A's translocation into epithelial cells and are associated with developing peptic ulcers. Vac A is another cytotoxin that inhibits the lysosomal and autophagy killing of these bacterial cells.[522] Outer membrane vesicles (OMVs) such as phosphatidylglycerol, phosphatidylethanolamine, phosphatidylcholine, cardiolipin, lipopolysaccharides, and some bacterial virulence factors, such as proteases, adhesins, and toxins promote infection, impair cellular function and modulate host immune defenses through IL-10.[521] H. pylori γ-glutamyl transpeptidase generates reactive oxygen species, and cause causes damage.[521] H. pylori prevents autophagy which is the first line of defense in immunity. H. pylori causes chronic inflammation and oxidative stress generated in gastric mucosa. H. pylori infection is crucial to gastric carcinogenesis.

Helicobacter pylori eradication

Multiple antibiotic regimens have been tried. Clarithromycin-based regimens have a reasonable eradication rate of as high as 90%. Recent clarithromycin resistance has been noted in up to 30% of patients. The most common regimens are amoxicillin and clarithromycin with PPI for 14 days. When given for 14 days, most regimens showed a higher eradication rate than 10 days or fewer days. Sequential therapy with amoxicillin followed by metronidazole and clarithromycin showed similar eradication rates. Amoxicillin is thought to prime the h. pylori cell wall leads to a better action of metronidazole and clarithromycin. With resistance occurring, newer regimens called quadruple therapy are becoming popular (PBMT – PPI, Bismuth, Metronidazole, Tetracycline; PAMC – PPI, Amoxicillin, Metronidazole, Clarithromycin).[524] Newer treatment modalities have shown promise, such as synthesized silver ultra-nanoclusters (SUNCs) alone or combined with metronidazole.[525] Probiotics such as lactobacillus reuteri are known to form clumps with H. pylori and get excreted in stools.[526] H. pylori eradication prevents gastric and duodenal ulcer formation and decreases the risk of developing gastric cancer. H. pylori eradication leads to better absorption of medications such as L-thyroxine.[527]

Primary prevention

Gastric cancer can be prevented by H. pylori testing and eradication. In the USA, H. pylori testing is recommended for individuals with a family history of gastric cancer in first-degree relatives and immigrants from high H. pylori prevalence regions. All individuals with positive tests should be offered H. pylori eradication therapy.

Secondary prevention

Endoscopic screening with biopsies should be recommended beginning at the age of 50 years for individuals with a family history of gastric cancer in first-degree relatives e, and individuals in highly endemic areas such as East Asia, Eastern Europe, and Andean Latin America. AGA recommends that patients with gastric intestinal metaplasia (GIM) be tested and treated for H pylori to reduce the risk of gastric cancer. In light of current evidence gaps, the AGA suggests routine use of short-interval repeat endoscopy with biopsies may not benefit as there is no clear-cut evidence. Still, it recommends that physicians selectively advocate surveillance in these patients.[528]

Conclusion

Gastric cancers, especially non-cardiac ones, can arise secondary to H. pylori infection and the progression to chronic active gastritis and gastric cancer. It is demonstrated that h. pylori induce several mechanisms of tumorigenesis. H. pylori eradication has decreased the incidence of gastric cancer in highly endemic areas. However, there is still a debate that it might augment the risk of other diseases and increase antibiotic resistance. Maintaining normal body weight, adopting healthy dietary choices, limiting consumption of salt-preserved foods and alcohol, and smoking abstinence can reduce the development of gastric cancer.

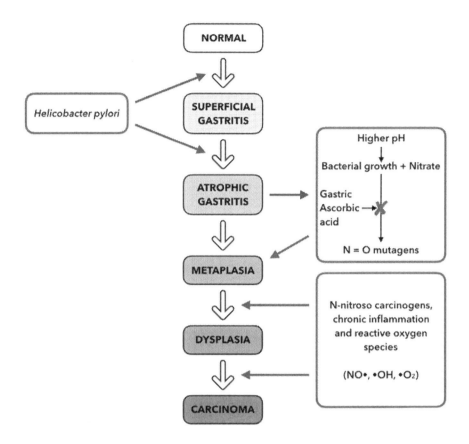

Figure 1: Model for progression of gastric cancer. [519]

24

PANCREATIC CANCER: IS IT PREVENTABLE?

Dr. Nagesh N S

Introduction

The pancreas (pan- all and Creas – flesh) (Meaning All Flesh) is a large gland in the retroperitoneum, nestling behind the stomach and lying across the spine. It has both endocrine and exocrine components making up the parenchyma.

It is divided into three parts: the head (including the neck and uncinate process), body, and tail. The head is wrapped on its lateral side by the second part of the duodenum, and the tail lies near the splenic hilum (Fig 1).

The main pancreatic duct runs throughout the entire pancreas and joins the common bile duct in the head region. The resultant common channel opens via the Ampulla of Vater into the second part of the duodenum.

The superior mesenteric vein and the splenic vein converge just behind the neck of the pancreas to form the portal vein.

The pancreas's primary function is to aid digestion and maintain blood glucose levels. The secretion of pancreatic enzymes does the former, while the latter is by the secretion of hormones like insulin and glucagon.

Statement of problem

Cancer, in general, is a public health problem worldwide. Pancreatic cancer is among the leading causes of cancer-related mortality. As per the global cancer statistics, 2020, the incidence is nearly 4,95,773 patients per year,[529] 13 the among all cancers afflicting the human race and affecting almost one in every 519 patients in India.[530] In the list of cancer-related deaths, pancreatic cancer ranks 7 (fig 2).[529]

The worldwide incidence of pancreatic cancer seems to increase with age and has a male preference.[531] With advancing technology and the advent of highly sensitive imaging modalities, the rate of early detection and hence the incidence of pancreatic cancer can rise.

The etiology of pancreatic cancer is diverse and multifactorial. Hereditary/genetic factors[532] and tobacco usage are the major contributors to pancreas cancer.

Cancer in the pancreas can occur in the exocrine (adenocarcinoma) and endocrine (neuroendocrine) components. Ductal adenocarcinoma accounts for more than 2/3rd. One of the reasons for garnering much attention and research worldwide is the dismal prognostic implications of developing pancreatic adenocarcinoma. When the disease is localized, the 5-year survival rate is about 42% and drastically drops to 14% with the regional spread of the disease.[533]

In its early stages, the disease shows no overt symptoms and tends to be missed. In due time with the progression of the disease patient presents with jaundice, weight loss, clay-colored stools, fatigue, and abdominal pain. Cancers arising in the body and tail region remain asymptomatic until they have metastasized to other parts ruling out the curative intent of treatment.

Traditionally surgery and chemotherapy have been the primary modalities to attempt to cure with a subset of patients requiring radiotherapy.

However, with ongoing research and analysis, a multi-modality approach seems the best way to tame this deadly disease. We are still a long way from our goal.

With such a deadly disease amongst us, it is only imperative that we all are aware of the causes of pancreatic cancer and do all we can to keep this at bay and protect ourselves and our loved ones.

Etiology

The etiology of pancreatic cancer is the subject of extensive studies and can be broadly categorized into modifiable and non-modifiable risk factors.[534]

Table 1

Modifiable risk factors	Non modifiable risk factors
Tobacco	Gender
Alcohol	Age
Obesity	Ethnicity
Dietary	Diabetes Mellitus
Exposure to toxic chemicals	Genetic factors
Periodontol disease	Family history
	Chronic infections
	Non O blood group
	Chronic pancreatitis

Tobacco

Cigarette smoking and tobacco consumption is the most critical risk factor for pancreatic cancer. The International Agency has also confirmed the causal association between the two for Research On Cancer[535,536] and other studies.[537–542]

The risk of pancreatic cancer increases with the duration of smoking and the number of daily cigarettes. The risk is nearly twice in smokers than non-smokers.[543–545]

In 2012, the European Prospective Investigation into Cancer (EPIC) study showed that the risk of pancreatic cancer increases for every five cigarettes smoked daily. The same study showed that passive smoking can increase the risk of pancreatic cancer by 50%.[540,542] With rising awareness regarding tobacco's potentially harmful effects, smoking has declined in many countries. Still, it is upward in some developing countries and among women.

The causal association tends to be high even after accounting for confounding factors such as alcohol consumption.

Alcohol

The risk of pancreatic cancer is increased with regular high alcohol consumption. Smokers who consume alcohol tend to be at an increased risk vis-à-vis non-smokers drinking alcohol. Even low to moderate alcohol intake in smokers ups the risk of malignancy.[546]

Obesity

Obesity and a sedentary lifestyle are risk factors for various diseases, including pancreatic cancer. A higher BMI during early adulthood is associated with higher disease-related mortality.[547]

Dietary factors

There is some evidence that increased consumption of red meat or processed meat and dairy products is associated with pancreatic cancer,[548,549] but a few studies have also found no association.[550]

However, it is only logical to assume that an organ closely associated with digestion is bound to be influenced by dietary factors. Cholesterol-rich foods, fried food, and processed meat containing nitrosamines (used as a preservative) are known risk factors for gastric malignancy and pancreatic cancer.[551]

At the other end of the spectrum, consuming fresh vegetables and fruits rich in antioxidants and citrus provides a protective cover.

Exposure to toxic chemicals

Exposure to chemicals and heavy metals such as beta-naphthylamine, benzidine, pesticides, asbestos, benzene, and chlorinated hydrocarbons has increased the incidence of pancreatic cancer.[552,553] Nickel, found in an occupational setting, is usually with polychlorinated biphenyls, which are known to interfere with DNA repair, induce apoptosis by inducing Reactive Oxygen Species (ROS) formation and increase DNA methylation.[554–557]

Exposure to cadmium and arsenic also increases the risk of pancreatic cancer as cadmium is known to accumulate in the pancreatic cells and inhibits DNA repair, and causes genomic instability.[554,558] It is also known to cause transdifferentiation of pancreatic cells and regulates the activity of several oncogenes and tumor suppressor genes expressed in pancreatic cells.[559,560]

Selenium, a micronutrient, is a protective element antagonistic to cadmium, arsenic and lead. It boosts p53 activity enhancing DNA repair. Selenoproteins are known to be effective in scavenging ROS.

Periodontal diseases

Studies also demonstrated a positive correlation between periodontal diseases, edentulism, and pancreatic cancer. The association persisted despite adjusting for other confounding variables such as gender, alcohol consumption, tobacco, higher BMI and diabetes mellitus. The exact reason for this causality is yet to be ascertained however the changes in oral microbiome lend a plausible explanation.[561]

Non-modifiable risk factors

Gender

According to the global cancer statistics of 2020, pancreatic cancer has a male predilection. The mortality rates, too, are skewed against the male population. A possible explanation could be higher exposure to the "modifiable" risk factors mentioned above. Is it only lifestyle changes or does the female population have genetic protection against this deadly disease is not known now. (fig 3 and 4).

Age

The incidence increases with age, with most patients above 50 at diagnosis—the highest peak between 60 and 80.[531,562,563] With environmental factors and toxic exposure having a cumulative effect, it is hypothesized that this is the reason for such a late peak in incidence.

Ethnicity

Like most diseases, different genetic make-up, different environmental exposure, and different lifestyles contribute to the disparity among races for the incidence of pancreatic cancer. According to 2020 statistics, the incidence is highest among Asians, followed by Europeans.

Some population-based studies also opine that differential exposure to toxic agents can explain not all differences between races. Other factors, such as genetic factors acquired mutations from known toxins, e.g., the ability to detoxify tobacco products, oncogene mutation and biomarker immune expression, may contribute to the increased risk of pancreatic cancer.[564,565] This genetic diversity also explains the different outcomes post-surgery/treatment among other races.

Diabetes Mellitus

The association between the two assumes significance because recent onset Type 2 DM has traditionally been a marker of pancreatic neoplasm.[38–40] Lending credibility to this is the reversal of diabetes post-surgery in these patients.[569]

The risk of pancreatic cancer progressively decreases with a longer duration of diabetes presence. However, an excess risk to 30% persists for decades after the diagnosis of T2DM.[570]

Family History

Approximately 10% of cases seem to have a familial component.[541,571–573] A retrospective review of 175 such families demonstrated a genetic mutation in 28%.[574] Familial pancreatic cancer is when a parent, sibling or child is diagnosed in a family with pancreatic cancer. The more first-degree relatives afflicted with the disease, the higher the chance of acquiring it. These families tend to have individuals getting diagnosed at an earlier age (< 50 years) and also have a higher risk of extrapancreatic malignancies and premalignant lesions of the pancreas.[575] The earlier the disease onset higher the chance of other family members acquiring it.

Genetic Factors

Germline mutations tend to increase the risk of cancer. Some of the well-researched mutations of hereditary pancreatic cancer include *BRCA1*, *BRCA2*, *PALB2*, *ATM*, *CDKN2A*, *APC*, *MLH1*, *MSH2*, *MSH6*, *PMS2*, *PRSS1* and *STK11*.

Familial cancer syndromes such as the hereditary non-polyposis colon cancer (Lynch syndrome)(MSH2, MLH1, MSH6, PMS2), the familial atypical multiple mole melanoma syndromes (CDKN2A), Peutz-Jeghers syndrome(STK11), hereditary breast and ovarian cancer syndrome, familial adenomatous polyposis (APC) and Li-Fraumeni syndrome have pancreatic malignancies.

Nearly 5-17% of patients with familial pancreatic cancer syndromes have a germline mutation of the BRCA 2 gene.[576]

Chronic infections

Helicobacter pylori is an established causative agent of gastric malignancies. Its role in pancreatic cancer is under scrutiny, with data supporting and refuting the causality.[577,578]Association of hepatitis B and C viruses have also been proposed, but no conclusive data has emerged.

ABO Blood group

The antigens A, B, and O are expressed not only on the cell surface of RBCs but on many other tissues in the body. Their expression and association with various malignancies are now well-established.

Different regions of the world report higher incidence in a particular blood group (A, B or AB) but agree on a lesser incidence amongst O blood group individuals. Survival rates are also better amongst O blood group patients.[579] The affinity of H pylori to A and B antigens also adds credence to this hypothesis.

Chronic pancreatitis

Pancreatitis is inflammation of the pancreatic parenchyma, which causes glandular damage, loss of parenchyma, and fibrosis when it occurs repeatedly. This leads to decreased digestive enzyme secretion and resultant malabsorption and malnutrition.

This repeated inflammation process causes ROS generation and provides a fertile bed for mutations. Chronic pancreatitis per se has a lot of etiological factors, the most common being alcohol consumption.

Hereditary pancreatitis also occurs in patients with cationic trypsinogen gene (PRSS1) mutation and Serine protease inhibitor kajal type 1 (SPINK1). These mutations increase the risk of malignancies by 50-60 fold.[580]

The EUROPAC study on hereditary pancreatitis also confirmed the higher risk and incidence of pancreatic malignancies in this patient cohort.[581]

Screening and prevention

One effective way to mitigate the dismal prognosis of such a deadly disease is to have strategies that enable early detection. Tumor markers, screening strategies, and better-resolution imaging technology are some steps in this direction. Screening large populations, however, is not feasible; hence, most research is directed toward the early detection of premalignant lesions.

The best-case scenario would be if we can prevent the disease from occurring altogether. To do this, we must understand the etiology and other high-risk behavior.

Lifestyle behavioral changes are the best and most effective strategy to prevent this cancer. Tobacco usage is associated with a high incidence of pancreatic cancer; nearly 30% of these can be prevented by smoking cessation.[582] After ten years of smoking cessation, the risk levels equalise that of a non-smoker.

Dietary modification, such as avoiding red and processed meat and increasing consumption of fruits, vegetables, and nuts is found to be protective.[583,584] A well-balanced and nutritious diet can help us achieve risk reduction.

Ensuring a minimum physical activity period daily, lower saturated fat consumption and adequate doses of vitamins avoid sedentary life and help reduce the risk of obesity.

Avoidance/ limitation of alcohol intake reduces the immediate risk of pancreatic cancer and the component of pancreatitis and, thereby, a malignant change.

The effects of non-modifiable risk factors are hard to mitigate. But a multi-disciplinary approach to the high-risk group (involvement of genetic testing groups, counselors, medical oncologist, GI radiologist, medical and surgical gastroenterologist, and GI nursing team) can be an effective way to make an early diagnosis. Effective screening strategies for these sub-groups could be Endoscopic ultrasound, higher resolution CT and MR imaging, etc.

In a nutshell, cancer is not entirely preventable. Still, with the proper knowledge of etiology, the right intent, and a high index of suspicion in high-risk groups, the problem of pancreatic cancer can be downsized and eventually tided over.

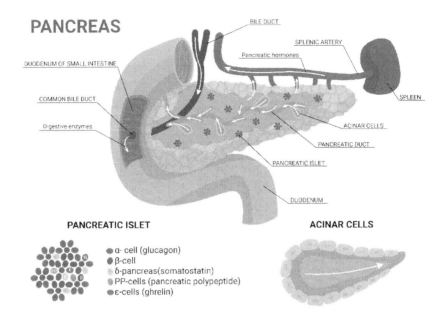

Figure 1: Normal pancreatic anatomy

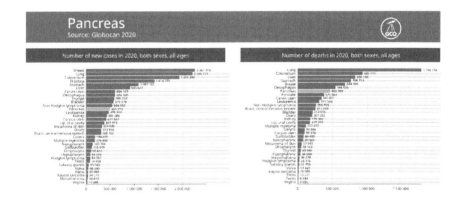

Figure 2: Reproduced from gco.iarc.fr

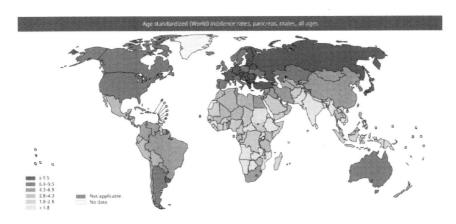

Figure 3: Reproduced from gco.iarc.fr

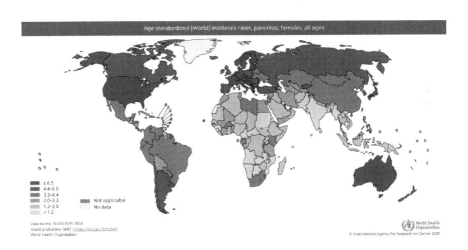

Figure 4: Reproduced from gco.iarc.fr

25

OVARIAN CANCER PREVENTION AND ROLE OF HORMONES

Dr. Monika Pansari

Ovarian cancer- risk factors and types

Ovarian cancer is the fourth most common cancer among Indian women as per GLOBOCAN 2012 and is the fifth most common cancer globally.[585] It is the most lethal among all gynecological malignancies and ranks 4th for cancer-related mortality among women.[586] The disease peaks during 50-78 years of a woman's life,[587] with 50% of cases diagnosed among post-menopausal women. The high mortality rate is attributed to the diagnosis of the disease in its advanced stages. The lack of early-stage diagnosis is primarily attributed to asymptomatic disease, and another primary reason is the lack of effective screening strategies. Of all the ovarian cancer cases, less than 15% are diagnosed in stage I, with 5-year survival rates of 94%. Most (almost 62% of cases) are diagnosed in stages III and IV, where the 5-year survival rate is less than 30%   globally.[588,589] The disease outcomes and mortality worsen with an increase in age at diagnosis.[590] From 1980 to date, there has been an improvement in the survival rates of these patients with advances in treatment strategies and a multidisciplinary approach.[590,591] The common risk factors for ovarian cancer are age, obesity, infertility, BRCA1/BRCA2 mutations, tobacco use, exposure to asbestos, etc.

A few factors that protect against ovarian cancer are oral contraceptives, increasing parity, breastfeeding, etc. Table 1 summarises the epidemiological characteristics and their strength of risk associated with epithelial ovarian cancers. A few symptoms that could help in ovarian cancer diagnosis are a pain in the lower abdomen, irregular periods, bleeding after menopause, loss of appetite, urination, signs of intestinal obstruction, and change of menstrual cycle in cases of pre-menopausal women and abdominal swelling. The presence of mutations in BRCA genes and other genes warrants initiation of screening even in young women aged between 35-40 years. The screening methodology involves transvaginal ultrasound coupled with CA-125 levels in the blood.[592]

Ovarian cancer is a heterogeneous and joint disease that originates in the ovary, fallopian tubes, and peritoneal cavity (Figure 1). Based on the origin, ovarian cancers can be classified into three types: non-epithelial (sex cord-stromal), epithelial, and germ cell.[593] According to WHO, epithelial ovarian cancers constitute 60% of all ovarian cancers.[594] Based on histology, ovarian cancer is broadly classified into two types. Type I are typically low-grade and less aggressive and often arise from lesions originating from endometriosis or benign tumors. They harbor somatic mutations predominantly in KRAS, PTEN and BRAF genes and lack TP53 mutations. Low-grade endometrioid, clear cell, low-grade serous, and mucinous cancer belong to type I. Type II cancers are high-grade, aggressive, and characterized by mutations in TP53, BRCA1 and BRCA2 genes.[595] Ovaries are both primary and metastatic sites for mucinous cancers.[596] However, mucinous cancers are more often metastasized cancers to the ovary that primarily originate from the gastrointestinal tract, including the stomach, colon, and appendix.[13] Endometrioid and clear-cell ovarian cancers are derived from the cervix or the uterus, likely due to retrograde menstruation from the endometrium.[598,599]High-grade serous ovarian cancers originate in the distal fallopian tubes or the surface of the ovary.[600-602]

Table 1

Hormonally related epidemiological factors associated with EOC risk

	Strength of relationship
Factors associated with increased EOC	
Reproductive factors	
Nulliparity	+++
Exogenous hormone use	
Combined HRT	+
Estrogen-only HRT	++
Androgens	+
Reproductive disorders	
Endometriosis	++[a]
PCOS	+/0
Infertility	++
Other	
Age	+++
Factors associated with decreased EOC risk	
Reproductive factors	
Pregnancy	− − −
Breast-feeding	−
Twinning and other non-singleton births (note 3)	−
Tubal ligation	− − −
Hysterectomy	− −
Exogenous hormone use	
Oral contraceptive use	− − −
High vs low progestin OCs	−
High vs low estrogen OCs	0
Factors not associated with EOC risk	
Reproductive factors	
Early menarche	0
Late menopause	0
Exogenous hormone use	
Fertility drug use	0

+, positively associated with EOC; −, negatively associated with EOC; 0, no association with EOC.

[a]Endometrioid and clear cell subtype only.

Adapted from Modugno et al EndocrRelat Cancer. 2012

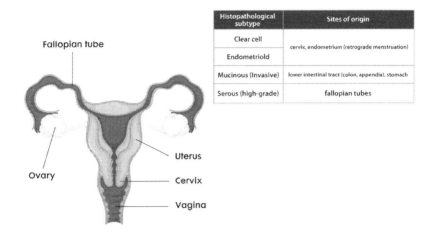

Histopathological subtype	Sites of origin
Clear cell	cervix, endometrium (retrograde menstruation)
Endometrioid	
Mucinous (Invasive)	lower intestinal tract (colon, appendix), stomach
Serous (high-grade)	fallopian tubes

Figure 1: Cellular origins of ovarian cancer

The connection between hormones and ovarian cancer

The hormones shown to have a conspicuous role in ovarian tumor development are estrogen, progesterone, androgens, and gonadotropins, either as tumor promoters or suppressors. The epidemiological evidence and data from cell lines suggest a role for estrogen and androgen in the initiation of epithelial ovarian cancers. At the same time, progesterone is protective against ovarian cancer, although data from prospective trials are missing.[603]

An inverse relationship exists between the use of oral contraceptives and ovarian cancer incidence. Oral contraceptives are known to reduce the risk of incidence of ovarian cancer.[604,605] Both long-term and short-term usage of oral contraceptives is known to confer protective effects.[606] An analysis of 45 epidemiological studies revealed that oral contraceptives reduce the risk of ovarian cancer incidence, and the longer the use, the higher the protection. Moreover, the protective effect persisted until 30 years of the cessation of oral contraceptives.[607] Although the data on oral contraceptives was consistent, the HRT (hormone replacement therapy) information was not. Few recent studies, such as Women's Health Initiative (WHI)[608] and the Million Women Study,[609] reported an increase in the risk of ovarian cancer for both estrogen-only (ET) and estrogen-progestin (EPT) formulations. However, the risk associated with EPT was lower than that of ET.

In corroboration with these reports, another study that conducted a meta-analysis of 14 published studies found that the risk of ovarian cancer increases by 22% with five years of ET compared with only 10% with EPT use, suggesting the risk of cancer incidence differs by regimen.[610] Androgens taken exogenously are also known to be associated with epithelial ovarian cancer (EOC), although results from multiple studies are contradictory. One case-control study found that Danazol, a synthetic androgen commonly used in the treatment of endometriosis, significantly increased EOC risk,[611] although another study did not end with similar findings.[612] Another hormone, testosterone, is also known to be associated with ovarian cancer. Testosterone is present in some daily-use products like tablets, patches, troches, or creams which is associated with a threefold increase in EOC.[612]

Role of Estrogens

High estrogen levels are associated with an increased risk of ovarian cancer, although the evidence is not robust, with mixed results from multiple studies. Estrogen executes its activity by binding to its estrogen receptor (ER) receptor. ER receptor exists in two forms, ERa and ERb. Interestingly both these forms of ER have a contradictory role in ovarian cancer; ERa acts as a tumor promoter and ERb as a tumor suppressor.[613] ERa expression promotes cell migration and invasion processes by promoting EMT (epithelial-mesenchymal transition), a hallmark of cancer progression; on the other hand, ERβ is known to inhibit these processes.[614] ERβ is highly expressed throughout the normal ovary, including in granulosa cells, theca cells, corpora lutea, and oocytes,[615-618] however, its expression is progressively lost during ovarian cancer development and progression.[619-622] While this loss of function of ERβ has been associated with loss at the genetic level. There is increasing evidence that lower expression of ERβ per se can also result from epigenetic changes, namely hypermethylation of its promoter.[623-625] In contrast, ERα expression is maintained or even increased in a subset of ovarian tumors.[622-626] As a result, there is an increase in the ERα/ERβ ratio with malignant progression of the ovary.[627,628] However, when these two ER forms are co-expressed, their interactions and effects on one another are poorly understood in vivo conditions. Nevertheless, in ovarian cancer cell line models, the expression of antagonists and agonists of ER is known to suppress tumor growth. Agonists of ERa and Antagonists of ERb induce tumor growth.[629]

With this data, anti-estrogen treatments such as aromatase inhibitors and tamoxifen represent viable options for ER-positive patients as they are well-tolerated and inexpensive.

Role of Progesterones

A substantial amount of epidemiological data suggests a protective role for progesterone and progestins against ovarian carcinogenesis.[630-632] Progesterone deficiencies due to increasing age, infertility, or a genetic LOH (loss of heterozygosity) at the progesterone receptor gene locus are associated with an increased risk of ovarian cancer.[633,634] In line with this, elevated progesterone levels decreased the risk of ovarian cancer. PR expression was higher in low-grade tumors, and high PR expression was associated with improved survival.[630] The protective effect of pregnancy has been documented in Asian, European, and North American populations.[635] Hormonal oral contraceptive use, either in estrogen and progesterone combination or progesterone alone, has been consistently associated with reduced risk. A meta-analysis involving 20 epidemiological studies conducted between 1970 and 1991 showed that using oral contraceptives reduces the risk incidence by 35%.[606] Additionally, the data indicated that the decrease in the risk of ovarian cancer is correlated with the duration of oral contraceptive use: a 10–12% decrease in the risk with one year of use and a 50% decrease with five years of use in both nulliparous and parous women.[606]

Progesterone's protective effect on cancer induction in ovarian cells is by reducing ovulation through elevated progesterone levels from oral contraceptive use or during pregnancy (pregnancy is characterized by high progesterone levels that are required for fetal development, breast development for lactation, maintenance of uterine/placental integrity, and myometrial quiescence).[636] Furthermore, PR expression (two forms of PR exist-PRa and PR-b), PR-b specifically[637-639] is a favorable prognostic marker associated with more prolonged progression-free survival.[637,640-645] Women with mutations in BRCA1/2 genes are known to be at higher risk of breast and ovarian cancer. Studies on mice carrying a BRCA1 mutation in ovarian granulosa (i.e., hormone-producing) cells[646-648] and humans with either aBRCA1 or BRCA2 mutation[649] demonstrated that these mice or humans had elevated levels of circulating hormones, both estrogen and progesterone.

However, ultimately little mechanistic information related to the impact of these hormones on the prevention and pathogenesis of ovarian cancer exists.

The molecular mechanisms of progesterone's protective role in ovarian cancer are not well understood, but the data suggest that the antiproliferative actions of progesterone are primarily through the induction of apoptosis.[650-652]

PR isoform-specific (PR-a and PR-b) actions are largely undefined in ovarian cancer. PR-b appears to be a more potent driver of ovarian cancer cell senescence relative to PR-a. Hormone-driven breast and gynecological cancers frequently exhibit upregulated protein kinases, such as MAPK,[653] CDK2,[654] and CK2,[655] which directly phosphorylate and modulate PR-b target gene selectivity. The use of progestins alone (megestrol acetate and medroxyprogesterone acetate) as ovarian cancer prevention therapeutics has been examined in several relatively small phase II clinical trials with variable inclusion criteria that resulted in modest response rates.[656] However, retrospective studies evaluating the association between total PR expression and progression-free disease survival[637,640-643,645,657] support the concept that the subsets of PR-positive ovarian tumors are susceptible to hormones and thus more likely to respond to endocrine therapy. While all this data advocates the anti-tumorigenic properties of progesterone in the context of ovarian cancer, one report contradicts these findings. In vivo, experiments were conducted with genetically modified mice (removal of genes responsible for cancer) where cancer in fallopian tubes was induced and injection of progesterone but not estrogen promoted metastasis in the peritoneum.[658] Further evidence is required to substantiate these findings and evaluate if PR could be explored as a druggable target for ovarian cancer prevention.

Nevertheless, a multi-analysis of 53 clinical trials that investigated the efficacies of endocrine therapies in epithelial ovarian cancers indicated a clinical benefit in 41% of patients with improved survival rates. This benefit was more prominent in patients positive for ER/PR. Thus, anti-endocrine therapies offer a promising strategy in the management of ovarian cancer in the front-line and recurrent settings.[659]

Role of Androgens

Androgen belongs to the family of steroid hormones that act via binding to its receptor, androgen receptor, AR. AR is a ligand-inducible transcription factor belonging to the steroid hormone receptor superfamily.[660,661] The biological actions of androgens, including testosterone and dihydrotestosterone, as well as those primarily derived from the adrenal gland and ovary (dehydroepiandrosterone (DHEA) and its sulfated form (DHEA-S), androstenedione, androstenediol), are usually mediated through the AR. Some evidence from in vitro studies suggests that androgens affect gene expression, growth, invasion, and survival in an ovarian cancer cell line.[662] Transcriptional activation of AR by its ligand (androgen) binding has been shown to induce cell invasion in ovarian cancer.[663,664] Epidemiological studies involving 1484 women showed that 12 who developed ovarian cancer had lower levels of DHEA, androsterone, and etiocholanolone in the urine compared to control subjects.[665] Studies investigating blood plasma levels of various kinds of androgens in ovarian cancer patients versus control subjects and data generated in post-menopausal women yielded controversial results. Although the studies suggested that androgen from the ovarian origin, rather than free circulating hormones contributes to ovarian tumorigenesis in pre-menopausal women.[666,667] Even the results on the correlation between expression of AR (by immunohistochemistry) and survival outcomes are also controversial, few studies have shown AR expression linked to clinically better outcomes while few studies contradicted these findings.[668] Transcriptional activity of AR in ovarian cancer cells: One of the regulatory mechanisms by which its transcriptional activity is regulated is by its nucleotide sequence. The *AR* gene contains a polymorphic CAG repeat segment coding for a polyglutamine sequence in exon 1. The length of the CAG repeats has been shown to correlate inversely with AR transcriptional activity in various types of cells, including ovarian cancer cells.[669-671] In primary cultures established from ovarian epithelium, CAG repeat lengths were significantly shorter in cancer cells than in normal cells.[672] However, robust data that relates CAG repeats with survival needs to be improved.

AR signaling in ovarian cancer cells: AR, as an inactive form, locates in the cytoplasm, coupling with heat shock proteins (HSP). Upon binding of androgens, AR is released from the HSP proteins, forms a homodimer, and is translocated into the nucleus where it, along with co-regulators, binds to an androgen response element, leading to transcriptional regulation of various target genes listed (red and blue molecules). IL-6, IL-8, and VDR (blue) have dual functions in ovarian cancer cells. They are not only the downstream effectors of the AR signaling pathway but are also upstream regulators in ovarian cancer cells (Figure 2).[668]

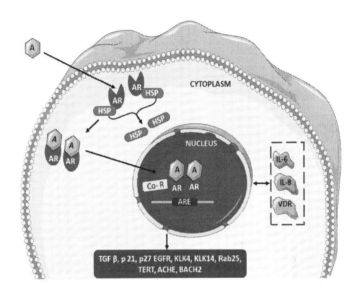

Figure 2: AR signaling in ovarian cancer cells (Adapted from Mizushima T et al., Cells 2019)

A = androgen; ACHE = acetylcholinesterase; AR = androgen receptor; ARE = androgen response element; BACH2 = basic leucine zipper transcription factor 2; Co-R = co-regulator; EGFR = epidermal growth factor receptor; HSP = heat shock protein; IL = interleukin; KLK = kallikrein; TERT = telomerase reverse transcriptase; TGF-β1 = transforming growth factor-β1; VDR = vitamin D receptor.

All this data points out the tumorigenic function of AR, and therapies aiming at the inactivation of AR (anti-androgens) could serve as a promising therapeutic approach for ovarian cancer patients.

Another significant area left unexplored is the role of these hormones in predicting the chemotherapy response in ovarian cancer patients. Platinum-based chemotherapy with or without taxanes (another form of chemotherapy) is the standard of care for these patients, along with surgery. The patients with aggressive disease would receive additional targeted therapies like bevacizumab (targets VGEF), PARP inhibitors (patients with BRCA mutations) like olaparib, etc. But unfortunately, most patients (more than 50%-- at least 80% of high-grade serous carcinoma) develop resistance to this therapy with cancer relapse, because of which these patients have low five-year survival rates of less than 30%. It would be interesting to explore whether any of these hormones could predict chemotherapy response in these patients. A recent report mentioned the significant positive prognostic association of all three hormone receptors, ER, PR, and AR. The expression of hormone receptors predicts survival and platinum sensitivity of high-grade serous ovarian cancer.[673]

Diagnosis of cancer in its early stages improves the survival of the patients to a great extent. Ovarian cancer patients diagnosed with stage-I have a survival rate of up to 90% when surgery and chemotherapy are offered as a standard of care.[674] Although it might not be possible to prevent ovarian cancer, some measures could reduce the incidence of ovarian cancer.

Ovarian cancer risk-reducing measures-In in general

The following measures could reduce the risk:

1. Mutations in BRCA genes pose a greater risk for ovarian cancer incidence. National Comprehensive Cancer Network (NCCN) recommends risk-reducing salpingo-oophorectomy (RRSO) in women with BRCA1/2 mutations after 35 years of age. The guidelines suggest that transvaginal ultrasound, combined with serum CA-125, could be considered at the clinician's discretion from 30–35 years in women not undergoing RRSO (NCCN Guidelines Version 3.2019).

2. Giving birth and Breastfeeding: Giving birth and breastfeeding reduce the frequency of ovulation and thus exposure to hormones. Parous women (women having given birth) compared to nulliparous (who did not give birth) women have a 30-40% lower risk of developing ovarian cancer.[675] A pooled analysis that compared ordinary women and women

with ovarian cancer revealed that breastfeeding significantly reduces the risk of incidence of ovarian cancer. Breastfeeding for a shorter duration, 1-3 months, also resulted in a risk reduction of 18%.[676]

3. Use of oral contraceptives: Oral contraceptives reduce risk even in women with BRCA mutations. Five-year or more use of oral contraceptives reduces the risk by 50%.

4. Tubal ligation (getting the fallopian tubes tied, also known as sterilization): As most ovarian cancers originate in fallopian tubes, when these tubes are tied up, the movement of tumor cells from these tubes to the ovary is obstructed. Tubal ligation is known to reduce the risk of ovarian cancer, as reported in multiple previous analyses.[677] Tubal ligation reduces the risk even in women with BRCA mutations.

5. Surgical procedures involving removal of both ovaries, hysterectomy.

26

PREVENTION OF CERVICAL CANCER: AN OVERVIEW

Dr. Poonam B Maurya, Prof. (Dr.) Vishwanath Sathyanarayanan, Mr. Aryaan Iqbal Shoaib

Introduction

Cervical cancer is the fourth most common cancer among women worldwide, with approximately 600,000 new cases and 342,000 deaths in 2020 alone.[678] The incidence and mortality rates are higher in low-income areas of the world compared to high-income countries, where it has almost halved due to access to resources and good healthcare services. If detected in the precancerous stage, we could prevent the aggressive form of cancer. The leading cause of almost all cervical cancers is human papillomavirus (HPV), a sexually transmitted disease. However, there are multiple strategies and screening tests to prevent the disease. Vaccination is the most common method of preventing HPV infection, and screening is done to assess whether it is present. In this chapter, we will discuss the prevention of cervical cancer.

Burden

In 2020, an estimated 604,127 new cases of cervical cancer were found, and 341,831 deaths were recorded among women worldwide.[678] Most high-income countries do not have high incidence or mortality rates compared to less-developed countries, which do not have developed screening programs and limited resources.[679] Around 254,672 deaths occur annually due to cervical cancer, in which 87% of those deaths happen in less-developed countries with essentially non-existent screening programs. [680] If there were good quality screening programs and resources, incidence and mortality rates could be reduced by almost 90% in these impoverished areas of the world.[680] Cervical cancer usually occurs early in women ages 21-67 years.[680] The median age of diagnosis is approximately 38-46 years. At the time of diagnosis, many of these women being in the advanced stage of the disease.[679]

India bears the burden of 23% of the world's cervical cancer cases. The development of cervical cancer in these women is within the range of 19-26 years. India has approximately 130,000 new cases and 74,000 deaths annually, accounting for 33% of global cervical cancer deaths.[681] The lack of screening programs, financial resources, and overall poor awareness of cervical cancer have caused this preventable disease to be the most common across the country, leading to higher mortality and reduced survival rates.

Risk Factors

The most common cause of cervical cancer is the human papillomavirus (HPV), which spreads through sexual contact. There are various types of HPV; more than 80 and around 30 of these subtypes can infect the cervix. [682] However, the immune system can fight against HPV infection, and only a tiny percentage of women develop cervical cancer. Other risk factors include being overweight, smoking habits, living an unhealthy lifestyle, and economic status, along with others. However, due to HPV being the most common cause, there are risk factors associated with being infected with HPV.[679]

A weakened immune system due to the human immunodeficiency virus (HIV) puts people at risk for HPV infections. Women infected with HIV at an early age would readily develop invasive cancer because of the immunocompromised system, which destroys cancer cells and slows their growth.[683] Those infected with HIV are at a higher risk of having high-risk HPV infections compared to HIV-negative women.[680] Cohen et al. (2019) stated that HIV infections introduced complications in the management of cervical cancer within women. The interaction between the tumor and HIV can lead to T-cells dysfunction. This dysfunction can increase the risk of latent infections during systemic treatment. Thrombocytopenia associated with HIV can increase difficulties with surgery and chemotherapy.[679] The correlation between the prevalence of HIV and HPV infection was positive, as regions with a higher rate of HIV infections were more likely to get HPV.[680] Cohen et al. (2019) found that 70% of HIV infections occurred in sub-Saharan Africa. An increase in cervical cancer was found in South Africa between 2001 and 2009, with an increase in HIV cases.[679] However, the carcinogenic transformation of being infected with HPV to invasive cancer takes 10-20 years, which provides an extended time frame to detect the disease at a relatively early stage with highly effective treatment.[680]

Sexual history can also increase the risk of cervical cancer by increasing the chance of being exposed to HPV. Being sexually active from a young age increases these chances, especially with multiple sexual partners. It may be hard to tell or know when someone has the HPV infection since many people have it and don't know themselves. [684] The risk increases by having sex with someone infected with HPV. This can be avoided by having sex with a single partner or screening partners for HPV. Using condoms can help, but they do not provide 100% protection from HPV. However, they can help protect someone from sexually transmitted diseases like HIV or Chlamydia. Chlamydia infection is another common risk factor for cervical cancer, infecting the reproductive system.[683] In addition, it was found that the Chlamydia bacteria can help the HPV infection to grow and live in the cervical area, increasing the chance of cervical cancer. However, it is almost impossible for a whole population to abstain from sexual activities, which is why other forms of prevention are more effective.[683]

Consistently smoking increases the chances of developing cervical cancer due to cancer-causing chemicals that affect multiple organs.[683] When these harmful chemicals in cigarettes enter your lungs and bloodstream, they end up in the mucus on the cervix. These chemicals and tobacco by-products damage the cervix cells' DNA and harm the immune system. These damages make it more difficult to fight off HPV infections and contributes to the development of cervical cancer.[683]

Low-income women who do not have access to good healthcare services, like cervical cancer screening, tend to be at a higher risk for cervical cancer.[684] While there are programs for low-cost screening, the quality may not be up to standard to catch the early stages of cervical cancer.[680] The limited options of a well-balanced diet increase the chance of cervical cancer without essential foods with vitamins A, C, and E and carotene.[684]

Prevention

Primary Prevention

The most effective and efficient method of primary prevention is HPV vaccination. Other prevention methods include monogamy or using condoms. However, they are not as effective as HPV vaccines since there is no clear evidence that these methods provide 100% protection from the HPV infection.[679] There are two types of vaccinations, bivalent (Cervarix™) and quadrivalent (Gardasil™) HPV vaccines. Each is at least 90% effective in preventing type 16 and 18 HPV. [685] Kaarthigeyan (2012) explained in detail the development of HPV vaccines; recombinant DNA technology is utilized to express the L1 major capsid protein of HPV in yeast, creating virus-like particles (VLPs).[681] These VLPs have a similar protein coat as HPV but without the genetic material; therefore, VLPs can be used as antigens to signal an immune response to coat the virus and prevent it from releasing the genetic material.[681] Kaarthigeyan (2012) stated that Cervarix™ had shown 90% efficacy globally against type 16 and 18 HPV types and that this bivalent vaccine only protects against cervical cancer. Kaarthigeyan (2012) further found that Gardasil™ showed 100% efficacy rates against the same type of HPV and that it protects against both genital warts and cervical cancer.[681] Both vaccines are safe, effective in preventing HPV infections, and immunogenic.[685] In follow-up cases where HPV vaccines are prevalent, there have been substantial decreases in cervical cancer cases. In countries where at least 50% of women were vaccinated, HPV infections decreased by almost 70%.[679] Cohen et al. (2019) stated that in Australia in 2007, as an HPV vaccine program, the Gardasil™ vaccine was administered to more than 70% of children. This resulted in almost a 40% reduction of cervical dysplasia in women under 18.[679] However, the result of an overall decrease in cervical cancer cases might not be established for another few years in countries where vaccination coverage is less than 50%.[679] Furthermore, introducing vaccination programs has been somewhat challenging due to cost restrictions, cultural barriers, lack of awareness, and difficulties contacting the target audience.[679] To increase vaccine coverage, cost-efficient HPV vaccines must be distributed to developing countries to address cervical cancer cases.

The two previously mentioned vaccines were prophylactic; there is another type called a therapeutic vaccine.[686] These vaccines aid in clearing HPV infections by generating T-cell immunity against HPV types E6 and E7 antigens. However, it is only effective in the trial stages.[686]

Secondary Prevention

It is crucial to detect HPV early when treatment and prevention are highly effective. Multiple screening tests exist to obtain an early diagnosis before HPV transforms into invasive cancer.[687] Obtaining samples for screening tests to analyze cervical cancer is simple and painless; the most common test is Papanicolaou Stain (Pap smear).[680] This procedure requires a small brush to collect a cell sample from the surface cervix, which is stained with Pap stain and examined for any abnormalities.[688] Further screening is done through an HPV test if any abnormalities are present. The DNA or RNA is tested for certain types of HPV infection that may cause cervical cancer.[688] This type of screening using a Pap smear and HPV test is known as a Pap/HPV co-test.[688] Consistent findings have shown that Pap smear as an HPV-based screening is more effective when compared with cytology.[680] It was found that women who undergo Pap smear screening over cytology were more likely to be diagnosed with a significantly lower likelihood of cervical dysplasia.[680] However, the Pap smear is not as helpful for women younger than 21 or older than 65 and women who have had a total hysterectomy.[688]

While screening for cervical cancer is necessary and practical, not all screening tests are helpful and may have some risks. Some risks include unnecessary follow-up tests, and false positive or false negative test results can occur.[688] Receiving a false positive result can cause a patient to be unnecessarily stressed and may be followed up with more tests and procedures. This can cause lots of anxiety and has also been linked with increased risks of issues with fertility or pregnancy in young women.[688] False positive results are more common when a co-test is done since HPV tests may find infections unrelated to cervical dysplasia or cancer. If a patient is given a false negative result, their condition may appear normal when cervical cancer is present. A false negative result can provide women with a false image of their situation and will delay the process of seeking necessary medical attention when she has symptoms of cervical cancer. It is essential to seek medical advice from a doctor about the risks of cervical cancer and what types of screening must be done to prevent the disease.[688]

To conclude, cervical cancer is preventable in most situations by the above methods, which can significantly lower incidence and mortality due to this disease.

27

PREVENTION OF LUNG CANCER AND IMPACT OF AWARENESS

Dr. Rajeev Vijayakumar

Cancer Prevention as a Clinical Oncology Discipline

Until recently, clinical oncology has been defined as a medical specialty that attempts to intervene to slow or reverse the final stage of the cancer process. Until now, Oncology has been involved in identifying and treating cancer of all backgrounds and kinds. Cancer evolution is a long process, starting from molecular alterations, progressing to a stepwise carcinogenic progression, leading to loss of cellular functions and changes in the morphology of the cell.

It is recognized that cancer is a continuum and hence oncologists are delving into various lifestyle behaviors related to cancer. They include diet and exercise, risk assessment, screening, and other preventive interventions designed to delay or reverse the cancer process.

Chemoprevention- cancer risk-reducing agents

Chemoprevention is a synonym for Cancer risk reduction. It is the use of a range of interventions, from drugs to isolated dietary components to whole-diet modulation, to block, reverse, or prevent the development of invasive cancer.

Lung Cancer Screening

Lung cancer screening programs using chest X-rays and sputum cytology began in the early 19th century. These programs led to an increase in the number of cancers detected, especially at an early stage. It translated into more patients living beyond five years.

A low-dose chest CT (LDCT) scan is an appealing strategy for lung cancer screening. It uses an average of 1.5 mSv radiation to perform a lung scan in 15 minutes. Conventional CT uses eight mSv of radiation and takes a few minutes. The LDCT image is not as sharp as the traditional image, but sensitivity and specificity for detecting lung lesions are similar.

LDCT works best in the high-risk population. The NLST (National Lung cancer screening Trial) was one of the first RCTs conducted in the USA. Two cohorts were randomized, one receiving LDCT thrice a year vs. group 2 receiving Chest X-rays.

Current and ex-smokers with > 30 pack years between 55 and 74 years were included. With a median follow-up of 6.5 years, 13% more lung cancers were diagnosed, and a 20% relative reduction in lung cancer mortality was observed in the LDCT arm compared to the chest x-ray arm. Another important finding from the NLST was a 6.7% decrease in death from any cause in the LDCT group. Further analysis of the NLST showed that screening prevented the most significant number of lung cancer deaths among participants at the highest risk but prevented very few deaths among those at the lowest risk. The pitfalls are an increased false positivity rate (almost 96%) leading to increased anxiety, tests, biopsies, and surgeries, which may, on many occasions, be excessive. The ideal inclusion criteria for LDCT are Age 55-75, a 30-pack year history, current or ex-smokers who quit in the last 15 years.

We can conclude that there is moderate certainty that annual screening for lung cancer with LDCT is of reasonable net benefit in asymptomatic persons at high risk for lung cancer based on age, total cumulative exposure to tobacco smoke, and years since quitting.

Cancer prevention by vegetables- Numerous constituents found in vegetables, including micronutrients (nutritive compounds, e.g., carotenoids, vitamins C and E, folic acid, and selenium), dietary fiber and phytochemicals (non-nutritive bioactive compounds with no known nutritional value, e.g., flavonoids, indoles, isothiocyanates, and glucosinulates) and interactions among these constituents might contribute to the ability of these foods to reduce cancer risk. Evidence for the anticancer properties comes from in vitro studies on animal models. It acts directly (free radical scavenging) and indirectly using complex pathways involving metabolic processes. Anti-carcinogenic agents work in synergy rather than alone.

As cancer is a multistep process, there are multiple stages where it may be reversed or stopped.

Vegetables are postulated to work by:

1. They prevent mutations.

II. Suppression of promotion, progression, invasion, and metastases.

Anticancer Mechanism of vegetables —

a) Dietary fibers – prevent carcinogen uptake by adsorption of carcinogens.

6. Vitamin C scavenges nitrite to avoid the formation of nitrosamines.

7. Flavonoids/isothiocyanates from cruciferous vegetables inhibit 'non-enzymatic' endogenous carcinogen formation.

d) Carotenoid's block and scavenge reactive metabolites and protect DNA. FAQs:

2. What are the chances that I will develop lung cancer?

3. The #1 cause of lung cancer is exposure to tobacco smoke. Your chances increase with the amount you smoke and the years you have smoked. The more you smoke or are exposed to smoke from others (second-hand smoke), the greater your chances of developing lung cancer. People who have never smoked may develop lung cancer, but their chance is much less than those who smoke or used to smoke. What can I do to decrease my risk of developing lung cancer?

The best way to lower your risk is to avoid tobacco smoke. It is never too late to stop smoking, but the sooner you stop, the better. Even if you can't quit altogether, cutting back on the number of cigarettes, you smoke can help, but cutting down is not as good as leaving altogether.

4. Are there other ways to decrease my risk of getting lung cancer?

Many things may reduce your risk, but none have been proven. These include:

a) Eating plenty of fruit.

b) Getting regular exercise.

c) Regular use of aspirin or celecoxib (Brand name Celebrex).

d) Regular use of inhaled corticosteroids (used for emphysema and asthma).

5. Are there things that increase my chances of getting lung cancer?

We know several things increase your risk of getting lung cancer. Other things may increase your risk, but we don't have enough information to say. These things increase your risk for lung cancer and should be avoided if possible:

a) Tobacco smoke.

b) Exposure to or working with hazardous chemicals such as silica, cadmium, arsenic, beryllium, chromium, diesel fumes, nickel, coal smoke and soot.

c) Exposure to particle pollution—like exhaust smoke.

d) Asbestos, a mineral formerly used in building materials that is still in some environments and products like old brake pads.

e) Radon, a radioactive gas that can be found in the environment. You can have levels checked if you live in a high-risk area.

f) High doses of supplemental beta-carotene (a pigment found in plants and fruits) above the Recommended Daily Allowance. The risk with high levels is mainly seen in former and current smokers.

28

PREVENTION OF UROLOGICAL CANCERS AND EARLY DETECTION OF PRECANCEROUS CONDITIONS

Dr. Raghunath S.K

Introduction

The etiology of cancer is multifactorial. Some risk factors have direct causal relationships, whereas few remain behind the curtain & may not have a direct causal relationship in cancer pathophysiology. The complex interplay between causative factors and cancer incidence makes formulating a common & strong preventive strategy challenging. For example, smoking is a vital risk factor for kidney and lung cancer; however, not all who smoke develop these cancers, and not all patients have a smoking history. Understanding this complexity helps us focus on multiple levels of cancer prevention. Broadly cancer prevention is a 3-step approach. Primary prevention is disease prevention by reducing individuals' exposure to risk factors and subsequently avoiding illness. Secondary prevention is the early detection and treatment of disease by screening activities. Tertiary prevention is using treatment and rehabilitation programs to improve the disease outcome amongst the affected. This review is mainly focused on discussing the first two steps.Except for testicular cancers & some pediatric cases, most urological cancers are usually diagnosed in the aging population. The morbidity of urological cancers is higher as they get diagnosed at an advanced stage, particularly in developing countries, due to a lack of awareness and limited screening programs. On the other hand, malignancies of the kidney & prostate are diagnosed late, as it doesn't give any symptoms in the early stages. The social stigma associated with penile lesions and testicular mass delays hospital visit which results in the disease getting diagnosed in advanced stages.

Pathophysiology of cancer

The theories of carcinogenesis are diverse, and science has not proved one theory as a final theory at this point. Recent advances in molecular science have come up with much new information. However, it will take time for data to mature to conclude. The somatic mutation theory (SMT) of carcinogenesis has been in the literature for over 60 years.[689]

It is based on the following premises:

1) Cancer is derived from a single somatic cell that successively has accumulated multiple DNA mutations (monoclonality).

2) Those mutations occur on genes that control cell proliferation and the cell cycle.

3) *Quiescence* is the default state of cell proliferation in metazoa.[690]

On the other hand, in 1999, an alternative theory, the *tissue organization field theory* (TOFT), was proposed. Its premises are significantly different from those of the SMT, namely:

1) Carcinogenesis is a problem of tissue organisation, comparable to organogenesis during early development.

2) *Proliferation* is the default state of all cells.[691,692]

Along with these mainstream theories, the role of mitochondrial dysfunction and oxidative stress leading to carcinogenesis has also been studied. [693,694] More research in these theories is directing the scientific community away from classical SMT theory & leaning towards changes that happen in the tissue microenvironment. Molecular research has helped us to understand that stromal-epithelial interactions and various architectural factors play a role in carcinogenesis. This leads us to the theory that cancer is a developmental process similar to organogenesis, which has been misdirected.[690]

In a nutshell, SMT is cell-based, and TOFT is tissue-based, and central to both these theories is genetic alteration, which alters cell proliferation or the tissue microenvironment. Irrespective of the view one believes, there is a common consensus that these internal changes are initiated/triggered by external factors like viruses, environmental causes, occupational exposure, radiation, dietary factors & many more. In preventive oncology, it is essential to understand these external causative factors so that exposure to these factors is prevented or effective measures like vaccines can be administered to treat the causative factor.

Etiology and risk factors in Urological cancers

Kidney

The incidence of Renal cell carcinoma (RCC) is on the rise. RCC accounts for 3 % of all adult malignant neoplasms & it is the most lethal tumor among common urological cancers.[695] The most common environmental factor associated with the incidence of RCC is tobacco products. The relative risk (RR) ranges from 1.4 to 2.5 in various studies & it is directly related to the duration of smoking and cumulative exposure (Pack-years).[696] The other two established risk factors are hypertension (HTN) and obesity. The RR of HTN for RCC is up to 2.48. The effect of HTN may cause structural and molecular changes, which may increase carcinogenic exposure. It is also suggested that RCC risk is unrelated to the medicine used for HTN.[697] Obese individuals are also likely to be at higher risk of RCC.[698] However, obese individuals are likely to have low-grade tumors & better cancer-specific survival; a phenomenon called the 'Obesity paradox'.[699] The potential mechanism for RCC in obese individuals is higher insulin-like growth factor expression, local inflammation & arterial nephrosclerosis.[700] End-stage renal disease (ESRD) patients who develop acquired cystic renal disease are at higher risk of developing RCC and should be monitored periodically for the same.[701] Recently, diabetes has also been detrimental to RCC.[702] The literature on various dietary and occupational factors remains inconclusive.[700,702] Around 5-8 % of RCC patients have hereditary risk factors.[703]

Bladder cancer & Urothelial cancer

The whole urothelium is exposed to environmental carcinogens and excreted in the urine. The bladder, a storage organ with the largest urothelial surface, has a maximum incidence of urothelial carcinoma. Aromatic amines are the main causative agents in carcinogen-induced bladder cancer, and the two most frequent sources are tobacco smoking and occupation exposure. It is estimated that 30-40 % of cases are attributed to tobacco smoking, and approximately 10 % of patients can be linked to occupational exposure.[704,705] Industries associated with paint, dye, metal & petroleum products increase occupational exposure. Drinking chlorinated water and water with a high level of arsenic have also been associated with bladder cancer.[705,706] Though minimal evidence suggests a hereditary component in bladder cancer, alteration in N-acetyltransferase (NAT2) and Glutathione S-Transferase (GSTM1) genes can decrease one's ability to detoxify aromatic amines. This can indirectly increase the risk of urothelial cancer. Besides this, ionizing radiation, pioglitazone & cyclophosphamide therapy can increase bladder cancer risk.[705,707,708] Chronic inflammation due to the indwelling catheter, recurrent urinary tract infection, bladder calculi, schistosomiasis infestation, etc., are also associated with higher urothelial and non-urothelial cancers of the bladder.[705,709,710] The literature about metabolic factors and their association with bladder cancer is scarce and shows poor association.[711] Apart from environmental exposure, specific risk factors for upper tract urothelial carcinoma (UTUC) are worth mentioning. Hereditary nonpolyposis colorectal carcinoma (HNPCC) or Lynch syndrome is a known risk factor for UTUC.[712] Exposure to aristocholic acid is also a known risk factor for UTUC & it can be either environmental contamination of agricultural products (Balkan endemic nephropathy)[713] or ingestion in herbal medicines, seen in China & Taiwan (Chinese herb nephropathy).[714] The analgesic use was also a risk factor for UTUC in past.[715]

Prostate cancer

Considering the high incidence in men, the aetiology of Prostate (PC) is one of the most researched topics. Despite the amount of literature it carries, many questions remain unanswered. With recent research, genetic predisposition emerges as one of the most substantial and most defined risk factors for PC. High-risk inherited genetic factors are estimated to cause approximately 5-10% of PC cases. For an individual with a family history of PC, the relative risk of getting PC is between 1.92 to 4.39 compared to the general population & it depends on the number of family members affected, the degree of relatedness & the age at which it was diagnosed.[716] Familial cancers are diagnosed early by 6-7 years but otherwise with similar clinical course. A particular subset of patients with genetic alteration in BRCA 1/BRCA2 is at increased risk of aggressive cancers.[717] None of the dietary factors is defined as causative factors for PC. Smoking, metabolic factors and obesity are associated with a higher incidence of aggressive disease, advanced presentation & poor oncological outcomes.[718,719] Various exogenous & environmental factors, estrogenic carcinogens, cadmium exposure & night shift at work are also associated with PC.[720–723]

Testicular cancer

The risk factors for testicular cancers are well-defined. These include white race, cryptorchidism, personal & family history of testicular cancer, and intratubular germ cell neoplasia.[724]

Penile cancer

Penile cancer is relatively rare, with an incidence of < 1 % of all cancers diagnosed in men. Incidences in high-income countries are even rare. Despite low incidence, Multiple factors are well studied as etiological factors. Human Papilloma virus (HPV) esp. HPV 16,18,31 & 33 are associated with penile cancer.[725,728] Premalignant lesions associated with HPV are also associated with invasive penile cancers.[727] Phimosis and chronic inflammatory condition, Lichen sclerosis, have been implicated in the development of penile cancer in various studies.[728] Malignant transformation can happen in 4-8 % of Lichen sclerosis.[729] Like other urological malignancies, Tobacco usage, obesity & poor penile hygiene is associated with invasive penile cancer.[730,731] Geographical areas with lower socioeconomic class have more prevalence due to inadequate education, poor hygiene, high HPV infections and lack of circumcision.[732] Higher incidence is also noted in patients with psoriasis who undergo treatment with psoralen UV – phototherapy (PUVA).[733]

Premalignant conditions in Urological Cancers

The emotional play in patients diagnosed with cancer always raises common questions; Am I late in cancer diagnosis? Could it be diagnosed earlier with some test? Where does cancer start? Etc. This is a familiar concept that cancer starts from 'something' variably termed as 'precancerous' or 'premalignant' lesions. Cancer patients always have this thought if it could have been diagnosed very early, and the general population is always searching for the answer to a more common question 'how can I prevent cancer?' In a nutshell, identifying a 'premalignant' condition is essential to cancer prevention. The definition of 'Premalignant' per the national cancer institute dictionary is a condition that may (or is likely to) become cancer.[734] However, it may not be this simple to interpret it. These lesions carry specific genetic alterations, giving them certain morphological features. But, It is essential to understand that progression to neoplasm is not a prerequisite for a lesion to be termed a 'premalignant'. There is a likely possibility of overdiagnosis and overtreatment if the clinical significance is not defined. Here, we discuss a few premalignant conditions in urological cancers, which may have clinical relevance & can be addressed accordingly for prevention strategies.

Kidney cancer

Out of all the Urological malignancies, premalignant lesions of the kidney are less defined. Limited usage of diagnostic biopsy & practically imperceptible lesions in radiology makes these lesions mysterious and of doubtful clinical value. Typically three lesions are described in the literature: atypical cyst, papillary adenoma & renal intraepithelial neoplasia (RIN).[735] Atypical cysts are uni/multilocular, lined by multi-layered epithelium or papillary projections, low-grade nuclear features and without any solid/nodular lesions. The lining of this cyst may harbour cytogenetic alterations like loss of 3p & trisomy of 7 or 17. In von-Hippel-Lindau (VHL) disease, there can be ciliary dysfunction due to loss of VHL gene function, leading to the development of innumerable cysts and RCC. The atypical cysts are pathologically differentiated by simple cysts with single epithelial lining without atypia later. Atypical cysts on imaging may be better termed complex cysts on radiology, should be classified as per the Bosniak classification system, and should be managed accordingly.[736] The second lesion is a papillary adenoma, defined by encapsulated papillary/tubulopapillary projections of less than or equal to 15mm size with minimal cytological changes.[737]) It shares cytogenetic alterations similar to papillary RCC. However, they rarely have invasive features. The third lesion RIN is controversial & very scarcely mentioned in modern literature, as its diagnostic and prognostic values still need to be defined. This lesion usually occurs within or close to the tumor with surgical specimens.

Bladder cancer & Urothelial cancer

2004 WHO classification of urothelial carcinoma classifies pre-malignant conditions as urothelial hyperplasia, reactive atypia, urothelial atypia of unknown significance (AUS) & urothelial dysplasia. [738] Urothelial hyperplasia is simply a thickening of urothelium with ten or more cell thicknesses (average is 4-7 cells) without nuclear atypia. It may be a precursor to low-grade papillary lesions. Reactive atypia is characterized by nuclear abnormalities in the background of inflamed urothelium and is usually associated with chronic inflammation/irritation of urothelium due to various stimuli. It may be associated with voiding symptoms. AUS is said when it is unclear whether the findings are pre-malignant or reactive. Urothelial dysplasia is considered to be genuinely pre-malignant. It is a normal-thickness urothelium with an altered cytological appearance of urothelial cells. It can result in carcinoma in situ or invasive urothelial carcinoma in up to 19% of the patient's[739] & it warrants close surveillance and treatment as required. Since hyperplasia to dysplasia to frank carcinoma is a pathological continuum for urothelial carcinoma, it is wise to act on these findings in the form of stringent surveillance to detect cancer in its early stage. Treating any condition that can produce chronic inflammation in urothelium by stabilising these changes is also appropriate as a preventive strategy.

Prostate cancer

Prostatic intra-epithelial neoplasia (PIN) and atypical small acinar proliferation (ASAP) are precancerous PC lesions. A PIN is architecturally benign acini or ducts lined by cytologically atypical cells. ASAP can be defined as focal changes suggestive of carcinoma; however, cytological, histochemical and architectural findings are insufficient to establish cancer diagnosis. It is worthwhile to note that PIN and ASAP are pathological findings & don't manifest themselves by physical examination or elevated PSA. The incidence of high-grade PIN (HGPIN) on routine biopsy is around 4-5 %, while finding ASAP is between 0.5-23 %.[740]

Finding these precancerous lesions on biopsy doesn't warrant immediate treatment. However, these findings pose a risk of finding significant PC on subsequent biopsies. The cancer detection on repeat biopsy ranges from 25-79% for HGPIN and 21-51% for ASAP.[741] Considering its significance, it is recommended that finding multifocal HGPIN or ASAP (Even a single foci) needs a repeat biopsy to rule out invasive cancer in 6 months. It is also to understand that these findings on biopsy don't imply that PC is inevitable. These lesions may remain stable and not get a cancer diagnosis in repeat biopsies. Even if a repeat biopsy finds cancer, it may likely be low-grade (ISUP grade group I) cancer in around 80 % of the patients.[742] Finally, as a preventive measure, the literature doesn't support any pharmacotherapy or dietary modification for treating these lesions apart from monitoring by repeat biopsies.

Testicular cancer

Germ cell neoplasia in situ (GCNIS) is a precursor lesion to the testis's post-pubertal seminomatous and non-seminomatous germ cell tumors (GCTs). It is prevalent in patients with disorders of sex development & various testicular dysgenesis syndromes. Since progression to the invasive tumor is almost 50 % at five years, identifying it on testicular biopsy is essential in high-risk and suspected cases. In a pathological dilemma where the tumor is entirely & spontaneously regressed & differentiating teratoma from the benign cyst, the presence of GCNIS in nearby areas can suggest a diagnosis of malignancy.[735]

Penile cancer

Penile intraepithelial neoplasia (PeIN) or carcinoma of situ (CIS) of the penis is a known pathological entity with a strong association with squamous cell carcinoma of the penis. PeIN includes three entities; erythroplasia of Queyrat (EQ), Bowen's disease (BD) & Bovanoid papulosis (BP).[743] EQ is CIS of glans and prepuce. If CIS involves the penile shaft & rest of the genitalia, it is BD. BP, though considered pre-malignant, it has a benign course. If not treated, this lesion can progress into invasive carcinoma in 5 - 33% of the patients.[744,745] However, these lesions rarely progress to metastasis.[746] Apart from PeIN, other Human papillomaviruses (HPV) related lesions like condylomata acuminate & Buschke-Lowenstein tumor & non-HPV related lesions like penile horn & lichen sclerosis have variable associations with progression to invasive cancer.

Specific prevention strategies & screening programs in urological cancers

Kidney Cancer: As noted before, tobacco smoking, obesity and hypertension are RCC's three most potent risk factors. All three elements are adjustable, and a quick and simple answer is a healthy lifestyle. Smoking cessation is protective against kidney cancer, as past smokers may have some protective effects from current smokers.[747] Regular physical activities can prevent obesity, metabolic syndrome and hypertension, which in turn may have protective effects against kidney cancer. Moderate physical activity can provide a protective effect against RCC independent of other risk factors.[748]This has been studied and confirmed in research. Diet has been linked with RCC. Diet rich in carbohydrates & fat content is hazardous in general. A diet inflammatory index has been developed to understand the relationship between diet and its association with inflammation in the body.[749] It is noted that avoiding a pro-inflammatory diet may reduce the risk factor for RCC.[750] Diet rich in fruits and vegetables, caffeinated coffee consumption, and moderated alcohol drinking habits can also decrease the risk of RCC.[751–753]

For secondary prevention of RCC, the result of past studies about screening could be more encouraging. However, increasing incidence, a high proportion of individuals in the asymptomatic stage at diagnosis and high mortality from RCC are a few solid reasons for detecting RCC by screening strategies. RCC currently meets a few but not all of the criteria for screening. There are inconclusive ideas about the benefit of early diagnosis, and starting early therapy, cost-effectiveness, ideal screening population, and strategies. However, targeted screening of high-risk individuals would be the most cost-effective strategy to gain maximum benefit and reduce the harms of screening & future research should focus on more precise risk assessment tools.[754]

A few conditions & effective preventive strategies need to be mentioned here. Patients with ESRD are at high risk of RCC development, which is 5-20 % higher than the general population.[755] The concerns to screening this population are relatively short life expectancy, higher adenoma incidence, altered imaging due to acquired cystic disease, and related costs. The wise approach would be to screen younger individuals with minimum co-morbidities from 3rd year of dialysis. Considering the high risk for native kidneys after transplantation, continuous periodic screening with imaging has been suggested for these individuals.[756] Individuals with a genetic predisposition to familial/hereditary RCC, like VHL disease, Tuberous sclerosis, and other familial forms, should also undergo regular screening by imaging. Genetic counseling and germline mutation testing are recommended in individuals < 46 years of age with kidney cancer & in patients with multifocal and bilateral tumors.[703]The risk of recurrence and cancer-specific mortality is always a concern in patients treated for RCC. Strict surveillance after primary treatment will detect recurrences early & its treatment will benefit overall survival.[757] Compared to low-risk localized disease, high-risk/ locally advanced pathology would have higher chances of recurrence. Individualised and risk-based models are developed based on various prognostic factors to suggest optimum follow-up.[758] Adjuvant therapy has been recommended to prevent recurrence and increase cancer-specific survival in RCC. Though there is increased disease-free survival in patients receiving tyrosine kinase inhibitors, there is no significant increase in overall survival when adding drug toxicity. A better suggestion to give adjuvant treatment is to identify a subset of the population which benefits the most.[759]

Bladder cancer & Urothelial carcinoma: Since most factors causing bladder cancer are modifiable, it is possible to prevent it primarily. Smoking cessation can decrease the risk of bladder cancer significantly. Smokers who quit smoking have a lower risk of bladder cancer than current smokers. It is estimated that there would be a 25 % risk reduction ten years after smoking cessation.[760] Apart from this, prevention of obesity, higher physical activity, vitamin A & D supplementation, a diet rich in fruits and vegetables & higher fluid intake can reduce bladder cancer incidence significantly.[761] Occupational health measures in various occupations like the tobacco industry, metal, dye & textile industry, farming, etc., can decrease bladder cancer incidence & morbidity by reducing exposure and periodic screening of this population. Combining all these, smoking cessation, lifestyle modification, and occupational health measures can decrease bladder cancer incidence significantly. As we all know, the prognosis of bladder cancer mainly depends on stage and grade. The progression of the stage is time-dependent, which means; early detection can help prevent morbidity and mortality from bladder cancer. Even though there are no established screening programs, early detection in high-risk populations (with environmental and occupational exposure) makes it worthwhile. One of the common reasons for bladder cancer screening is that no test is perfect for screening. However, combining these tests in high-risk populations can yield good results. There is a clear need for early detection to reduce morbidity and mortality.[762] As noted earlier, Lynch syndrome is associated with upper tract urothelial carcinoma. It is estimated that the risk is 22 times higher than the general population & it's 3rd malignancy after colon and endometrium in this population.[712] It is advised in the literature that any patient with UTUC & age less than 65 years and any personal or family history of Lynch spectrum cancers should undergo genetic counseling and germline testing. A positive result can trigger screening of the family and appropriate screening for early detection.[763]

Prostate Cancer: Of all urological cancers, PC is probably the most studied cancer from prevention aspects. Considering its incidence, mortality & changing landscape of the pathological spectrum, it's always a catchy question, how can a PC be prevented? The main risk factors for PC are non-modifiable, and the precursor lesion and pathological changes are obviously way earlier than clinical cancer; it's a good target for chemoprevention. The primary prevention strategy for PC has minimal directions as most modifiable risk factors show a limited cause-effect relationship. Smoking cessation/ avoidance has been suggested, as smoking is mainly associated with poor oncological outcomes. Various dietary factors have been studied, but no specific recommendation can be made. Selenium and vitamin E have been studied but didn't show any protective effect.[764] Other dietary factors showed no significant protective effect. For chemoprevention, 5-alpha-reductase inhibitors (5-ARI) have been studied in two landmark trials. PC prevention trial (PCPT) used finasteride as a chemo-preventive agent versus placebo. The key finding from this trial[765] was that it reduces the incidence of PC diagnosis by around 25 %. It also increases the sensitivity of digital rectal examination (DRE) and PSA for cancer detection in the treatment arm. The treatment arm detected 43 % less low-grade PC. However, it revealed a relatively higher diagnosis of Gleason pattern 7-10 compared to the placebo arm. The reasons for this finding have been discussed extensively, and the data suggest that it may need to be revised. For any cancer, the preventive strategy needs to reduce the mortality rate. However, data from PCPT doesn't show the survival benefit of finasteride on PC-specific survival. Since reducing the incidence and detecting low-grade cancer was achieved, this chemo-preventive strategy may be cost-effective. The long-term data outcome also suggests that taking finasteride for very long is safe without any significant side effects. Another landmark trial (REDUCE) also showed a 23 % risk reduction for PC over four years.[766] However, the FDA committee believed that the results of both trials showed a significant increase in the diagnosis of Gleason pattern 8 to 10 & they concluded that 5-ARIs might not have a favorable risk-to-benefit ratio.[767] Since then, 5-ARIs are not used for chemoprevention in routine urology practice. PSA-based screening for PC has been a matter of debate for the last two decades. PSA-based screening has been noted to have doubled the incidence with a marginal decrease in mortality. The two most extensive randomized trials, PLCO and ESRPC, confirmed these results.[768,769] Based on these results, US preventive services task force (USPSTF) recommended against PSA screening in 2012.[770] However, revisiting these results with other statistical models predicted a 37-43 % reduction in PC-specific mortality. It is also noted that there would be a 46-57% rise in the metastatic presentation if PSA-based screening is wholly abandoned.[771] In 2017, USPSTF revised the policy and gave grade C recommendations for PSA-based screening in men between 55 and 69 years. Currently, in most of the world, PSA-based screening is offered to asymptomatic men in this age group with an informed decision. Various international guidelines mention starting PSA screening in high-risk populations aged 45-50. This population includes men with a family history of PC & those with BRCA germline mutations.

Testicular cancer: Patients with undescended testicles should undergo timely orchiopexy to preserve testicular function and to reduce the future risk of malignancy. With age, the chances of testicular malignancy increase in undescended testicles & it is recommended that after 12 years with a normal contralateral testicle, it is better to go for an orchidectomy.[773] There is no evidence that screening for testicular cancer is beneficial. Adults with risk factors should be made aware and be explained about the regular self-examination of testicles.[774,775] There is a recommendation against routine screening of testicular cancer. Testicular microlithiasis has been linked with testicular cancer. However, the literature doesn't support it. It has been recommended that isolated microlithiasis may not have any implications. However, co-occurrences of risk factors warrant regular follow-up until age 55.[776]

Penile cancer: Despite low incidence, etiological factors are well studied, and preventive strategies are discussed effectively to prevent invasive cancer. Primary prevention includes smoking cessation, better hygiene & education about sexual exposure & how to be cautious. Childhood and adolescent circumcision have long been discussed as a preventive measure against penile cancer.[728] Circumcision can benefit in multiple ways. Exposed glans can detect cancer early. Removing the foreskin can reduce the area for cancer development.[777] Regarding neonatal circumcision, it is discussed that it may benefit poor-income countries and the geographical regions where the hygienic practice is not up to the mark.[777] Vaccination against HPV is one way to prevent HPV-related lesions and penile cancer. A bivalent and quadrivalent vaccine has been administered to avoid HPV-related benign and malignant problems. It was primarily started for cervical cancer aimed at pre-pubertal females. Initial female-only programs are being converted to gender-neutral vaccination programs since they are highly effective (> 90%) in preventing HPV-related problems. The total dose (3 injections) needs to be administered before the commencement of sexual activity for the vaccine to be effective.[777] Identification and treatment of premalignant lesions are crucial. Surgical excision with circumcision, application of 5 –

FU/imiquimod & laser ablation has been described as effective treatment to prevent these lesion from malignant transformation.[777]

Vaccines in Urological cancer prevention

Immune-based treatment & its outcomes in RCC and bladder cancer have opened a new avenue in treating advanced urological cancers. Much research has happened on cancer vaccines to treat advanced malignancies. Peptide-based vaccines are designed to elicit specific T cells against antigens expressed by tumor cells. It may have a survival advantage with limited side effects on normal tissue. However, peptide vaccines as monotherapy have failed in most phase 3 trials & combination therapy is being developed to gain clinically significant outcomes. The best combination would be immunomodulators, which can amply T cell expansion and increase the vaccine effect for extended periods.[778] Sipuleucel-T was the first cancer vaccine approved for the treatment of CRPC in 2010 by the FDA. Similarly, various peptide-based vaccines are tried in phase 1/phase two trials for renal and bladder cancers. HPV-related vaccination has been discussed earlier.

Conclusion

As we understand, cancer is a multifactorial entity. Apart from basic pathophysiology, our gradual understanding of external factors, genetics, and other molecular factors made us go in various directions to find a solution to this deadly disease with variable success. However, except few preventive strategies, we are short of what we would like to achieve primarily due to ever-changing cancer biology. In the future, more research is required to understand high-risk groups for particular cancer & to develop a sensitive non-invasive test to apply preventive measures more effectively. Not only science, but we as a community also need to adopt a healthy lifestyle for our biological systems and find ways to make our daily activities more environmentally friendly. A general awareness in the community and active measures and incentives by various authorities to curb tobacco usage will go a long way toward preventing urological cancers.

29

DETECTION OF PRECANCEROUS CONDITIONS AND PREVENTION OF HEPATOBILIARY CANCERS

Dr. Ashwini Kumar Kudari

Chronic fibrotic liver diseases such as viral hepatitis eventually develop liver cirrhosis, which causes the occurrence of hepatocellular carcinoma (HCC). Given the limited therapeutic efficacy in advanced HCC, preventing HCC development could be an effective strategy for improving patient prognosis. However, there is still no established therapy to meet the goal. Studies have elucidated various molecular mechanisms and signaling pathways involved in HCC development. Genetically engineered or chemically-treated experimental models of cirrhosis and HCC have been developed and shown their potential value in investigating molecular therapeutic targets and diagnostic biomarkers for HCC prevention. It is estimated that roughly 1-2% of the population is affected by liver cirrhosis, and the risk of HCC increases according to the severity of liver fibrosis and dysfunction. Regular tumor surveillance for cirrhotic patients has enabled efficient early detection of

HCC tumors to be eligible for potentially curative treatments: surgical resection, local ablation, and liver transplantation. However, complete tumor removal is not equivalent to a cure because of persisting cirrhosis in the remnant liver. Repeated tumor recurrences are observed in nearly 80% of the patients, limiting the improvement of 5-year survival up to 70-80%. Once the tumor reaches an advanced stage, there is no curative treatment option; even a multi-kinase inhibitor, sorafenib, could yield survival benefits for only up to several months. The refractory nature of HCC suggests that prevention of its development in high-risk patients is the most effective strategy to improve mortality substantially.

Risk factors and molecular mechanisms of HCC development

A wide range of etiological agents contributes to hepatocarcinogenesis through specific molecular mechanisms, indicating the necessity to develop strategies for HCC prevention accordingly. Chronic infection of the hepatitis B virus (HBV) is the most common global cause of HCC, affecting more than 350 million individuals (6% of the world population) and being the dominant etiology, especially in China and Africa. HBV proteins and HBV DNA integration into the host genome have been suggested to possess a direct carcinogenic effect by activating cis and trans oncogenic signals in host hepatocytes. Inconsistent, high serum HBV DNA level, indicative of increased viral replication, is predictive of HCC development, which is not necessarily accompanied by advanced liver fibrosis. It has been suggested that certain HBV strains, e.g., genotype C in the Asian population and genotype F in the Alaskan population, or mutations in the HBV genome, e.g., within pre-core and basal core promoter regions, increase the risk of HCC. Superinfection with hepatitis delta virus (HDV) is associated with severe hepatitis, accelerated fibrosis progression, and increased risk of HCC.

Hepatitis C virus

Hepatitis C virus (HCV) affects 170 million individuals worldwide, has been the major risk factor for HCC in many industrialized countries, and contributes to the increasing HCC incidence in the US. Clinically, the incidence of HCV-related HCC increases according to the severity of liver fibrosis. In contrast to HBV-related HCC, patients with minimal fibrosis rarely develop HCC, suggesting that the cirrhotic microenvironment is the primary driver.

Exposure to environmental carcinogens

Dietary contamination with the potent hepatocarcinogen, aflatoxin B1 (AFB1, a natural mycotoxin produced by Aspergillus fungi) is observed in some tropical regions with warm and humid climates, especially in Eastern and Southeastern Asia and sub-Saharan Africa, where HBV infection is prevalent. AFB1 causes a loss-of-function mutation in the "hotspot" codon 249 (G to T transversion) of exon 7 in the TP53 tumor suppressor gene and exhibits a remarkable synergistic hepatocarcinogenic effect with HBV. Food or water contamination with other fungal toxins such as fumonisin, blue-green algae-derived microcystins, nitrosamine, inorganic arsenic, and betel quid chewing are also suggested to increase HCC risk.

Alcohol

Liver cirrhosis induced by long-term, excessive intake of alcohol is a well-established risk factor of HCC. It is one of the major causes in North America and Western Europe. Alcohol likely has an indirect carcinogenic effect through the establishment of cirrhosis.

Non-alcoholic fatty liver disease, obesity, and Type 2 Diabetes

Recent studies have suggested that many HCC cases developed in so-called cryptogenic cirrhosis may be attributable to non-alcoholic fatty liver disease (NAFLD), including non-alcoholic steatohepatitis (NASH). Epidemiological data have suggested a tight association of NAFLD/NASH with visceral obesity and diabetes accompanied by insulin resistance, which was also independently reported as a risk factor for HCC development.

Hepatic iron overload disorders: Hemochromatosis

Genetic hemochromatosis (GH) is mainly caused by homozygous mutations in the hemochromatosis (HFE) gene, especially C282Y (more common in Caucasians) and, to a lesser extent, H63D, which abnormally increase iron absorption and accumulation mainly in the liver, heart, and pancreas. Established cirrhosis is an HCC risk factor in GH.

Genetic risk factors

Recent studies have identified etiology-specific or independent host genetic polymorphisms associated with increased risk of HCC in patients with chronic liver diseases. A single nucleotide polymorphism (SNP) in the epidermal growth factor (EGF) gene (SNP rs4444903) was associated with increased EGF expression and elevated risk of HCC development in cirrhotic patients.

Other risk factors

HCC risk in primary biliary cirrhosis (PBC) with stage 4 cirrhosis is about the same as in HCV-related cirrhosis. HCC occurs less frequently in autoimmune hepatitis (AIH) only after the establishment of cirrhosis, suggesting that inflammation alone is insufficient. Only scarce epidemiological evidence exists for other rare forms of chronic liver diseases, such as alpha 1-antitrypsin deficiency. There is conflicting evidence regarding the association of smoking with HCC risk, for which the confounding effect of alcohol abuse cannot be entirely excluded. Human immunodeficiency virus (HIV) co-infection increases the risk of HCC in patients with chronic viral hepatitis.

Approaches To HCC Prevention

Cancer prevention is grouped into the following categories:

(1) "Primary prevention" to prevent exposure to risk factors.

(2) "Secondary prevention" to prevent cancer development in patients with risk factors.

(3) "Tertiary prevention" to prevent cancer recurrence in patients curatively treated for initial cancer but not for the risk factor.

Primary prevention has been proven effective, but no established secondary and tertiary prevention therapies exist. Interferon has been extensively tested in viral hepatitis-related HCC as proof-of-principle therapy, although there is still a need for more potent and less toxic treatment.

338

Primary prevention

Primary prevention aims to eliminate or reduce exposure to etiological agents and could be immediately effective, especially in developing countries.

Viral hepatitis-related HCC

One prominent success is the population-based universal infant vaccination for HBV, which has shown to be effective in preventing neonatal HBV infection from infected mother (vertical transmission).

Non-viral hepatitis-related HCC

Eliminating food contamination may be an effective public health strategy to reduce HCC. The post-harvest intervention was effective in lowering AFB1 intake in West Africa. However, such intervention, which requires water and sanitation infrastructure, may be practically infeasible in many resource-poor countries. Strategies to reduce other risk factors, such as alcohol abuse, obesity, and diabetes, are also needed, especially in developed countries. Dietary iron overload as a result of drinking habits may also be preventable.

Secondary prevention

Secondary prevention aims to prevent HCC in individuals chronically affected by the etiological agents. This approach is grouped into two categories:

(1) Eradication of the etiological agents (curative treatment).

(2) Blockade of carcinogenesis progression in the presence of etiological agents (non-curative treatment).

Complete eradication of HBV and HCV is still challenging once the chronic infection is established. There are already more than a half billion people with chronic infection, rationalizing the non-curative approach as a practical option. Secondary prevention should be "less toxic" to be well tolerated for long-term treatment to asymptomatic patients and "inexpensive" considering the long duration of the treatment and the large size of the target patient population, mainly residing in developing countries. Regular tumor surveillance in patients at high risk of HCC is vital for secondary prevention and has improved patient survival.

HBV-related HCC

Alpha interferon, nucleoside, and nucleotide analogs, suppressing HBV replication, are clinically available as antiviral therapies. A series of studies collectively suggested that interferon therapy lessens the risk of HCC development. Prolonged suppression of HBV replication by a nucleoside , lamivudine, reduced the risk of HBV-related HCC.

HCV-related HCC

Meta-analyses of retrospective and relatively small prospective clinical trials of interferon-based treatment have shown that sustained viral response (SVR) is consistently associated with a lower risk of HCC and improved patient survival. However, SVR is achieved in only up to 50-60% of patients. Irrespective of viral clearance, it has been suggested that suppression of hepatic inflammation could delay disease progression and reduce HCC risk; biochemical response, i.e., normalization of liver enzymes such as alanine aminotransferase (ALT), achieved by either interferon, glycyrrhizin, or ursodeoxycholic acid (UDCA), have been suggested to reduce HCC risk.

Aflatoxin B1-related HCC

Chlorophyllin, water-soluble salts of natural chlorophylls, acts as an interceptor molecule forming tight molecular complexes, reduces the carcinogenic activity of AFB1 in vivo, acts as an antioxidant, and serves as a potent inhibitor of cytochrome P450 enzymes from bioactivation of the carcinogen. A clinical trial in Qidong, China, confirmed that chlorophyllin reduced the urinary level of aflatoxin-N7-guanine adducts, a biomarker of the biological effectiveness of the therapy, warranting further assessment of its long-term effect and safety profile in a larger patient cohort. A supplementary diet with chlorophyll-rich foods such as spinach and leafy green vegetables may be an alternative.

Alcohol- and metabolic disorder-related HCC

It is unclear whether termination of alcohol abuse reduces HCC risk in alcoholic cirrhosis despite survival benefits. There is also no clear evidence that correction of obesity and diabetes reduces HCC, suggesting the need to determine the usefulness of lifestyle adjustment, weight loss, bariatric surgery, and treatment of diabetes on HCC risk.

Iron overload-related HCC

A cohort study with long-term clinical observation showed that phlebotomy/venesection (iron depletion therapy) could effectively reduce HCC incidence and prolong survival in GH.

Tertiary prevention

HCC recurrence targeted by tertiary prevention is categorized into two types:

(1) Dissemination of primary tumor cells mostly observed within 1-2 years after curative treatment as "early" recurrence.

(2) De novo carcinogenesis arising from the remnant cirrhotic liver that appears as "late" recurrence independently from the treated primary tumor. Theoretically, the latter is divided into:

(2-a) Promotion/growth of (pre)neoplastic clones that already exist but are not detected at the time of curative treatment.

(2-b) De novo initiation of (pre)neoplastic clones that are not present at the time of treatment.

Phytochemicals And Nutritional Supplements

Phytochemicals, plant-derived bioactive chemicals, and other dietary substances have been increasingly recognized as potential treatment options in HCC prevention. Together with other food-derived agents and nutritional supplements, this class of drugs is called complementary and alternative medicine (CAM). Some exert a pleiotropic effect in preventing carcinogenesis, although mechanisms are unknown. A few of them, such as glycyrrhizin, are incorporated into clinical practice in specific countries.

Gallbladder and bile duct cancers

Gallbladder cancer (GBC) is an uncommon but highly fatal malignancy; fewer than 5000 new cases are diagnosed yearly in the United States. Most are found incidentally in patients undergoing exploration for cholelithiasis; a tumor will be found in 1 to 2 percent of such cases. The poor prognosis associated with GBC is thought to be related to the advanced stage at diagnosis due to the gallbladder's anatomic position and the vagueness and non-specificity of symptoms.

Epidemiology

Worldwide, prominent geographic variability in GBC incidence correlates with the prevalence of cholelithiasis. High rates of GBC are seen in South American countries, particularly Chile, Bolivia, and Ecuador, as well as some areas of northern India, Pakistan, Japan, Korea, and Poland. In Chile, mortality rates from GBC are the highest in the world. These populations share a high prevalence of gallstones and salmonella infection which are recognized risk factors for GBC [6-8]. Both genetic factors and socioeconomic issues that delay or prevent access to cholecystectomy for gallstones are considered contributory.

Risk factors

Several risk factors have been identified for GBC, many of which share a common characteristic of chronic gallbladder inflammation.

Gallstone disease — Gallstone disease is present in 70 to 90 percent of patients with GBC, and a history of gallstones appears to be one of the most substantial risk factors for developing GBC. Despite the increased risk of GBC in patients with gallstones, the overall incidence of GBC in patients with cholelithiasis is only 0.5 to 3 percent. The risk is higher with larger gallstones and a longer duration of cholelithiasis (particularly over 40 years).

Porcelain gallbladder — Porcelain gallbladder is an uncommon manifestation of chronic cholecystitis characterized by intramural calcification of the gallbladder wall. It is associated with cholelithiasis in more than 95 percent of cases. As with other gallstone-related conditions, these patients are at increased risk of GBC. The reported incidence of GBC in patients with a porcelain gallbladder ranges from 0 to 60 percent, with more recent studies suggesting a rate of approximately 2 to 3 percent. The increased risk may be confined to patients with selective mucosal calcification or incomplete mural calcification.

Gallbladder polyps — Gallbladder polyps are outgrowths of the gallbladder mucosal wall that are usually found incidentally on ultrasonography or after cholecystectomy. They are classified as benign or malignant, and benign lesions are classified as nonneoplastic (e.g., cholesterol and inflammatory polyps, adenomyomas) or neoplastic (e.g., adenomas, leiomyoma). The most common benign neoplastic lesion is an adenoma, a glandular tumor composed of cells resembling biliary tract epithelium. It is unclear whether adenomatous polyps represent a premalignant lesion and, if so, with which frequency they progress to carcinoma. Unlike GBC, gallbladder polyps tend not to occur in patients with cholelithiasis, chronic inflammation is generally absent, and cancer-related molecular changes seen in GBCs have not been identified in adenomas. Nevertheless, larger polyps are more likely to contain foci of invasive cancer, and some (but not all) studies suggest a correlation between gallbladder polyps and the risk of GBC.

Primary sclerosing cholangitis — A higher risk of gallbladder mass lesions is reported in the chronic inflammatory state associated with primary sclerosing cholangitis. In a study of 286 patients, 6 percent of cases were found to have gallbladder masses, of which 56 percent were GBCs. Therefore, an annual screening ultrasound of the gallbladder is recommended for these patients.

Chronic infection

Salmonella — In endemic settings, approximately 1 to 4 percent of acutely infected individuals become chronic asymptomatic carriers of Salmonella typhi. Several reports and a meta-analysis of 17 case-control and cohort studies suggest an association between chronic S. Typhi carriage and elevated risk of GBC. Because chronic carriage occurs more often in individuals with cholelithiasis, gallstones are thought to represent a potential nidus for ongoing infection.

Helicobacter — Helicobacter colonization of the biliary epithelium (particularly Helicobacter bilis) has been implicated in the pathogenesis of gallbladder disease, including GBC, based on the detection of Helicobacter-derived cytotoxins and surface proteins using sensitive molecular and immunohistochemical techniques. The strength of this association requires further clarification. Congenital biliary cysts are cystic dilatations that may occur singly or multiply throughout the bile ducts. They were initially termed choledochal cysts (involving the extrahepatic bile duct), but the clinical classification was revised in 1977 to include intrahepatic cysts. Biliary cysts may be congenital or acquired and are associated with various anatomic abnormalities. An anomalous pancreaticobiliary duct junction is present in approximately 70 percent of patients with biliary cysts. Like anomalous pancreaticobiliary duct junction, biliary cysts are persistent in Asian populations. Abnormal pancreaticobiliary duct junction — Anomalous pancreaticobiliary duct junction is a rare anatomic variation in which the pancreatic duct drains into the common bile duct, resulting in a long common channel (usually over 2 cm in length). This condition may represent the embryological ducts' failure to fully migrate into the duodenum. This condition is most prevalent in Asian populations, primarily Japanese. Anomalous pancreaticobiliary duct junction appears to increase the risk of biliary and pancreatic malignancy, even in patients without a biliary cyst or ductal dilation. GBC is the most common malignancy in patients with an anomalous pancreaticobiliary duct junction and no bile duct cysts. As a result, prophylactic cholecystectomy is recommended in affected patients.

Medications — Some drugs have also been implicated in biliary carcinogenesis, including methyldopa, oral contraceptives/menopausal hormone therapy, and isoniazid. Others have found no convincing evidence for an association between oral contraceptive use and GBC.

Carcinogen exposure — Evidence accumulates that carcinogen exposure may also be involved in the etiology of GBC. An increased risk of GBC has been described in workers in the industries manufacturing or working on oil, paper, chemical, shoe, textile, and cellulose acetate fiber. An increased risk is also seen among miners exposed to radon,cigarette smokers and possibly in those with high exposure to aflatoxin. Aflatoxin is a mycotoxin that commonly contaminates corn, soybeans, and peanuts, and associated with hepatocellular cancer risk.

Obesity — Obesity has been consistently associated with an increased risk for GBC. Biliary tract cancers were traditionally divided according to their primary anatomical site into cancers of the gallbladder, the extrahepatic ducts, and the ampulla of Vater. At the same time, intrahepatic tumors of the bile system were classified as primary liver cancers. More recently, cholangiocarcinoma has been used to refer to bile duct cancers arising in the intrahepatic, perihilar, or distal (extrahepatic) biliary tree, exclusive of the gallbladder or ampulla of Vater.Anatomically, intrahepatic cholangiocarcinomas originate from small intrahepatic ductules (peripheral cholangiocarcinomas) or large intrahepatic ducts proximal to the right bifurcation and left hepatic ducts. The extrahepatic bile ducts are divided into the perihilar (including the confluence) and distal segments. The transition occurs where the common bile duct lies posterior to the duodenum, proximal to the insertion of the cystic duct into the common bile duct. Generally, perihilar disease represents approximately 50 percent; distal disease, 40 percent; and intrahepatic disease, less than 10 per cent of cholangiocarcinoma cases. As a general rule, the incidence of biliary tract cancers increases with age; the typical patient with cholangiocarcinoma is between 50 and 70. However, patients with cholangiocarcinomas arising in primary sclerosing cholangitis (PSC) and those with choledochal cysts were present nearly two decades earlier. In contrast to gallbladder cancer, where the female gender predominates, the incidence of cholangiocarcinoma is slightly higher in men. The higher incidence of PSC in men is probably a reason for this higher incidence.

Risk factors

Several risk factors for cholangiocarcinoma have been recognized, although a specific risk factor cannot be identified for many patients. The main risk factors in the United States and Europe are primary sclerosing cholangitis (PSC) and fibropolycystic liver disease (e.g., choledochal cysts). A clear and strong association exists between chronic intrahepatic stone disease (hepatolithiasis, also called recurrent pyogenic cholangitis) and cholangiocarcinoma. Chronic liver disease (cirrhosis and viral infection) is now recognized as a risk factor, particularly for intrahepatic cholangiocarcinoma. In certain regions (e.g., Thailand), chronic infection with liver fluke is the driving risk factor. Finally, at least four genetic conditions, Lynch syndrome, BRCA-associated protein-1 (BAP1) tumor predisposition syndrome, cystic fibrosis, and biliary papillomatosis, appear to increase the risk for cholangiocarcinoma.

Primary hepatobiliary disease

Primary sclerosing cholangitis — PSC is an inflammatory disorder of the biliary tree that leads to fibrosis and stricturing of the intrahepatic and extrahepatic bile ducts. PSC is strongly associated with inflammatory bowel disease, notably ulcerative colitis (UC); approximately 40 to 50 percent of patients have symptomatic colitis, while the incidence of colitis is around 90 percent in patients with PSC.

Fibropolycystic liver disease — Congenital abnormalities of the biliary tree (Caroli syndrome, congenital hepatic fibrosis, choledochal cysts) carry an approximately 15 percent risk of malignant change in the adult years (average age at diagnosis 34. Choledochal cysts are congenital cystic dilatations of the bile ducts. At the same time, Caroli disease is a variant of choledochal cyst disease characterized by multiple cystic dilations of the intrahepatic biliary ducts. The overall incidence of cholangiocarcinoma in patients with untreated cysts is as high as 28 percent.Cholelithiasis, cholecystitis, and hepatolithiasis — While cholelithiasis is a well-described vital risk factor for gallbladder cancer, the association between gallstones and cholangiocarcinoma is less well-established. However, four epidemiologic studies note an increased risk for cholangiocarcinoma among patients with symptomatic gallstone disease or cholecystitis, but of a lower magnitude than for gallbladder cancer. A clear and strong association exists between chronic intrahepatic stone disease (hepatolithiasis, also called recurrent pyogenic cholangitis) and cholangiocarcinoma. A stone disease affecting only the intrahepatic bile ducts is exceedingly rare in the West but is endemic in certain parts of Southeast Asia.

Chronic liver disease — Hepatitis B virus (HBV) and hepatitis C virus (HCV), and liver cirrhosis, regardless of etiology, have been examined as risk factors for intrahepatic cholangiocarcinoma.

Viral hepatitis — An association between HCV infection and cholangiocarcinoma was initially suggested in 1991. Since then, several reports have noted a higher-than-expected rate of HCV-associated cirrhosis in patients with cholangiocarcinoma, although the risk is much lower than for hepatocellular cancer.

Precursor (intraductal) lesions — There are three known precursors to invasive cholangiocarcinoma: intraductal papillary neoplasm of the bile ducts], the rare intraductal tubulopapillary neoplasm of the bile ducts, and the much more common biliary intraepithelial neoplasia.

Genetic disorders — At least four genetic disorders are associated with an increased risk of cholangiocarcinoma:

a)   Lynch syndrome (hereditary nonpolyposis colorectal cancer).

b)   BAP1 tumor predisposition syndrome.

c)   Cystic fibrosis.

d)   A rare inherited disorder called multiple biliary papillomatosis.

Infections

Parasitic infection — In Asia (particularly Thailand), infection with liver flukes of the genera Clonorchis and Opisthorchis is associated with cholangiocarcinoma of the intrahepatic bile ducts. Humans are infected by consuming undercooked fish, with the adult worms inhabiting and laying eggs in the biliary system. These organisms induce a chronic inflammatory state in the proximal biliary tree, presumably leading to malignant transformation of the lining epithelium. Carcinogens produced by bacteria in fish and other foods, smoking, alcohol, and HBV infection might also act as cofactors.

Prevention of risk factors whenever possible, screening of people with risk factors, early diagnosis, and treatment are required to prevent and better manage patients with established diseases.

References:

Chapter 1

1. *DeVita, Hellman and Rosenberg's Cancer, Principles and Practice of Oncology 11th Ed.*
2. *Abeloff's Clinical Oncology 5th Ed.*
3. *IARC monographs on the identification of carcinogenic hazards to humans (Accessed via https://monographs.iarc.who.int/.*
4. *Cell phones and Cancer risk: National Cancer Institute (Accessed via https://www..gov/about-/causes-prevention/risk/radiation/cell-phones-fact-sheet).*

Chapter 2

5. *Epstein MA, Achong BG, Barr YM. Virus particles in cultured lymphoblasts from Burkitt's lymphoma. Lancet. 1964;1:702–703*

6. *Stehelin D, Varmus HE, Bishop JM, Vogt PK. DNA related to the transforming gene(s) of avian sarcoma viruses is present in normal avian DNA. Nature. 1976; 260:170–3.*

7. *Chang Y, Moore PS, Weiss RA. Human oncogenic viruses: nature and discovery. Phil. Trans. R. Soc. B 2017;372: 20160264. http://dx.doi.org/10.1098/rstb.2016.0264*

8. *de Martel C, Georges D, Bray F, Ferlay J, Clifford GM. Global burden of Cancer attributable to infections in 2018: a worldwide incidence analysis. Lancet Glob Health. 2020;8:e180-e190. doi: 10.1016/S2214-109X(19)30488-7.*

9. *IARC. Schistosomes, Liver Flukes and Helicobacter pylori; IARC Working Group on the Evaluation of Carcinogenic Risks to Humans; IARC: Lyon, France, 1994; Volume 61, pp. 1–241.*

10. *IARC. Biological Agents. Volume 100 B. A Review of Human Carcinogens; IARC: Lyon, France, 2012; Volume 100, pp. 1–441.*

11. *Liu J, Yang HI, Lee MH, Hsu WL, Chen HC, Chen CJ. Epidemiology of Virus Infection and Human Cancer. In: Shurin M, Thanavala Y, Ismail N. (eds) 2015. Infection and Cancer: Bi-Directorial Interactions. Springer, Cham. https://doi.org/10.1007/978-3-319-20669-1_3*

12. *Wong Y, Meehan MT, Burrows SR, Doolan DL, Miles JJ. Estimating the global burden of Epstein-Barr virus-related Cancers. J Cancer Res Clin Oncol. 2022;148:31-46. doi: 10.1007/s00432-021-03824-y.*

13. *De Leo A, Calderon A, Lieberman PM. Control of Viral Latency by Episome Maintenance Proteins. Trends Microbiol. 2020;28:150-162. doi: 10.1016/j.tim.2019.09.002.*

14. *Lau KCK, Burak KW, Coffin CS. Impact of Hepatitis B Virus Genetic Variation, Integration, and Lymphotropism in Antiviral Treatment and Oncogenesis. Microorganisms. 2020;8:1470. doi: 10.3390/microorganisms8101470.*

15. *Tsukuda S, Watashi K. Hepatitis B virus biology and life cycle. Antiviral Res. 2020;182:104925. doi: 10.1016/j.antiviral.2020.104925.*

16. Groves IJ, Coleman N. *Human papillomavirus genome integration in squamous carcinogenesis: what have next-generation sequencing studies taught us?* J Pathol. 2018;245:9-18. doi: 10.1002/path.5058.

17. Cosper PF, Bradley S, Luo L, Kimple RJ. *Biology of HPV Mediated Carcinogenesis and Tumor Progression.* Semin Radiat Oncol. 2021;31:265-273. doi: 10.1016/j.semradonc.2021.02.006.

18. Ahmed MM, Cushman CH, De Caprio JA. *Merkel Cell Polyomavirus: Oncogenesis in a Stable Genome.* Viruses. 2021;14:58. doi: 10.3390/v14010058.

19. Luo Y, Liu Y, Wang C, Gan R. *Signaling pathways of EBV-induced oncogenesis.* Cancer Cell Int. 2021;21:93. doi: 10.1186/s12935-021-01793-3.

20. Maksimova V, Panfil AR. *Human T-Cell Leukemia Virus Type 1 Envelope Protein: Post-Entry Roles in Viral Pathogenesis.* Viruses. 2022;14:138. doi: 10.3390/v14010138.

21. Tempera I, Lieberman PM. *Oncogenic Viruses as Entropic Drivers of Cancer Evolution.* Front Virol. 2021;1:753366. doi: 10.3389/fviro.2021.753366.

22. Huda MN, Nurunnabi M. *Potential Application of Exosomes in Vaccine Development and Delivery.* Pharm Res. 2022;1–37. doi: 10.1007/s11095-021-03143-4.

23. Bui JD, Schreiber RD. *Cancer immunosurveillance, immunoediting and inflammation: independent or interdependent processes?* Curr Opin Immunol. 2007;19:203-8. doi: 10.1016/j.coi.2007.02.001.

24. Hanahan D, Coussens LM. *Accessories to the crime: functions of cells recruited to the tumor microenvironment.* Cancer Cell. 2012;21:309-22. doi: 10.1016/j.ccr.2012.02.022.

25. Hanahan D. *Hallmarks of Cancer: New Dimensions.* Cancer Discov. 2022;12:31-46. doi: 10.1158/2159-8290.CD-21-1059.

26. Mesri EA, Feitelson MA, Munger K. *Human viral oncogenesis: a Cancer hallmarks analysis.* Cell Host Microbe. 2014;15:266-82. doi: 10.1016/j.chom.2014.02.011.

27. Krump NA, You J. *Molecular mechanisms of viral oncogenesis in humans.* Nat Rev Microbiol. 2018;16:684-698. doi: 10.1038/s41579-018-0064-6.

28. Vescovo T, Pagni B, Piacentini M, Fimia GM, Antonioli M. *Regulation of Autophagy in Cells Infected With Oncogenic Human Viruses and Its Impact on Cancer Development.* Front Cell Dev Biol. 2020;8:47. doi: 10.3389/fcell.2020.00047.

29. Jayshree, R. S., and Kumar, R. V. *"Contribution of the Gut and Vaginal Microbiomes to Gynecological Cancers,"* in Preventive Oncology for the Gynecologist (Springer Singapore), 2019; 399–416. doi:10.1007/978-981-13-3438-2_31.

30. van Tong H, Brindley PJ, Meyer CG, Velavan TP. *Parasite Infection, Carcinogenesis and Human Malignancy.* E Bio Medicine. 2017;15:12-23. doi: 10.1016/j.ebiom.2016.11.034.

31. Béziat V, Jouanguy E. *Human inborn errors of immunity to oncogenic viruses.* Curr Opin Immunol. 2021;72:277-285. doi: 10.1016/j.coi.2021.06.017.

32. Somasundaram A, Rothenberger NJ, Stabile LP. *The Impact of Estrogen in the Tumor Microenvironment.* Adv Exp Med Biol. 2020;1277:33-52. doi: 10.1007/978-3-030-50224-9_2.

33. Jayshree R.S. *The Immune Microenvironment in Human Papilloma Virus-Induced Cervical Lesions-Evidence for Estrogen as an Immunomodulator.* Front Cell Infect Microbiol. 2021;11:649815. doi: 10.3389/fcimb.2021.649815.

34. Shimizu I, Kohno N, Tamaki K, Shono M, Huang HW, He JH, et al. *Female hepatology: Favorable role of estrogen in chronic liver disease with hepatitis B virus infection.* World J Gastroenterol 2007;13:4295-4305. http://www.wjgnet.com/1007-9327/13/4295.asp

35. Ruggieri A, Gagliardi MC, Anticoli S. *Sex-Dependent Outcome of Hepatitis B and C Viruses Infections: Synergy of Sex Hormones and Immune Responses?* Front Immunol. 2018;9:2302. doi: 10.3389/fimmu.2018.02302.

36. Kang Y, Cai Y, Yang Y. *The Gut Microbiome and Hepatocellular Carcinoma: Implications for Early Diagnostic Biomarkers and Novel Therapies.* Liver Cancer. 2021;11:113-125. doi: 10.1159/000521358.

37. Luo W, Guo S, Zhou Y, Zhao J, Wang M, Sang L, et al. *Hepatocellular Carcinoma: How the Gut Microbiota Contributes to Pathogenesis, Diagnosis, and Therapy.* Front Microbiol. 2022;13:873160. doi: 10.3389/fmicb.2022.873160.

38. Cao W, Yu P, Yang K, Cao D. *Aflatoxin B1: metabolism, toxicology, and its involvement in oxidative stress and Cancer development.* Toxicol Mech Methods. 2022;32:395-419. doi: 10.1080/15376516.2021.2021339.

39. Lin CL, Kao JH. *Natural history of acute and chronic hepatitis B: The role of HBV genotypes and mutants.* Best Pract Res Clin Gastroenterol. 2017;31:249-255. doi: 10.1016/j.bpg.2017.04.010.

40. Tornesello AL, Tagliamonte M, Buonaguro FM, Tornesello ML, Buonaguro L. *Virus-like Particles as Preventive and Therapeutic Cancer Vaccines.* Vaccines (Basel). 2022;10:227. doi: 10.3390/vaccines10020227.

41. World Health Organization. *WHO guideline for screening and treatment of cervical pre-Cancer lesions for cervical Cancer prevention, 2nd ed.* 2021. World Health Organization. https://apps.who.int/iris/handle/10665/342365.

42. Lichter K, Krause D, Xu J, Tsai SHL, Hage C, et al. *Adjuvant Human Papillomavirus Vaccine to Reduce Recurrent Cervical Dysplasia in Unvaccinated Women: A Systematic Review and Meta-analysis.* Obstet Gynecol. 2020;135:1070-1083. doi: 10.1097/AOG.0000000000003833.

43. *Training Modules on Hepatitis B and C Screening, Diagnosis and Treatment.* World Health Organization, 28th July 2020. https://www.who.int/publications/i/item/9789290227472

44. Premkumar M, Chawla YK. *Should We Treat Immune Tolerant Chronic Hepatitis B? Lessons from Asia.* J Clin Exp Hepatol. 2022;12:144-154. doi: 10.1016/j.jceh.2021.08.023.

45. Yang YC, Yang HC. *Recent Progress and Future Prospective in HBV Cure by CRISPR/Cas.* Viruses. 2021;14:4. doi: 10.3390/v14010004.

46. Bhattacharjee C, Singh M, Das D, Chaudhuri S, Mukhopadhyay A. *Current therapeutics against HCV.* Virusdisease. 2021;32:228-243. doi: 10.1007/s13337-021-00697-0.

47. Stinco M, Rubino C, Trapani S, Indolfi G. Treatment of hepatitis B virus infection in children and adolescents. World J Gastroenterol. 2021;27:6053-6063. doi: 10.3748/wjg.v27.i36.6053.

Chapter 3

48. Aravind Gopal, Sunita Mondal, Asha Gandhi, Sarika Arora Effect of integrated yoga practices on immune response in examination stress – A preliminary study. 10.4103/0973-6131.78178.

49. Martin, E. I., Ressler, K. J., Binder, E., and Nemeroff, C. B. (2009). The neurobiology of anxiety disorders: brain imaging, genetics and psychoneuroendocrinology. Psychiatr. Clin. North Am. 32, 549–575. doi: 10.1016/j.psc.2009.05.004

50. Lawrence S Sklar et al. , Carleton university, Ottawa, Ontario, Canada. Stress and Cancer. 0033-2909/81/8903-0369.

51. Livea Dornela Godoy, Matheus Teixeira Rossignoli et al. A comprehensive overview on stress neurobiology: Basic concepts and clinical implications. 10.3389/fnbeh.2018.00127

52. Pacheco R, Contreras F, Prado C (2012) Cells, molecules and mechanisms involved in the neuro-immune interaction. Cell Interact 2012:139–166

53. Selye, H. (1950). Stress and the general adaptation syndrome. Br. Med. J. 1, 1383–1392.

54. Herbert TB, Cohen S. Stress and immunity in humans: a meta-analytic review. Psychosom Med. 1993;55(4):364-379.

55. Dantzer R, Kelley KW. Stress and immunity: an integrated view of relationships between the brain and the immune system. Life Sci. 1989;44(26):1995-2008.

56. Dunn, G. P., L. J. Old, R. D. Schreiber 2004. The three Es of Cancer immunoediting. Annu. Rev. Immunol. 22: 329–360.

57. Burnet F.M. Immunological surveillance. London: Pergamon Press, 1970.

58. Schmale, A.H., Jr and Iker, HP. The psychological setting of uterine cervical Cancer. Annals of the New York Academy of Sciences. 1966,125,807-813.

59. Rogentine, G.N., et al. Psychological factors in the prognosis of Malignant melanoma. Psychosomatic medicine. 1979, 41,647-655

60. Furth, J.Hormones as etiological agents in neoplasia. In F.F Becker (Ed), Cancer: A comprehensive treatise (Vol 1). New York: Plenum Press,1975

61. Welsch, C.W, & Nagasawa, H. Prolactin and murine mammary tumorigenesis: A review. Cancer Research, 1977,37,951-963

62. Burnet, M. 1957. Cancer; a biological approach. I. The processes of control. Br. Med. J. 1: 779–786.

63. Gallois PH, Forzy G, Dhont JL. Hormonal changes during relaxation. Encephale 1984;10:79-82. French.

64. Burnet, M. 1957. Cancer; a biological approach. I. The processes of control. Br. Med. J. 1: 779–786.

65. Dunn, G. P., L. J. Old, R. D. Schreiber 2004. The three Es of Cancer immunoediting. Annu. Rev. Immunol. 22: 329–360.

66. Kumar, Abbas, Fausto; Robbins and Cotran: Pathologic Basis of Disease; Elsevier, 7th ed.

67. Everett E. Vokes • Harvey M. Golomb (Eds.) Oncologic Therapies

68.   Iannello A et al, J Leukoc Biol. 2008;84(1):1-26. doi:10.1189/jlb.0907650

69.   Smyth MJ, Hayakawa Y, Takeda K, Yagita H (November 2002). "New aspects of natural-killer-cell surveillance and therapy of Cancer." Nature Reviews. Cancer. 2(11): 850–61.

70.   Vinay DS, Ryan EP, Pawelec G, et al. Immune evasion in Cancer: Mechanistic basis and therapeutic strategies. Semin Cancer Biol. 2015;35 Suppl:S185-S198. doi:10.1016/j.semCancer.2015.03.004.

Chapter 6

71.   https://www.ncbi.nlm.nih.gov/pmc/articles/PMC4048459/

72.   https://pubmed.ncbi.nlm.nih.gov/24857081/

73.   https://pubmed.ncbi.nlm.nih.gov/24857081/

74.   https://www.ncbi.nlm.nih.gov/pmc/articles/PMC526387/

75.   https://www.Cancer.gov/news-events/Cancer-currents-blog/2020/lung-Cancer-treating-mental-health-longer-survival

76.   https://www.Cancer.org/treatment/survivorship-during-and-after-treatment/long-term-health-concerns/recurrence/can-i-do-anything-to-prevent-Cancer-recurrence.html

77.   (https://www.mdpi.com/2077-0383/11/3/653/htm)

78.   (https://www.ncbi.nlm.nih.gov/pmc/articles/PMC7793079/)

79.   (https://www.Cancer.org/treatment/survivorship-during-and-after-treatment/be-healthy-after-treatment/nutrition-and-physical-activity-during-and-after-Cancer-treatment.html)

80.   https://www.ncbi.nlm.nih.gov/pmc/articles/PMC5862633/

81.   Exercise : https://www.Cancer.org/treatment/survivorship-during-and-after-treatment/be-healthy-after-treatment/physical-activity-and-the-Cancer-patient.html.

Chapter 7

82. - Nunez P, Srinivasan R..Electroencephalogram. Scholarpedia. 2007; 2(2): 1348.

83. - Klimesch W. EEG alpha and theta oscillations reflect cognitive and memory performance: a review and analysis. Brain ResRev. 1999. April; 29 (2–3): 137–296.

84 - Clément F, Belleville S. Effect of disease severity on neural compensation of item and associative recognition in mild cognitive impairment. J Alzheimers Dis. 2012; 29 (1): 109-123.

85 - S.-T. Lin, P. Yang, C.-Y. Lai, Y.-Y. Su, Y.-C. Yeh, M.-F. Huang, and C.-C. Chen, "Mental Health Implications of Music: Insight from Neuroscientific and Clinical Studies," Harvard Review of Psychiatry, 2011.

86 - M. A. Phipps, D. L. Carroll, and A. Tsiantoulas, "Music as a Therapeutic Intervention on an Inpatient Neuroscience Unit," Complementary Therapies in Clinical Practise, 2010.

87 - M. M. Stanczyk, "Music Therapy in Supportive Cancer Care," Reports of Practical Oncology and Radiotherapy, 2011.

88 - Ros Shilawani S. Abdul Kadir, Mohd Hafizi Ghazali, Zunairah Hj. Murat, Mohd Nasir Taib, H. A. Rahman, and S. A. M. Aris, "The Preliminary Study On The Effect Of Nasyid Music And Rock Music On

Brainwave Signal Using EEG," (ICEED 2010) , 2nd International Congress on Engineering Education, pp. 58 - 63, Kuala Lumpur, Malaysia, 2010.

89 - T. McCaffrey, J. Edwards, and D. Fannon, "Is There a Role for Music Therapy in the Recovery Approach in Mental Health?," The Arts in Psychotherapy, 2011.

90 - R. Maddick, "Naming the unnameable and communicating the unknowable : Reflections on a combined music therapy/social work program," The Arts in Psychotherapy, 2011.

91 - T.-Y. Chang, C.-S. Liu, B.-Y. Bao, S.-F. Li, T.-I. Chen, and Y.-J. Lin, "Characterization of road traffic noise exposure and prevalence of hypertension in central Taiwan," Science of the total environment, 2011.

92 - C. Padungtod, C. Ekpanyaskul, P. Nuchpongsai, N. Laemun, T. Matsui, and K. Hiramatsu, "Aircraft Noise Exposure and Its Effects on Quality of Life and Cognitive Function Among Thai Residents," Epidemiology, vol. 22, pp. 29-185, 2011.

93 - Hoffman, "Brain Training Against Stress: Theory, Methods and Results from an Outcome Study," 2005.

94 - Z. H. Murat, M. N. Taib, Z. M. Hanafiah, S. Lias, R. S. S. A. Kadir, and H. A. Rahman, "Initial Investigation of Brainwave Synchronization After Five Sessions of Horizontal Rotation

Intervention Using EEG," 5th International Colloquium on Signal Processing & Its Applications (CSPA 2009), pp. 350 - 354, 2009.

95 - C. Spironelli and A. Angrilli, "EEG delta band as a marker of brain damage in aphasic patients after recovery of language," Neuropsychologia, vol. 47, pp. 988-994, 2009.

96 - P. Jemmer. (2009). Getting in a (Brain-wave) State through Entrainment, Meditation, and Hypnosis.

97 - M. Teplan, "Fundamentals Of EEG Measurement," Measurement Science Review, 2002.

98. Aldridge A. Music therapy research. A review of references in the medical literature. Arts in Psychotherapy. 1993;20:11–35. [Google Scholar].

99. Pothoulaki M., McDonald R., Flowers P. Methodological issues in music interventions in oncology settings. A systematic literature review. Arts in Psychotherapy. 2006;33:446–455.

100. Beck S. The therapeutic use of music for Cancer-related pain. Oncology Nursing Forum. 1991;18(8):1327–1337.

101. Magill-Levreault L. The use of music therapy to address the suffering in advanced Cancer pain. Journal of Palliative Care. 2001;17(3):167–172.

102. Zimmerman L., Pozehl B., Duncan K., Schmitz R. Effect of music in patients who had chronic pain. Western Journal of Nursing Research. 1989;11(3):298–309.

103. Koelsch S, Siebel WA. Towards a neural basis of music perception. Trends Cogn Sci 2005;9:578-84.

104. Boso M, Politi P, Barale F, Enzo E. Neurophysiology and neurobiology of the musical experience. Funct Neurol 2006;21:187-91.

105. Lin ST, Yang P, Lai CY, Su YY, Yeh YC, Huang MF, et al. Mental health implications of music: Insight from neuroscientific and clinical studies. Harv Rev Psychiatry 2011;19:34-46.

106. Limb CJ. Structural and functional neural correlates of music perception. Anat Rec A Discov Mol Cell Evol Biol 2006;288:435-46.

107. Kemper KJ, Danhauer SC. Music as therapy. South Med J 2005;98:282-8.

108. Chan MF. Effects of music on patients undergoing a C-clamp procedure after percutaneous coronary interventions: A randomized controlled trial. Heart Lung 2007;36:431-9.

109. Bernardi L, Porta C, Sleight P. Cardiovascular, cerebrovascular, and respiratory changes induced by different types of music in musicians and non-musicians: The importance of silence. Heart 2006;92:445-52.

110. Rickard NS, Toukhsati SR, Field SE. The effect of music on cognitive performance: Insight from neurobiological and animal studies. Behav Cogn Neurosci Rev 2005;4:235-61.

111. Levitin DJ, Menon V. Musical structure is processed in "language" areas of the brain: A possible role for Brodmann area 47 in temporal coherence. Neuroimage 2003;20:2142-52.

112. Levitin DJ. The World in Six Songs: How the Musical Brain Created Human Nature. New York: Penguin; 2008.

113. Levitin DJ, Tirovolas AK. Current advances in the cognitive neuroscience of music. Ann N Y Acad Sci 2009;1156:211-31.

114. Menon V, Levitin DJ. The rewards of music listening: Response and physiological connectivity of the mesolimbic system. Neuroimage 2005;28:175-84.

115. Colleoni M, Mandala M, Peruzzotti G, et al. Depression and degree of acceptance of adjuvant cytotoxic drugs. Lancet. 2000;356:1326–1327. doi: 10.1016/S0140-6736(00)02821-X.

116. Pinquart M, Duberstein PR. Depression and Cancer mortality: a meta-analysis. Psychol Med. 2010;40:1797–1810. doi: 10.1017/S0033291709992285.

117. Mishel MH, Hostetter T, King B, Graham V. Predictors of psychosocial adjustment in patients newly diagnosed with gynecological Cancer. Cancer Nurs. 1984;7:291–299. doi: 10.1097/00002820-198408000-00003.

118. Linden W, Vodermaier A, Mackenzie R, Greig D. Anxiety and depression after Cancer diagnosis: prevalence rates by Cancer type, gender, and age. J Affect Disord. 2012;141:343–351. doi: 10.1016/j.jad.2012.03.025.

119. Brintzenhofe-Szoc KM, Levin TT, Li Y, Kissane DW, Zabora JR. Mixed anxiety/depression symptoms in a large Cancer cohort: prevalence by Cancer type. Psychosomatics. 2009;50:383–391. doi: 10.1176/appi.psy.50.4.383.

120. Colleoni M, Mandala M, Peruzzotti G, et al. Depression and degree of acceptance of adjuvant cytotoxic drugs. Lancet. 2000;356:1326–1327. doi: 10.1016/S0140-6736(00)02821-X. [PubMed] [CrossRef] [Google Scholar].

121. Pinquart M, Duberstein PR. Depression and Cancer mortality: a meta-analysis. Psychol Med. 2010;40:1797–1810. doi: 10.1017/S0033291709992285. [PMC free article] [PubMed] [CrossRef] [Google Scholar].

122. Satin JR, Linden W, Phillips MJ. Depression as a predictor of disease progression and mortality in Cancer patients: a meta-analysis. Cancer. 2009;115:5349–5361. doi: 10.1002/cncr.24561. [PubMed] [CrossRef] [Google Scholar].

123. Lemon J, Edelman S, Kidman AD. Perceptions of the "Mind-Cancer" Relationship Among the Public, Cancer Patients, and Oncologists. J Psychosoc Oncol. 2004;21:43–58. doi: 10.1300/J077v21n04_03. [CrossRef] [Google Scholar].

Chapter 8

124. "NCI Dictionary of Cancer Terms" National Cancer Institute. 2011-02-02. Retrieved 2018-03-28.)

125. Aberle DR, Allegra CJ, Ganschow P, Hahn SM, Lee CN, Millon-Underwood S, Pike MC, Reed SD, Saftlas AF, Scarvalone SA, Schwartz AM, Slomski C, Yothers G, Zon R: NIH State-of-the-Science Conference Statement: Diagnosis and Management of Ductal Carcinoma In Situ (DCIS). NIH Consens State Sci Statements 2009;26:1–27.And Ernster VL, Ballard-Barbash R, Barlow WE, Zheng Y, Weaver DL, Cutter G, Yankaskas BC, Rosenberg R, Carney PA, Kerlikowske K, Taplin SH, Urban N, Geller BM: Detection of ductal carcinoma in situ in women undergoing screening mammography. J Natl Cancer Inst 2002; 94:1546–1554.

126. Mittra I, Mishra G A, Dikshit R P, Gupta S, Kulkarni V Y, Shaikh H K A et al. Effect of screening by clinical breast examination on breast Cancer incidence and mortality after 20 years: prospective, cluster randomised controlled trial in Mumbai BMJ 2021; 372 :n256 doi:10.1136/bmj.n256.

127. Lee SM, Goo JM, Park CM et-al. A new classification of adenocarcinoma: what the radiologists need to know. Diagn Interv Radiol. 2012;18 (6): 519-26. doi:10.4261/1305-3825.DIR.5778-12.1 - Pubmed citation

128. Recommendations for the Management of Subsolid Pulmonary Nodules Detected at CT: A Statement from the Fleischner Society David P. Naidich, Alexander A. Bankier, Heber MacMahon, Cornelia M. Schaefer-Prokop, Massimo Pistolesi, Jin Mo Goo, Paolo Macchiarini, James D. Crapo, Christian J. Herold, John H. Austin, and William D. Travis Radiology 2013 266:1, 304-317.

129. Fischerova D, Zikan M, Dundr P, Cibula D. Diagnosis, treatment, and follow-up of borderline ovarian tumors. Oncologist. 2012;17(12):1515-33. doi: 10.1634/theoncologist.2012-0139. Epub 2012 Sep 28. PMID: 23024155; PMCID: PMC3528384).

130. Shaheen, Nicholas J. MD, MPH1; Falk, Gary W. MD, MS2; Iyer, Prasad G. MD, MS3; Souza, Rhonda F. MD4; Yadlapati, Rena H. MD, MHS (GRADE Methodologist)5; Sauer, Bryan G. MD, MSc (GRADE Methodologist)6; Wani, Sachin MD7. Diagnosis and Management of Barrett's Esophagus: An Updated ACG Guideline. The American Journal of Gastroenterology: April 2022 - Volume 117 - Issue 4 - p 559-587 doi: 10.14309/ajg.0000000000001680.

131. Farges O, Dokmak S: Malignant Transformation of Liver Adenoma: An Analysis of the Literature. Dig Surg 2010;27:32-38. doi: 10.1159/000268405.

132. Pryczynicz A, Bandurski R, Guzińska-Ustymowicz K, Niewiarowska K, Kemona A, Kędra B. Ménétrier's disease, a premalignant condition, with coexisting advanced gastric Cancer: A case report and review of the literature. Oncol Lett. 2014 Jul;8(1):441-445. doi: 10.3892/ol.2014.2141. Epub 2014 May 13. PMID: 24959292; PMCID: PMC4063657.

Chapter 9

133. *Vinay Kumar, MBBS, MD Frcp, Abul K. Abbas M, Jon C. Aster, MD P, Jerrold R. Turner, MD P. Neoplasia -Robbins & Cotran Pathologic Basis of Disease. 10th ed. Vinay Kumar, MBBS, MD Frcp, Abul K. Abbas M, Jon C. Aster, MD P, Jerrold R. Turner, MD P, editors. Elsevier; 2021. 267–338 p.*

134. *A. Diamantis M.D., Ph.D., E. Magiorkinis B.Sc., M.D., Ph.D., G. Androutsos M.D. PD. What's in a name? Evidence that Papanicolaou, not Babes, deserves credit for the PAP test. Diagn Cytopathol. 2010;38(7):473–6.*

135. *Leslie Foulds M.A. MD. The natural history of Cancer. J Chron Dis. 1958;8(9):2–37.*

136. *van der Waal I. Historical perspective and nomenclature of potentially malignant or potentially premalignant oral epithelial lesions with emphasis on leukoplakia—some suggestions for modifications. Oral Surg Oral Med Oral Pathol Oral Radiol [Internet]. 2018;125(6):577–81. Available from: https://doi.org/10.1016/j.oooo.2017.11.023*

137. *Wacholder S. Precursors in Cancer epidemiology: Aligning definition and function. Cancer Epidemiol Biomarkers Prev. 2013;22(4):521–7.*

138. *Eduardo L. Franco TER. Cancer Precursors- Epidemiology, Detectin and Prevention. 2002nd ed. Eduardo L. Franco TER, editor. Springer; 2002.*

139. *Berman JJ, Albores-Saavedra J, Bostwick D, DeLellis R, Eble J, Hamilton SR, et al. PreCancer: A conceptual working definition. Results of a Consensus Conference. Cancer Detect Prev. 2006;30(5):387–94.*

140. *Srivastava S, Koay EJ, Borowsky AD, Marzo AM De, Ghosh S, Wagner PD, et al. Cancer overdiagnosis: a biological challenge and clinical dilemma. Nat Rev Cancer. 2022;19(6):349–58.*

141. *Caporaso NE. Why Precursors Matter. Cancer Epidemiol Biomarkers Prev. 2013;22(4):518–20.*

142. *Hanahan D, Robert A. Weinberg. The Hallmark of Cancer. Cell. 2000;100(7):57–70.*

143. *Koss, Leopold G.; Melamed MRK. Diagnostic Cytology and Its Histopathologic Bases, Carcinoma of the Uterine Cervix and Its Precursors. 5th Editio. Koss, Leopold G.; Melamed MRK, editor. Phildelphia,Pennsylvania, USA: Lippincott Williams & Wilkins Squamous; 2006. Chapter 11-pg283-394.*

144. *Warnakulasuriya S. Oral Surgery, Oral Medicine, Oral Pathology and Oral Radiology. Oral Surg Oral Med Oral Pathol Oral Radiol [Internet]. 2018;125(6):582–90. Available from: https://doi.org/10.1016/j.oooo.2018.03.011*

145. *Ritu N, C WD. The Bethesda System for Reporting Cervical Cytology Defi nitions, Criteria, and Explanatory Notes International Publishing Switzerland 2015 No Title. Third Edit. Wilbur RN• DC, editor. Springer Cham Heidelberg New York Dordrecht London © Springer; 2014.*

146. *Sung H, Ferlay J, Siegel RL, Laversanne M, Soerjomataram I, Jemal A, et al. Global Cancer Statistics 2020: GLOBOCAN Estimates of Incidence and Mortality Worldwide for 36 Cancers in 185 Countries. CA Cancer J Clin. 2021;71(3):209–49.*

147. *Ellenson RJK• LH, Ronnett BM, editors. Blaustein's Pathology of the Female Genital Tract. 7th ed. Springer Nature Switzerland AG 2; 2019. 439–472 p.*

148. Schnitt SJ,: Schnitt SJ et al Purdie CA WDMEVSA. WHO classification of breast tumors. 5th ed. Dilani Lokuhetty, Valerie A. White, Reiko Watanabe IAC, editor. Lyon, France IARC: IARC; 2019. 11–24; 28–31;-71–81 p.

149. Lopez-Garcia MA, Geyer FC, Lacroix-Triki M, Marchió C, Reis-Filho JS. Breast Cancer precursors revisited: Molecular features and progression pathways. Histopathology. 2010;57(2):171–92.

150. Costa A, Zanini V. PreCancerous lesions of the breast. Nat Clin Pract Oncol. 2008;5(12):700–4.

151. Warnakulasuriya S, Kujan O, Aguirre-Urizar JM, Bagan J V., González-Moles MÁ, Kerr AR, et al. Oral potentially malignant disorders: A consensus report from an international seminar on nomenclature and classification, convened by the WHO Collaborating Centre for Oral Cancer. Vol. 27, Oral Diseases. 2021. 1862–1880 p.

152. Bostwick DG, Cheng L. Precursors of prostate Cancer. Histopathology. 2012;60(1):4–27.

153. Reibel J, Gale N, & Hille J. (2017). JKC, GIn: El-Naggar AK, Chanrandis JR, Takata T, Slootweg PPJ eds. . p. 11.-115. WHO Classification of Head and Neck Tumors-Oral potentially malignant disorders and oral epithelial dysplasia. 4th ed. In: El-Naggar AK, Chan JKC, Grandis JR, Takata T, Slootweg PPJ E, editor. Lyon, France,IARC.; 2017. 112–115 p.

154. Müller S. Oral epithelial dysplasia, atypical verrucous lesions and oral potentially malignant disorders: focus on histopathology. Oral Surg Oral Med Oral Pathol Oral Radiol [Internet]. 2018;125(6):591–602. Available from: https://doi.org/10.1016/j.oooo.2018.02.012

155. Rodrigues Neto EM, Teofilo Campos FM, Oliveira Meneses CA, Barbosa Calcia TB, Cetira Filho EL. Potentially Malignant Oral Lesions: A Mini Review. J Young Pharm. 2021;13(1):28–30.

156. Nankivell P, Williams H, Matthews P, Suortamo S, Snead D, McConkey C, et al. The binary oral dysplasia grading system: Validity testing and suggested improvement. Oral Surg Oral Med Oral Pathol Oral Radiol [Internet]. 2013;115(1):87–94. Available from: http://dx.doi.org/10.1016/j.oooo.2012.10.015

157. Kumaraswamy KL, Vidhya M, Rao PK, Mukunda A. Oral biopsy: Oral pathologist's perspective. J Cancer Res Ther. 2012;8(2):192–8.

158. Taylor PR, Abnet CC, Dawsey SM. Squamous dysplasia-The precursor lesion for esophageal squamous cell carcinoma. Cancer Epidemiol Biomarkers Prev. 2013;22(4):540–52.

159. Wang GQ, Abnet CC, Shen Q, Lewin KJ, Sun XD, Roth MJ, et al. Histological precursors of oesophageal squamous cell carcinoma: Results from a 13 year prospective follow up study in a high risk population. Gut. 2005;54(2):187–92.

160. Grady WM, Yu M, Markowitz SD, Chak A. Barrett's esophagus and esophageal adenocarcinoma biomarkers. Cancer Epidemiol Biomarkers Prev. 2020;29(12):2486–94.

161. Gullo I, Grillo F, Mastracci L, Vanoli A, Carneiro F, Saragoni L, et al. PreCancerous lesions of the stomach, gastric Cancer and hereditary gastric Cancer syndromes. Pathologica. 2020;112(3):166–85.

162. Dinis-Ribeiro M, Areia M, de Vries AC, Marcos-Pinto R, Monteiro-Soares M, O'Connor A, et al. Managment of preCancerous conditions and lesiond in the stomach (MAPS). Endoscopy [Internet]. 2012;44(1):74–94. Available from: http://www.ncbi.nlm.nih.gov/pmc/articles/PMC3367502/pdf/nihms-381287.pdf

163. Naini B V., Odze RD. Advanced preCancerous lesions (APL) in the colonic mucosa. Best Pract Res Clin Gastroenterol [Internet]. 2013;27(2):235–56. Available from: http://dx.doi.org/10.1016/j.bpg.2013.03.012

164. Cree IDNRDODKVPMRP.SKMWFCLA. WHO Classification of Digestive system. 5th edition. Nagtegaal ID, Odze RD, Klimstra D, Paradis V, Rugge M, Schirmacher P, et al., editors. Lyon, France; 2019. 30-36;65-71;163-174:221-229;300-319; p.

165. Frič P, Škrha J, Šedo A, Bušek P, Laclav M, Bunganič B, et al. Precursors of pancreatic Cancer. Eur J Gastroenterol Hepatol. 2017;29(3):E13–8.

166. Nakano M. Premalignant lesions of hepatocellular carcinoma. Nippon rinsho Japanese J Clin Med. 2001;59 Suppl 6:216–21.

167. McKenney JK. Precursor lesions of the urinary bladder. Histopathology. 2019;74(1):68–76.

168. Ximing J Yang, MD P. Preca prostate 2017. UpToDate 2022. p. 1.Ximing J Yang, MD, P. Preca prostate 2017. UpToD.

169. Nelson WG, De Marzo AM, Deweese TL, Lin X, Brooks JD, Putzi MJ, et al. Preneoplastic prostate lesions: An opportunity for prostate Cancer prevention. Ann N Y Acad Sci. 2001;952:135–44.

170. Mostofi FK, Sesterhenn IA, Davis CJ. A pathologist's view of prostatic carcinoma. Cancer. 1993;71(3 S):906–32.

Chapter 10

171. Global Burden of Disease 2019 Cancer Collaboration, Kocarnik JM, Compton K, Dean FE, Fu W, Gaw BL, J, et al. Cancer Incidence, Mortality, Years of Life Lost, Years Lived With Disability, and Disability-Adjusted Life Years for 29 Cancer Groups From 2010 to 2019: A Systematic Analysis for the Global Burden of Disease Study 2019. JAMA Oncol. 2022;8(3):420-444. doi: 10.1001/jamaoncol.2021.6987.

172. Kulothungan V, Sathishkumar K, Leburu S, Ramamoorthy T, Stephen S, Basavarajappa D, et al. Burden of Cancers in India - estimates of Cancer crude incidence, YLLs, YLDs and DALYs for 2021 and 2025 based on National Cancer Registry Program. BMC Cancer. 2022;22(1):527. doi: 10.1186/s12885-022-09578-1.

173. Chang CC, Lee WT, Hsiao JR, Ou CY, Huang CC, Tsai ST, et al. Oral hygiene and the overall survival of head and neck Cancer patients. Cancer Med. 2019;8(4):1854-1864. doi: 10.1002/cam4.2059.

174. O'Grady I, Anderson A, O'Sullivan J. The interplay of the oral microbiome and alcohol consumption in oral squamous cell carcinomas. Oral Oncol. 2020;110:105011. doi: 10.1016/j.oraloncology.2020.105011.

175. Koifman L, Barros R, Schulze L, Ornellas AA, Favorito LA. Myiasis associated with penile carcinoma: a new trend in developing countries? Int Braz J Urol. 2017;43(1):73-79. doi: 10.1590/S1677-5538.IBJU.2016.0084.

176. Larsen MN, Elbe AM, Madsen M, Madsen EE, Ørntoft C, Ryom K, Dvorak J, Krustrup P. An 11-week school-based 'health education through football programme' improves health knowledge related to hygiene, nutrition, physical activity and well-being-and it's fun! A scaled-up, cluster-RCT with over 3000 Danish school children aged 10-12 years old. Br J Sports Med. 2021;55(16):906-911. doi: 10.1136/bjsports-2020-103097.

177. Takeuchi Y, Ohara M, Kanto T. Nationwide awareness-raising program for viral hepatitis in Japan: the "Shitte kan-en" project. Glob Health Med. 2021;3(5):301-307. doi: 10.35772/ghm.2021.01063.

178. Osman A, Kowitt SD, Sheeran P, Jarman KL, Ranney LM, Goldstein AO. Information to Improve Public

Perceptions of the Food and Drug Administration (FDA's) Tobacco Regulatory Role. Int J Environ Res Public Health. 2018;15(4):753. doi: 10.3390/ijerph15040753

179. Bam TS, Chand AB, Shah BV. Evidence of the Effectiveness of Pictorial Health Warnings on Cigarette Packaging in Nepal. Asian Pac J Cancer Prev. 2021;22(S2):35-44. doi: 10.31557/APJCP.2021.22.S2.35.

180. Schoueri-Mychasiw N, Weerasinghe A, Vallance K, Stockwell T, Zhao J, Hammond D, et al. Examining the Impact of Alcohol Labels on Awareness and Knowledge of National Drinking Guidelines: A Real-World Study in Yukon, Canada. J Stud Alcohol Drugs. 2020;81(2):262-272. doi: 10.15288/jsad.2020.81.262.

181. Agide FD, Garmaroudi G, Sadeghi R, Shakibazadeh E, Yaseri M, Koricha ZB. Likelihood of Breast Screening Uptake among Reproductive-aged Women in Ethiopia: A Baseline Survey for Randomized Controlled Trial. Ethiop J Health Sci. 2019;29(5):577-584. doi: 10.4314/ejhs.v29i5.7.

182. Bernat JK, Hullmann SE, Sparks GG. Communicating breast Cancer risk information to young adult women: A pilot study. J Psychosoc Oncol. 2017 May-Jun;35(3):249-259. doi: 10.1080/07347332.2016.1277821.

183. Abu SH, Woldehanna BT, Nida ET, Tilahun AW, Gebremariam MY, Sisay MM. The role of health education on cervical Cancer screening uptake at selected health centers in Addis Ababa. PLoS One. 2020;15(10):e0239580. doi: 10.1371/journal.pone.0239580.

184. Wirtz C, Mohamed Y, Engel D, Sidibe A, Holloway M, Bloem P, et al. Integrating HPV vaccination programs with enhanced cervical Cancer screening and treatment, a systematic review. Vaccine. 2021;S0264-410X(21)01447-X. doi: 10.1016/j.vaccine.2021.11.013.

185. Choi Y, Oketch SY, Adewumi K, Bukusi E, Huchko MJ. A Qualitative Exploration of Women's Experiences with a Community Health Volunteer-Led Cervical Cancer Educational Module in Migori County, Kenya. J Cancer Educ. 2020;35(1):36-43. doi: 10.1007/s13187-018-1437-2.

186. Gabrielli S, Maggioni E, Fieschi L. Cervical Cancer prevention in Senegal: an International Cooperation Project Report. Acta Biomed. 2018;89(6-S):29-34. doi: 10.23750/abm.v89i6-S.7460.

187. Melvin CL, Vines AI, Deal AM, Pierce HO, Carpenter WR, Godley PA. Implementing a small media intervention to increase colorectal Cancer screening in primary care clinics. Transl Behav Med. 2019;9(4):605-616. doi: 10.1093/tbm/iby063.

188. Chan MW, Chean KY, Kader Maideen SF, Kow FP. The Intention and Uptake of Colorectal Cancer Screening after a Brief Health Education Program in a Malaysian Primary Care Setting: A Population-Based Study. Asian Pac J Cancer Prev. 2021;22(11):3475-3482. doi: 10.31557/APJCP.2021.22.11.3475.

189. Ferrante D, Chellini E, Merler E, Pavone V, Silvestri S, Miligi L et al. Italian pool of asbestos workers cohorts: mortality trends of asbestos-related neoplasms after long time since first exposure. Occup Environ Med. 2017;74(12):887-898. doi: 10.1136/oemed-2016-104100.

190. Womack DM, Kennedy R, Chamberlin SR, Rademacher AL, Sliney CD. Patients' lived experiences and recommendations for enhanced awareness and use of integrative oncology services in Cancer care. Patient Educ Couns. 2022;105(7):2557-2561. doi: 10.1016/j.pec.2021.11.018.

191. Bow EJ, Bourrier V, Phillips D, Winski G, Williams M, Kostiuk N, et al. Hand Hygiene Compliance at a Canadian provincial Cancer centre - the complementary roles of nurse auditor-driven and patient auditor-driven audit processes and impact upon practice in ambulatory Cancer care. Am J Infect Control. 2021;49(5):571-575. doi: 10.1016/j.ajic.2020.10.012.

Chapter 11

192. *Dialogues Clin Neurosci. 2016 Mar; 18(1): 33–43. doi: 10.31887/DCNS.2016.18.1/ksmith. Habit formation Kyle S. Smith, PhD*

193. *J Neurosci Res. 2020 Jun; 98(6): 986–997. Published online 2019 Nov 6. doi: 10.1002/jnr.24552*

194. *Freeze BS, Kravitz AV, Hammack N, Berke JD, Kreitzer AC (2013) Control of basal ganglia output by direct and indirect pathway projection neurons. J Neurosci 33:18531–18539.*

195. *Kouzarides T (2007) Chromatin modifications and their function. Cell 128:693– 705.*

196. *Renthal W, Nestler EJ (2009) Histone acetylation in drug addiction. Semin Cell Dev Biol 20:387–394.*

197. *Front. Psychol., 27 March 2020 Sec. Eating Behavior Volume 11 - 2020 | https://doi.org/10.3389/fpsyg.2020.00560*

198. *Consumption of red meat and processed meat and Cancer incidence: a systematic review and meta-analysis of prospective studies Maryam S Farvid 1 , Elkhansa Sidahmed 2 , Nicholas D Spence 3 , Kingsly Mante Angua 4 , Bernard A Rosner 5 , Junaidah B Barnett 2*

199. *Obesity and Cancer: Kathleen Y Wolin 1 , Kenneth Carson, Graham A Colditz DOI: 10.1634/theoncologist.2009-0285.*

200. *Indian J Med Paediatr Oncol. 2009 Apr-Jun; 30(2): 61–70. doi: 10.4103/0971-5851.60050*

201. *Smokeless tobacco and tobacco-related nitrosamines. Published: December, 2004 DOI:https://doi.org/10.1016/S1470-2045(04)01633-X.*

202. *Global burden of Cancer in 2020 attributable to alcohol consumption: a population-based study. July 13, 2021DOI:https://doi.org/10.1016/S1470- 2045(21)00279-5.*

203. *AntiCancer Agents Med Chem, 2013 Jan;13 (1):70-82. Vitamin D, sunlight and Cancer connection, Michael F Holick 1 PMID: 23094923.*

204. *Cancers (Basel). 2019 Aug; 11(8): 1041, 2019 Jul 24. doi: 10.3390/Cancers11081041.*

205. *Cancer screening and early detection in the 21st century Jennifer Loud, DNP, CRNP and Jeanne Murphy, PhD, CNM.*

206. *https://www.safecosmetics.org/get-the-facts/chemicals-of- concern/known-carcinogens.*

207. *https://www.Cancer.gov/about-Cancer/causes-prevention/risk/radiation/cell- phones-fact-sheet.*

Chapter 13

208. *Luciana Besedovsky & Tanja Lange & Jan Born, Sleep and immune function, Eur J Physiol (2012) 463:121– 137 DOI 10.1007/s00424-011-1044-0.*

209. *Gabriele Sulli, Michael Tun Yin Lam, Satchidananda Panda, Interplay between circadian clock and Cancer: new frontiers for Cancer treatment, Trends Cancer. 2019 August ; 5(8): 475–494. doi:10.1016/j.trecan.2019.07.002.*

Chapter 14

210. Schneider EL, Guralnik JM: The ageing of America: Impact on health care costs. JAMA 263: 2335-2340, 1990.

211. National Cancer Institute: Surveillance, Epidemiology, and End Results (SEER) 17 Registry (2000- 2003): Age-Adjusted Incidence Rates. Bethesda, MD, National Cancer Institute www.seer.Cancer .gov/csr.

212. The effect of a multidisciplinary approach to the geriatric oncology patient. Catherine Terret et al., journal of clinical oncology, volume 25, issue 14.

213. httpwww.aetnainternational.com/en/about-us/explore/future-health/ageing-population-graphics.htmlgraphics.html.

214. httpwww.aetnainternational.com/en/about-us/explore/future-health/ageing-population-graphics.htmlgraphics.html.

215. Noone, A.M.,). (2018). SEER Cancer statistics review, 1975–2015.

216. López-Otín C. The hallmarks of ageing. Cell. 2013 Jun 6;153(6):1194-217. Hanahan D, Weinberg RA. Hallmarks of Cancer: the next generation. Cell. 2011 Mar 4;144(5):646-74.

217. Surbone A, Kawaga-Singer M, Terret C, et al.: The illness trajectory of elderly Cancer patients across cultures: SIOG position paper. Ann Oncol [Epub ahead of print on October 6, 2006].

218. Steinman MA, Landefeld CS, Rosenthal JE, et al.: Polypharmacy and prescribing quality in older people. J Am Geriatr Soc 54:1516-1523, 2006.

219. 65. Zulian GB: Geriatric medical oncology in the care of elderly Cancer patients. Crit Rev Oncol Hematol 41:343-347, 2002.

220. Fried L, Ferrucci L, Darer J, et al.: Untangling the concepts of disability, frailty, and comorbidity: Implications for improved targeting and care. J Gerontol A Biol Sci Med Sci 59A:255-264, 2004.

Chapter 15

221. Ng M, Fleming T, Robinson M, Thomson B, Graetz N, Margono C, et al. Global, regional, and national prevalence of overweight and obesity in children and adults during 1980-2013: a systematic analysis for the Global Burden of Disease Study 2013. Lancet 2014;384:766–81.

222. NCD Risk Factor Collaboration (NCD-RisC). Trends in adult body-mass index in 200 countries from 1975 to 2014: a pooled analysis of 1698 population-based measurement studies with 19·2 million participants. Lancet. 2016 Apr 2;387(10026):1377-1396. doi: 10.1016/S0140-6736(16)30054-X. Erratum in: Lancet. 2016 May 14;387(10032):1998. PMID: 27115820.

223. NCD Risk Factor Collaboration (NCD-RisC). Worldwide trends in body-mass index, underweight, overweight, and obesity from 1975 to 2016: a pooled analysis of 2416 population-based measurement studies in 128·9 million children, adolescents, and adults. Lancet. 2017 Dec 16;390(10113):2627-2642. doi: 10.1016/S0140-6736(17)32129-3. Epub 2017 Oct 10. PMID: 29029897; PMCID: PMC5735219.

224. Arnold M, Pandeya N, Byrnes G, Renehan PAG, Stevens GA, Ezzati PM, et al. Global burden of Cancer attributable to high body-mass index in 2012: a population-based study. Lancet Oncol 2015;16:36–46.

225. Calle EE, Rodriguez C, Walker-Thurmond K, Thun MJ. Overweight, obesity, and mortality from Cancer in a prospectively studied cohort of U.S. adults. N Engl J Med. 2003; 348:1625–1638. [PubMed: 12711737].

226. Guh DP, Zhang W, Bansback N, Amarsi Z, Birmingham CL, Anis AH. The incidence of co-morbidities related to obesity and overweight: a systematic review and meta-analysis. BMC Public Health. 2009 Mar 25;9:88. doi: 10.1186/1471-2458-9-88. PMID: 19320986; PMCID: PMC2667420.

227. Arnold M, Leitzmann M, Freisling H, Bray F, Romieu I, Renehan A, Soerjomataram I. Obesity and Cancer: An update of the global impact. Cancer Epidemiol. 2016 Apr;41:8-15. doi: 10.1016/j.canep.2016.01.003. Epub 2016 Jan 14. PMID: 26775081.

228. Lim Y, Boster J. Obesity and Comorbid Conditions. 2021 Oct 25. In: StatPearls [Internet]. Treasure Island (FL): StatPearls Publishing; 2022 Jan–. PMID: 34662049.

229. Ritchie and Max Roser (2018) - "Causes of death." Published online at OurWorldInData.org. Retrieved from: 'https://ourworldindata.org/causes-of-death' [Online Resource].

230. Lauby-Secretan B, Scoccianti C, Loomis D, Grosse Y, Bianchini F, Straif K. Body fatness and Cancer—viewpoint of the IARC Working Group. N Engl J Med 2016;375:794–8.

231. Iyengar N, Kochhar A, Morris P, Zhou XK, Ghossein RA, Pino A, Mg F, Pfster DG, Patel SG, Boyle JO, Hudis CA, Dannenber AJ. Impact of obesity on survival of patients in early stage squamous cell carcinoma of the oral tongue. Cancer. 2014 doi: 10.1002/cncr.28532 [Epub ahead of print].

232. Berger NA. Cancer: Obesity-associated gastrointestinal tract Cancer, from beginning to end. Cancer. 2014 doi: 10.1002/cncr.28534.

233. Kyrgiou M, Kalliala I, Markozannes G, Gunter MJ, Paraskevaidis E, Gabra H, Martin-Hirsch P, Tsilidis KK. Adiposity and Cancer at major anatomical sites: umbrella review of the literature. BMJ. 2017 Feb 28;356:j477. doi: 10.1136/bmj.j477. PMID: 28246088; PMCID: PMC5421437.

234. Petrelli F, Cortellini A, Indini A, et al. Association of Obesity With Survival Outcomes in Patients With Cancer: A Systematic Review and Meta-analysis. JAMA Netw Open. 2021;4(3):e213520. doi:10.1001/jamanetworkopen.2021.3520.

235. Lennon, H., Sperrin, M., Badrick, E. et al. The Obesity Paradox in Cancer: a Review. Curr Oncol Rep 18, 56 (2016). https://doi.org/10.1007/s11912-016-0539-4.

236. *Othman EM, Leyh A, Stopper H. Insulin mediated DNA damage in mammalian colon cells and human lymphocytes in vitro. Mutat Res 2013;745-746:34–9.*

237. *Crosbie EJ, Zwahlen M, Kitchener HC, Egger M, Renehan AG. Body mass index, hormone replacement therapy, and endometrial Cancer risk: a meta-analysis. Cancer Epidemiol Biomark Prev 2010;19:3119–30.*

238. *Key TJ, Appleby P.N, Reeves GK, Roddam A, Dorgan JF, Longcope C, et al. Body mass index, serum sex hormones, and breast Cancer risk in postmenopausal women. J Natl Cancer Inst 2003;95:1218–26.*

239. *Zeleniuch-Jacquotte A, Afanasyeva Y, Kaaks R, Rinaldi S, Scarmo S, Liu M, et al.Premenopausal serum androgens and breast Cancer risk: a nested case-control study. Breast Cancer Res 2012;14:R32.*

240. *Dalamaga M, Diakopoulos KN, Mantzoros CS. The role of adiponectin in Cancer: a review of current evidence. Endocr Rev 2012;33:547–94.*

241. *Deng T, Lyon CJ, Bergin S, Caligiuri MA, Hsueh WA. Obesity, Inflammation, and Cancer. Annu Rev Pathol. 2016 May 23;11:421-49. doi: 10.1146/annurev-pathol-012615-044359. PMID: 27193454.*

242. *Goran MI, Alderete TL. Targeting adipose tissue inflammation to treat the underlying basis of the metabolic complications of obesity. Nestle Nutr Inst Workshop Ser. 2012;73:49-60; discussion p61-6. doi: 10.1159/000341287. Epub 2012 Oct 29. PMID: 23128765; PMCID: PMC4439096.*

243. *Himbert C, Delphan M, Scherer D, Bowers LW, Hursting S, Ulrich CM. Signals from the Adipose Microenvironment and the Obesity-Cancer Link-A Systematic Review. Cancer Prev Res (Phila). 2017 Sep;10(9):494-506. doi: 10.1158/1940-6207.CAPR-16-0322. PMID: 28864539; PMCID: PMC5898450.*

244. *Song M, Chan AT, Sun J. Influence of the Gut Microbiome, Diet, and Environment on Risk of Colorectal Cancer. Gastroenterology. 2020 Jan;158(2):322-340. doi: 10.1053/j.gastro.2019.06.048. Epub 2019 Oct 3. PMID: 31586566; PMCID: PMC6957737.*

245. *Sánchez-Alcoholado L, Ordóñez R, Otero A, Plaza-Andrade I, Laborda-Illanes A, Medina JA, Ramos-Molina B, Gómez-Millán J, Queipo-Ortuño MI. Gut Microbiota-Mediated Inflammation and Gut Permeability in Patients with Obesity and Colorectal Cancer. Int J Mol Sci. 2020 Sep 16;21(18):6782.*

246. *Loo TM, Kamachi F, Watanabe Y, Yoshimoto S, Kanda H, Arai Y, Nakajima-Takagi Y, Iwama A, Koga T, Sugimoto Y, Ozawa T, Nakamura M, Kumagai M, Watashi K, Taketo MM, Aoki T, Narumiya S, Oshima M, Arita M, Hara E, Ohtani N. Gut Microbiota Promotes Obesity-Associated Liver Cancer through PGE2-Mediated Suppression of Antitumor Immunity. Cancer Discov. 2017 May;7(5):522-538. doi: 10.1158/2159-8290.CD-16-0932. Epub 2017 Feb 15. PMID: 28202625.doi: 10.3390/ijms21186782. PMID: 32947866; PMCID: PMC7555154.*

247. *Lv J, Guo L, Liu JJ, Zhao HP, Zhang J, Wang JH. Alteration of the esophageal microbiota in Barrett's esophagus and esophageal adenocarcinoma. World J Gastroenterol. 2019 May 14;25(18):2149-2161. doi: 10.3748/wjg.v25.i18.2149. PMID: 31143067; PMCID: PMC6526156.*

248. *Uhlenhopp DJ, Then EO, Sunkara T, Gaduputi V. Epidemiology of esophageal Cancer: update in global trends, etiology and risk factors. Clin J Gastroenterol. 2020 Dec;13(6):1010-1021. doi: 10.1007/s12328-020-01237-x. Epub 2020 Sep 23. PMID: 32965635.*

249. Elliott JA, Reynolds JV. Visceral Obesity, Metabolic Syndrome, and Esophageal Adenocarcinoma. Front Oncol. 2021 Mar 12;11:627270. doi: 10.3389/fonc.2021.627270. PMID: 33777773; PMCID: PMC7994523.

250. Ma C, Avenell A, Bolland M, Hudson J, Stewart F, Robertson C, Sharma P, Fraser C, MacLennan G. Effects of weight loss interventions for adults who are obese on mortality, cardiovascular disease, and Cancer: systematic review and meta-analysis. BMJ. 2017 Nov 14;359:j4849. doi: 10.1136/bmj.j4849. PMID: 29138133; PMCID: PMC5682593.

251. Chlebowski RT, Luo J, Anderson GL, Barrington W, Reding K, Simon MS, Manson JE, Rohan TE, Wactawski-Wende J, Lane D, Strickler H, Mosaver-Rahmani Y, Freudenheim JL, Saquib N, Stefanick ML. Weight loss and breast Cancer incidence in postmenopausal women. Cancer. 2019 Jan 15;125(2):205-212. doi: 10.1002/cncr.31687. Epub 2018 Oct 8. PMID: 30294816; PMCID: PMC6890496.

252. Zhang X, Rhoades J, Caan BJ, Cohn DE, Salani R, Noria S, Suarez AA, Paskett ED, Felix AS. Intentional weight loss, weight cycling, and endometrial Cancer risk: a systematic review and meta-analysis. Int J Gynecol Cancer. 2019 Nov;29(9):1361-1371. doi: 10.1136/ijgc-2019-000728. Epub 2019 Aug 26. PMID: 31451560; PMCID: PMC6832748.Ritchie and Max Roser (2017) - "Obesity." Published online at OurWorldInData.org. Retrieved from: 'https://ourworldindata.org/obesity'[Online Resource]

253. Look AHEAD Research Group, Yeh HC, Bantle JP, Cassidy-Begay M, et al. Intensive Weight Loss Intervention and Cancer Risk in Adults with Type 2 Diabetes: Analysis of the Look AHEAD Randomized Clinical Trial. Obesity (Silver Spring). 2020 Sep;28(9):1678-1686. doi: 10.1002/oby.22936. PMID: 32841523; PMCID: PMC8855671.

254. O'Brien PE, Hindle A, Brennan L, Skinner S, Burton P, Smith A, Crosthwaite G, Brown W. Long-Term Outcomes After Bariatric Surgery: a Systematic Review and Meta-analysis of Weight Loss at 10 or More Years for All Bariatric Procedures and a Single-Centre Review of 20-Year Outcomes After Adjustable Gastric Banding. Obes Surg. 2019 Jan;29(1):3-14. doi: 10.1007/s11695-018-3525-0. PMID: 30293134; PMCID: PMC6320354.

255. Schauer DP, Arterburn DE, Livingston EH, Coleman KJ, Sidney S, Fisher D, O'Connor P, Fischer D, Eckman MH. Impact of bariatric surgery on life expectancy in severely obese patients with diabetes: a decision analysis. Ann Surg. 2015 May;261(5):914-9. doi: 10.1097/SLA.0000000000000907. PMID: 25844968; PMCID: PMC4388039.

256. Carlsson LMS, Sjöholm K, Jacobson P, Andersson-Assarsson JC, Svensson PA, Taube M, Carlsson B, Peltonen M. Life Expectancy after Bariatric Surgery in the Swedish Obese Subjects Study. N Engl J Med. 2020 Oct 15;383(16):1535-1543. doi: 10.1056/NEJMoa2002449. PMID: 33053284; PMCID: PMC7580786.

257. Byers T, Sedjo RL. Does intentional weight loss reduce Cancer risk? Diabetes Obes Metab. 2011 Dec;13(12):1063-72. doi: 10.1111/j.1463-1326.2011.01464.x. PMID: 21733057.

258. Luo J, Hendryx M, Manson JE, Figueiredo JC, LeBlanc ES, Barrington W, Rohan TE, Howard BV, Reding K, Ho GY, Garcia DO, Chlebowski RT. Intentional Weight Loss and Obesity-Related Cancer Risk. JNCI Cancer Spectr. 2019 Aug 9;3(4):pkz054. doi: 10.1093/jncics/pkz054. PMID: 31737862; PMCID: PMC6795232.

259. Ashrafian H, Ahmed K, Rowland SP, Patel VM, Gooderham NJ, Holmes E, et al. . Metabolic surgery and Cancer: protective effects of bariatric procedures. Cancer. (2011) 117:1788–99.

260. Deng T, Lyon CJ, Bergin S, Caligiuri MA, Hsueh WA. Obesity, inflammation, and Cancer. Annu Rev Pathol. (2016) 11:421–49.

261. Kim S, Karin M. Role of TLR2-dependent inflammation in metastatic progression. Ann N Y Acad Sci. (2011) 1217:191–206.

262. Pollak M. Insulin and insulin-like growth factor signaling in neoplasia. Nat Rev Cancer. (2008) 8:915–28.

263. Tsugane S, Inoue M. Insulin resistance and Cancer: epidemiological evidence. Cancer Sci. (2010) 101:1073–9.

264. Sjöholm K, Carlsson LMS, Svensson PA, Andersson-Assarsson JC, Kristensson F, Jacobson P, Peltonen M, Taube M. Association of Bariatric Surgery With Cancer Incidence in Patients With Obesity and Diabetes: Long-term Results From the Swedish Obese Subjects Study. Diabetes Care. 2022 Feb 1;45(2):444-450.

265. Ishihara BP, Farah D, Fonseca MCM, Nazario A. The risk of developing breast, ovarian, and endometrial Cancer in obese women submitted to bariatric surgery: a meta-analysis. Surg Obes Relat Dis. 2020 Oct;16(10):1596-1602.

266. Schauer DP, Feigelson HS, Koebnick C, Caan B, Weinmann S, Leonard AC, Powers JD, Yenumula PR, Arterburn DE. Bariatric Surgery and the Risk of Cancer in a Large Multisite Cohort. Ann Surg. 2019 Jan;269(1):95-101.

267. H Mackenzie, S R Markar, A Askari, O Faiz, M Hull, S Purkayastha, H Møller, J Lagergren, Obesity surgery and risk of Cancer, British Journal of Surgery, Volume 105, Issue 12, November 2018, Pages 1650–1657.

268. Wiggins T, Antonowicz SS, Markar SR. Cancer Risk Following Bariatric Surgery-Systematic Review and Meta-analysis of National Population-Based Cohort Studies. Obes Surg. 2019 Mar;29(3):1031-1039. doi: 10.1007/s11695-018-3501-8. PMID: 30591985.

269. Sjostrom L, Gummesson A, Sjostrom CD, et al. Effects of bariatric surgery on Cancer incidence in obese patients in Sweden (Swedish Obese Subjects Study): a prospective, controlled intervention trial. Lancet Oncol 2009;10:653-62.

270. Adams TD, Stroup AM, Gress RE, et al. Cancer incidence and mortality after gastric bypass surgery. Obesity (Silver Spring) 2009;17:796-802.

271. Sebastianelli L, Benois M, Vanbiervliet G, Bailly L, Robert M, Turrin N, Gizard E, Foletto M, Bisello M, Albanese A, Santonicola A, Iovino P, Piche T, Angrisani L, Turchi L, Schiavo L, Iannelli A. Systematic Endoscopy 5 Years After Sleeve Gastrectomy Results in a High Rate of Barrett's Esophagus: Results of a Multicenter Study. Obes Surg. 2019 May;29(5):1462-1469. doi: 10.1007/s11695-019-03704-y. PMID: 30666544.

272. Genco A, Soricelli E, Casella G, Maselli R, Castagneto-Gissey L, Di Lorenzo N, Basso N. Gastroesophageal reflux disease and Barrett's esophagus after laparoscopic sleeve gastrectomy: a possible, underestimated long-term complication. Surg Obes Relat Dis. 2017 Apr;13(4):568-574. doi: 10.1016/j.soard.2016.11.029. Epub 2016 Dec 9. PMID: 28089434.

273. Plat VD, Kasteleijn A, Greve JWM, Luyer MDP, Gisbertz SS, Demirkiran A, Daams F. Esophageal Cancer After Bariatric Surgery: Increasing Prevalence and Treatment Strategies. Obes Surg. 2021 Nov;31(11):4954-4962. doi: 10.1007/s11695-021-05679-1. Epub 2021 Sep 7. PMID: 34494230; PMCID: PMC8490213.

274. *Musella M, Berardi G, Bocchetti A, Green R, Cantoni V, Velotti N, et al. . Esophagogastric neoplasms following bariatric surgery: an updated systematic review. Obes Surg. (2019) 29:2660–9. 10.1007/s11695-019-03951-z*

275. *Sebastianelli L, Benois M, Vanbiervliet G, Bailly L, Robert M, Turrin N. Systematic endoscopy 5 years after sleeve gastrectomy results in a high rate of barrett's esophagus: results of a multicenter study. Obes Surg. (2019) 29:1462–9. 10.1007/s11695-019-03704-y*

276. *Bailly L, Fabre R, Pradier C, Iannelli A. Colorectal Cancer Risk Following Bariatric Surgery in a Nationwide Study of French Individuals With Obesity. JAMA Surg. 2020 May 1;155(5):395-402. doi: 10.1001/jamasurg.2020.0089. PMID: 32159744; PMCID: PMC7066530.*

277. *Taube M, Peltonen M, Sjöholm K, Palmqvist R, Andersson-Assarsson JC, Jacobson P, Svensson PA, Carlsson LMS. Long-term incidence of colorectal Cancer after bariatric surgery or usual care in the Swedish Obese Subjects study. PLoS One. 2021 Mar 25;16(3):e0248550. doi: 10.1371/journal.pone.0248550. PMID: 33764991; PMCID: PMC7993847.*

278. *Ciccioriccio MC, Iossa A, Boru CE, De Angelis F, Termine P, Giuffrè M, Silecchia G; CRIC-ABS 2020 GROUP. Colorectal Cancer after bariatric surgery (Cric-Abs 2020): Sicob (Italian society of obesity surgery) endorsed national survey. Int J Obes (Lond). 2021 Dec;45(12):2527-2531. doi: 10.1038/s41366-021-00910-6. Epub 2021 Jul 19. PMID: 34282268.*

279. *Almazeedi S, El-Abd R, Al-Khamis A, Albatineh AN, Al-Sabah S. Role of bariatric surgery in reducing the risk of colorectal Cancer: a meta-analysis. Br J Surg. 2020 Mar;107(4):348-354. doi: 10.1002/bjs.11494. Epub 2020 Jan 24. PMID: 31976551.*

280. *Bruno DS, Berger NA. Impact of bariatric surgery on Cancer risk reduction. Ann Transl Med. 2020 Mar;8(Suppl 1):S13. doi: 10.21037/atm.2019.09.26. PMID: 32309417; PMCID: PMC7154324.*

281. *Tee MC, Cao Y, Warnock GL, Hu FB, Chavarro JE. Effect of bariatric surgery on oncologic outcomes: a systematic review and meta-analysis. Surg Endosc. 2013 Dec;27(12):4449-56. doi: 10.1007/s00464-013-3127-9. Epub 2013 Aug 16. PMID: 23949484; PMCID: PMC4018832.*

Chapter 16

282. *Egiziano G, Bernatsky S, Shah AA Cancer and autoimmunity: Harnessing longitudinal cohorts to probe the link. Best Pract Res Clin Rheumatol. 2016;30.*

283. *Afferni, C., Buccione, C., Andreone, S., Galdiero, M. R., Varricchi, G., Marone, G., et al. (2018). The Pleiotropic immunomodulatory functions of IL-33 and its implications in tumour immunity. Front. Immunol. 9:2601. doi: 10.3389/fimmu.2018.02601.*

284. *Carsons S The association of malignancy with rheumatic and connective tissue diseases. Semin Oncol. 1997;24(3):360.*

285. *Balkwill F, Mantovani A. Inflammation and cancer: back to Virchow Lancet. 2001;357(9255):539–545. Simon TA, Thompson A, Gandhi KK, et al.: Incidence of malignancy in adult patients with rheumatoid arthritis: a meta-analysis, Arthritis Res Ther 17:212, 2015.*

286. *Franklin J, Lunt M, Bunn D, et al.: Incidence of lymphoma in a large primary care derived cohort of cases of inflammatory polyarthritis, Ann Rheum Dis 65:617, 2006.*

Gridley G, Klippel JH, Hoover RN, et al.: Incidence of cancer among men with Felty syndrome, Ann Intern Med 120:35, 1994.

287. Franklin J, Lunt M, Bunn D, et al.: Incidence of lymphoma in a large primary care derived cohort of cases of inflammatory polyarthritis, Ann Rheum Dis 65:617, 2006.

288. Gridley G, Klippel JH, Hoover RN, et al.: Incidence of cancer among men with Felty syndrome, Ann Intern Med 120:35, 1994.

289. Bernatsky S et al., Cancer risk in systemic lupus: an updated international multi-centre cohort study. J Autoimmun. 2013 May;42:130-5. Epub 2013 Feb 12.

290. Gayed M, Bernatsky S, Ramsey-Goldman R, et al.: Lupus and cancer, Lupus 18:479, 2009.

291. Dreyer L, Faurschou M, Mogensen M, Jacobsen S. High incidence of potentially virus-induced malignancies in systemic lupus erythematosus: a long-term follow-up study in a Danish cohort. Arthritis Rheum. 2011;63(10):3032–3037.

292. Goobie GC, Bernatsky S, Ramsey-Goldman R, Clarke AE. Malignancies in systemic lupus erythematosus: a 2015 update. Curr Opin Rheumatol. 2015;27(5):454–460.

293. Giannouli S, Voulgarelis M Predicting progression to lymphoma in Sjögren's syndrome patients. Expert Rev Clin Immunol. 2014 Apr;10(4):501-12

294. Derk CT, Rasheed M, Artlett CM, et al.: A cohort study of cancer incidence in systemic sclerosis, J Rheumatol 33:1113, 2006.

295. Bobba RK, Holly JS, Loy T, Perry MC. Scar carcinoma of the lung: a historical perspective. Clin Lung Cancer. 2011;12(3):148–154.

296. Fardet L, Dupuy A, Gain M, et al.: Factors associated with underlying malignancy in a retrospective cohort of 121 patients with dermatomyositis, Medicine 88:91, 2009.

297. Chang C-C, Chang C-W, Nguyen P-AA, et al.: Anklyosing spondylitis and the risk of cancer, Oncology Let 14:1315, 2017.

298. Shah AA, Casciola-Rosen L, Rosen A. Review: cancer-induced autoimmunity in the rheumatic diseases. Arthritis Rheumatol. 2015;67(2):317–326.

299. Shah AA, Rosen A, Hummers L, Wigley F, Casciola-Rosen L. Close temporal relationship between onset of cancer and scleroderma in patients with RNA polymerase I/III antibodies. Arthritis and rheumatism. 2010;62(9):2787–2795.

300. Houghton AN (1994) Cancer antigens: immune recognition of self and altered self. J Exp Med 180:1–4

301. Ernest Maningding, Tanaz A Karmani. Mimics of vasculitis Rheumatology, Volume 60, Issue 1, January 2021, Pages 34–47

302. Podjasek JO, Wetter DA, Pittelkow MR, Wada DA Cutaneous small-vessel vasculitis associated with solid organ malignancies: the Mayo Clinic experience, 1996 to 2009. J Am Acad Dermatol. 2012;66(2)

303. Lakhanpal S, Ginsburg WW, Michet CJ, Doyle JA, Moore SB Eosinophilic fasciitis: clinical spectrum and therapeutic response in 52 cases. Semin Arthritis Rheum. 1988;17(4):221.

304. Ehrenfeld M, Gur H, Shoenfeld Y Rheumatologic features of hematologic disorders. Curr Opin Rheumatol. 1999;11(1):62.

305. Georgescu L, Quinn GC, Schwartzman S, et al.: Lymphoma in patients with rheumatoid arthritis: association with the disease state or methotrexate treatment, Semin Arthritis Rheum 26:794, 1997.

306. Silman AJ, Petrie J, Hazleman B, et al.: Lymphoproliferative cancer and other malignancy in patients with rheumatoid arthritis treated with azathioprine: a 20-year follow-up study, Ann RheumDis 47:988, 1988.

307. Faurschou M, Sorensen IJ, Mellemkjaer L, Loft AG, Thomsen BS, Tvede N, et al. Malignancies in Wegener's granulomatosis: incidence and relation to cyclophosphamide therapy in a cohort of 293 patients. J Rheumatol. 2008;35(1):100–105.

308. Crane GM, Powell H, Kostadinov R, Rocafort PT, Rifkin DE, Burger PC, et al. Primary CNS lymphoproliferative disease, mycophenolate and calcineurin inhibitor usage. Oncotarget. 2015;6(32):33849–33866.

309. Alias A, Rodriguez EJ, Bateman HE, Sterrett AG, Valeriano-Marcet J. Rheumatology and oncology: an updated review of rheumatic manifestations of malignancy and anti-neoplastic therapy. Bull NYU Hosp Jt Dis. 2012;70(2):109–114.

310. Kostine M et al. Rheumatic disorders associated with immune checkpoint inhibitors in patients with cancer-clinical aspects and relationship with tumor response: a single-centre prospective cohort study. Ann Rheum Dis. 2018;77(3):393.

311. arga J, Haustein UF, Creech RH, Dwyer JP, Jimenez SA. Exaggerated radiation-induced fibrosis in patients with systemic sclerosis. JAMA. 1991;265(24):3292–3295.

Chapter 17

312. Meyskens Jr, F. L., Mukhtar, H., Rock, C. L., Cuzick, J., Kensler, T. W., Yang, C. S., … Alberts, D. S. (2016). Cancer Prevention: Obstacles, Challenges, and the Road Ahead. JNCI: Journal of the National Cancer Institute, 108(2), djv309.

313. https://doi.org/10.1093/jnci/djv309 Colditz, G. A., Sellers, T. A., & Trapido, E. (2006). Epidemiology — identifying the causes and preventability of cancer? Nature Reviews Cancer, 6(1), 75–83. https://doi.org/10.1038/nrc1784.

314. Prevention.

(Cancer control : knowledge into action : WHO guide for effective programmes ; module 2.)1.Neoplasms – prevention and control. 2.Health planning. 3.National health programs – organization and administration. 4.Health policy. 5.Guidelines. I.World Health Organization. II.Series. ISBN 92 4 154711 1 (NLM classification: QZ 200)

315. IARC Handbooks for cancer prevention -Preamble for primary prevention -2019.

316. https://edrn.nci.nih.gov/about-edrn/five-phase-approach-and-prospective-specimen-collection-retrospective-blinded-evaluation-study-design/.

317. https://www.cancer.gov/about-cancer/causes-prevention/hp-prevention-overview-pdq.

318. NATIONAL CANCER GRID (NCG) OF INDIA TATA MEMORIAL CENTER Consensus Evidence Based Resource Stratified Guidelines on Secondary prevention of Cervical, Breast & Oral Cancers NCG WORKING GROUP Resource Stratified guidelines for Preventive Oncology and Primary Care.

Chapter 18

319. Sung H, Ferlay J, Siegel RL, et al. Global Cancer Statistics 2020: GLOBOCAN Estimates of Incidence and Mortality Worldwide for 36 Cancers in 185 Countries. CA Cancer J Clin. 2021;71(3):209-249. doi:10.3322/caac.21660

320. Bodicoat, D.H., Schoemaker, M.J., Jones, M.E. et al. Timing of pubertal stages and breast cancer risk: the Breakthrough Generations Study. Breast Cancer Res 16, R18 (2014). https://doi.org/10.1186/bcr3613

321. Colditz GA, Baer HJ, Tamimi RM. Breast cancer. In: Schottenfeld D, Fraumeni JF, editors. Cancer Epidemiology and Prevention. 3rd ed. New York: Oxford University Press, 2006.

322. Russo J, Moral R, Balogh GA, Mailo D, Russo IH. The protective role of pregnancy in breast cancer. Breast Cancer Res. 2005;7(3):131-142. doi:10.1186/bcr1029

323. Britt K, Ashworth A, Smalley M. Pregnancy and the risk of breast cancer. Endocr Relat Cancer. 2007;14(4):907-933. doi:10.1677/ERC-07-0137

324. Ewertz M, Duffy SW, Adami HO, et al. Age at first birth, parity and risk of breast cancer: a meta-analysis of 8 studies from the Nordic countries. Int J Cancer. 1990;46(4):597-603. doi:10.1002/ijc.2910460408

325. Benz CC. Impact of aging on the biology of breast cancer. Crit Rev Oncol Hematol. 2008;66(1):65-74. doi:10.1016/j.critrevonc.2007.09.001

326. Nagrani R, Mhatre S, Rajaraman P, et al. Central obesity increases risk of breast cancer irrespective of menopausal and hormonal receptor status in women of South Asian Ethnicity. Eur J Cancer. 2016;66:153-161. doi:10.1016/j.ejca.2016.07.022

327. Lee CI, Chen LE, Elmore JG. Risk-based Breast Cancer Screening: Implications of Breast Density. Med Clin North Am. 2017;101(4):725-741. doi:10.1016/j.mcna.2017.03.005

328. Trentham-Dietz A, Newcomb PA, Nichols HB, Hampton JM. Breast cancer risk factors and second primary malignancies among women with breast cancer. Breast Cancer Res Treat. 2007;105(2):195-207. doi:10.1007/s10549-006-9446-y

329. Kurian AW, McClure LA, John EM, Horn-Ross PL, Ford JM, Clarke CA. Second primary breast cancer occurrence according to hormone receptor status. J Natl Cancer Inst. 2009;101(15):1058-1065. doi:10.1093/jnci/djp181

330. Bernstein JL, Thompson WD, Risch N, Holford TR. Risk factors predicting the incidence of second primary breast cancer among women diagnosed with a first primary breast cancer. Am J Epidemiol. 1992;136(8):925-936. doi:10.1093/oxfordjournals.aje.a116565

331. Miller ME, Muhsen S, Olcese C, Patil S, Morrow M, Van Zee KJ. Contralateral Breast Cancer Risk in Women with Ductal Carcinoma In Situ: Is it High Enough to Justify Bilateral Mastectomy?. Ann Surg Oncol. 2017;24(10):2889-2897. doi:10.1245/s10434-017-5931-2

332. Reiner AS, Lynch CF, Sisti JS, et al. Hormone receptor status of a first primary breast cancer predicts contralateral breast cancer risk in the WECARE study population. Breast Cancer Res. 2017;19(1):83. Published 2017 Jul 19. doi:10.1186/s13058-017-0874-x

333. Early Breast Cancer Trialists' Collaborative Group (EBCTCG). Effects of chemotherapy and hormonal therapy for early breast cancer on recurrence and 15-year survival: an overview of the randomised trials. Lancet. 2005;365(9472):1687-1717. doi:10.1016/S0140-6736(05)66544-0.

334. Kim SY, Cho N, Kim SY, et al. Supplemental Breast US Screening in Women with a Personal History of Breast Cancer: A Matched Cohort Study. Radiology. 2020;295(1):54-63. doi:10.1148/radiol.2020191691.

335. American Cancer Society. Breast Cancer Facts & Figures 2019-2020. Atlanta, Ga: American Cancer Society; 2019.

336. Singletary SE. Rating the risk factors for breast cancer. Ann Surg. 2003;237(4):474-482. doi:10.1097/01.SLA.0000059969.64262.87

337. Apostolou P, Fostira F. Hereditary breast cancer: the era of new susceptibility genes. Biomed Res Int. 2013;2013:747318. doi:10.1155/2013/747318

338. Armstrong, N., Ryder, S., Forbes, C., Ross, J., & Quek, R. G. (2019). A systematic review of the international prevalence of BRCA mutation in breast cancer. Clinical epidemiology, 11, 543. 10.2147/CLEP.S206949

339. Pathology of familial breast cancer: differences between breast cancers in carriers of BRCA1 or BRCA2 mutations and sporadic cases. Breast Cancer Linkage Consortium. Lancet. 1997;349(9064):1505-1510.

340. Collins A, Politopoulos I. The genetics of breast cancer: risk factors for disease. Appl Clin Genet. 2011;4:11-19. Published 2011 Jan 7. doi:10.2147/TACG.S13139

341. Greene MH. Genetics of breast cancer. Mayo Clin Proc. 1997;72(1):54-65. doi:10.4065/72.1.54

342. Snoj T. Hormones in Food as a Potential Risk for Human Reproductive and Health Disorders. Acta Veterinaria. 2019;69(2): 137-152. https://doi.org/10.2478/acve-2019-0011.

343. Ye H, Shaw IC. Food flavonoid ligand structure/estrogen receptor-a affinity relationships - toxicity or food functionality?. Food Chem Toxicol. 2019;129:328-336. doi:10.1016/j.fct.2019.04.008

344. Bao, P. P. et al. Fruit, vegetable, and animal food intake and breast cancer risk by hormone receptor status. Nutr. Cancer 64, 806–819 (2012).

345. Farvid, M. S. et al. Fruit and vegetable consumption in adolescence and early adulthood and risk of breast cancer: Population based cohort study. BMJ 353, 1–12 (2016).

346. Guo, J., Wei, W. & Zhan, L. Red and processed meat intake and risk of breast cancer: a meta-analysis of prospective studies. Breast Cancer Res. Treat. 151,191–198(2015).

347. Brinkman, M. T. et al. Consumption of animal products, their nutrient components and post-menopausal circulating steroid hormone concentrations. Eur. J. Clin. Nutr. 64, 176–183 (2010).

348. Shin, M. H. et al. Intake of dairy products, calcium, and vitamin D and risk of breast cancer. J. Natl. Cancer Inst. 94, 1301–1311 (2002).

349. Al Sarakbi, W., M. Salhab, and K. Mokbel, Dairy products and breast cancer risk: a review of the literature. Int J Fertil Womens Med, 2005. 50(6): p. 244-9

350. de Cabo, R., & Mattson, M. P. (2019). Effects of Intermittent Fasting on Health, Aging, and Disease. The New England journal of medicine, 381(26), 2541–2551.

351. Raffaghello, L. et al. (2008) Starvation-dependent differential stress resistance protects normal but not cancer cells against high-dose chemotherapy. Proc. Natl. Acad. Sci. U. S. A. 105, 8215–8220

352. Galluzzi L, Baehrecke EH, Ballabio A, Boya P, Bravo-San Pedro JM, Cecconi F, et al. Molecular definitions of autophagy and related processes. EMBO J. 2017;36(13):1811-36

353. Bernstein L, Henderson BE, Hanisch R, Sullivan-Halley J, Ross RK. Physical exercise and reduced risk of breast cancer in young women. J Natl Cancer Inst. 1994;86(18):1403-1408. doi:10.1093/jnci/86.18.1403

354. McTiernan A, Kooperberg C, White E, et al. Recreational physical activity and the risk of breast cancer in postmenopausal women: the Women's Health Initiative Cohort Study. JAMA. 2003;290(10):1331-1336. doi:10.1001/jama.290.10.1331

355. Warren MP. The effects of exercise on pubertal progression and reproductive function in girls. J Clin Endocrinol Metab. 1980;51(5):1150-1157. doi:10.1210/jcem-51-5-1150

356. Collaborative Group on Hormonal Factors in Breast Cancer. Breast cancer and hormonal contraceptives: collaborative reanalysis of individual data on 53 297 women with breast cancer and 100 239 women without breast cancer from 54 epidemiological studies. Lancet. 1996;347(9017):1713-1727. doi:10.1016/s0140-6736(96)90806-5.

357. Kumle M, Weiderpass E, Braaten T, Persson I, Adami HO, Lund E. Use of oral contraceptives and breast cancer risk: The Norwegian-Swedish Women's Lifestyle and Health Cohort Study. Cancer Epidemiol Biomarkers Prev. 2002;11(11):1375-1381.

358. Kawai M, Malone KE, Tang MT, Li CI. Active smoking and the risk of estrogen receptor-positive and triple-negative breast cancer among women ages 20 to 44 years. Cancer. 2014;120(7):1026-1034. doi:10.1002/cncr.28402

359. Xue, Fei & Willett, Walter & Rosner, Bernard & Hankinson, Susan & Michels, Karin. (2011). Cigarette Smoking and the Incidence of Breast Cancer. Archives of internal medicine. 171. 125-33. 10.1001/archinternmed.2010.503.

360. Terry MB, Zhang FF, Kabat G, et al. Lifetime alcohol intake and breast cancer risk. Ann Epidemiol. 2006;16(3):230-240. doi:10.1016/j.annepidem.2005.06.048

361. Hamajima N, Hirose K, Tajima K, et al. Alcohol, tobacco and breast cancer--collaborative reanalysis of individual data from 53 epidemiological studies, including 58,515 women with breast cancer and 95,067 women without the disease. Br J Cancer. 2002;87(11):1234-1245. doi:10.1038/sj.bjc.6600596

362. Seitz HK, Pelucchi C, Bagnardi V, La Vecchia C. Epidemiology and pathophysiology of alcohol and breast cancer: Update 2012. Alcohol Alcohol. 2012;47(3):204-212. doi:10.1093/alcalc/ags011

363. Hirko KA, Chen WY, Willett WC, et al. Alcohol consumption and risk of breast cancer by molecular subtype: Prospective analysis of the nurses' health study after 26 years of follow-up. Int J Cancer. 2016;138(5):1094-1101. doi:10.1002/ijc.29861

364. Shaukat N, Jaleel F, Moosa FA, Qureshi NA. Association between Vitamin D deficiency and Breast Cancer. Pak J Med Sci. 2017;33(3):645-649. doi:10.12669/pjms.333.11753

365. Köstner K, Denzer N, Müller CS, Klein R, Tilgen W, Reichrath J. The relevance of vitamin D receptor (VDR) gene polymorphisms for cancer: a review of the literature. Anticancer Res. 2009;29(9):3511-3536.

366. Goodwin PJ, Ennis M, Pritchard KI, Koo J, Hood N. Prognostic effects of 25-hydroxyvitamin D levels in early breast cancer. J Clin Oncol. 2009;27(23):3757-3763. doi:10.1200/JCO.2008.20.0725

367. Shin MH, Holmes MD, Hankinson SE, Wu K, Colditz GA, Willett WC. Intake of dairy products, calcium, and vitamin d and risk of breast cancer. J Natl Cancer Inst. 2002;94(17):1301-1311.

doi:10.1093/jnci/94.17.1301

368. Zhang SM, Willett WC, Selhub J, et al. *Plasma folate, vitamin B6, vitamin B12, homocysteine, and risk of breast cancer. J Natl Cancer Inst. 2003;95(5):373-380. doi:10.1093/jnci/95.5.373*

369. Wu K, Helzlsouer KJ, Comstock GW, Hoffman SC, Nadeau MR, Selhub J. *A prospective study on folate, B12, and pyridoxal 5'-phosphate (B6) and breast cancer. Cancer Epidemiol Biomarkers Prev. 1999;8(3):209-217.*

370. Matejcic M, de Batlle J, Ricci C, et al. *Biomarkers of folate and vitamin B12 and breast cancer risk: report from the EPIC cohort. Int J Cancer. 2017;140(6):1246-1259. doi:10.1002/ijc.30536*

371. Gray S. *Breast cancer and hormone-replacement therapy: The million women study. Lancet 2003;362:1332.*

372. Feig, B. W., & Ching, C. D. (2018). *The MD Anderson surgical oncology handbook, sixth edition. Wolters Kluwer Health Adis (ESP).*

373. Preston DL, Mattsson A, Holmberg E, Shore R, Hildreth NG, Boice JD Jr. *Radiation effects on breast cancer risk: a pooled analysis of eight cohorts [published correction appears in Radiat Res. 2002 Nov;158(5):666]. Radiat Res. 2002;158(2):220-235. doi:10.1667/0033-7587(2002)158[0220:reobcr]2.0.co;2*

374. Pijpe A, Andrieu N, Easton DF, et al. *Exposure to diagnostic radiation and risk of breast cancer among carriers of BRCA1/2 mutations: retrospective cohort study (GENE-RAD-RISK). BMJ. 2012;345:e5660. Published 2012 Sep 6. doi:10.1136/bmj.e5660*

375. Urbaniak C, Gloor GB, Brackstone M, Scott L, Tangney M, Reid G. *The microbiota of breast tissue and its association with breast cancer. Appl Environ Microbiol. (2016) 82:5039–48. doi: 10.1128/AEM.01235-16*

376. Suman S, Sharma PK, Rai G, et al. *Current perspectives of molecular pathways involved in chronic inflammation-mediated breast cancer. Biochem Biophys Res Commun. 2016;472(3):401-409. doi:10.1016/j.bbrc.2015.10.133*

377. Harper S, Lynch J, Meersman SC, Breen N, Davis WW, Reichman MC. *Trends in area-socioeconomic and race-ethnic disparities in breast cancer incidence, stage at diagnosis, screening, mortality, and survival among women ages 50 years and over (1987-2005). Cancer Epidemiol Biomarkers Prev. 2009;18(1):121-131. doi:10.1158/1055-9965.EPI-08-0679*

378. Li CI, Malone KE, Daling JR. *Differences in breast cancer hormone receptor status and histology by race and ethnicity among women 50 years of age and older. Cancer Epidemiol Biomarkers Prev. 2002;11(7):601-607.*

379. Sharma M, Sharma JD, Sarma A, et al. *Triple negative breast cancer in people of North East India: critical insights gained at a regional cancer centre. Asian Pac J Cancer Prev. 2014;15(11):4507-4511. doi:10.7314/apjcp.2014.15.11.4507.*

380. Priestman TJ, Priestman SG, Bradshaw C. *Stress and breast cancer. Br J Cancer. 1985;51(4):493-498. doi:10.1038/bjc.1985.71.*

381. Puertollano MA, Puertollano E, de Cienfuegos GÁ, de Pablo MA. *Dietary antioxidants: immunity and host defense. Curr Top Med Chem. 2011;11(14):1752-1766. doi:10.2174/156802611796235107.*

382. de Cabo, R., & Mattson, M. P. (2019). *Effects of Intermittent Fasting on Health, Aging, and Disease. The New England journal of medicine, 381(26), 2541–2551.*

383. Hewitt JA, Mokbel K, van Someren KA, Jewell AP, Garrod R. *Exercise for breast cancer survival: the effect on cancer risk and cancer-related fatigue (CRF). Int J Fertil Womens Med. 2005;50(5 Pt 1):231-239.*

384. Gopal, Aravind et al. "Effect of integrated yoga practices on immune responses in examination stress - A preliminary study." International journal of yoga vol. 4,1 (2011): 26-32. doi:10.4103/0973-6131.78178.

385. Shaukat N, Jaleel F, Moosa FA, Qureshi NA. Association between Vitamin D deficiency and Breast Cancer. Pak J Med Sci. 2017;33(3):645-649. doi:10.12669/pjms.333.11753.

386. Szyf M, Pakneshan P, Rabbani SA. DNA methylation and breast cancer. Biochem Pharmacol. 2004;68(6):1187-1197. doi:10.1016/j.bcp.2004.04.030.

387. Barak Y. The immune system and happiness. Autoimmun Rev. 2006;5(8):523-527. doi:10.1016/j.autrev.2006.02.010.

388. Besedovsky L, Lange T, Born J. Sleep and immune function. Pflugers Arch. 2012;463(1):121-137. doi:10.1007/s00424-011-1044-0.

Chapter 19

389. Andarieh MG, Delavar MA, Moslemi D, Ahmadi MH, Zabihi E, Esmaeilzadeh S. Infertility as a risk factor for breast cancer: Results from a hospital-based case-control study. Journal of Cancer Research and Therapeutics [Internet]. 2019 [cited 2023 Feb 8];15(5):976–80. Available from: https://pubmed.ncbi.nlm.nih.gov/31603097/ .

390. Barańska A, Błaszczuk A, Kanadys W, Malm M, Drop K, Polz-Dacewicz M. Oral Contraceptive Use and Breast Cancer Risk Assessment: A Systematic Review and Meta-Analysis of Case-Control Studies, 2009–2020. Cancers. 2021 Nov 12;13(22):5654.

391. Hall JM, Friedman L, Guenther C, Lee MK, Weber JL, Black DM, et al. Closing in on a breast cancer gene on chromosome 17q. American journal of human genetics [Internet]. 1992 [cited 2023 Feb 8];50(6):1235–42. Available from: https://www.ncbi.nlm.nih.gov/pmc/articles/PMC1682570/ .

392. Wooster R, Neuhausen S, Mangion J, Quirk Y, Ford D, Collins N, et al. Localization of a breast cancer susceptibility gene, BRCA2, to chromosome 13q12-13. Science. 1994 Sep 30;265(5181):2088–90.

393. Rojas K, Stuckey A. Breast Cancer Epidemiology and Risk Factors. Clinical Obstetrics and Gynecology [Internet]. 2016 Dec 1;59(4):651–72. Available from: https://insights.ovid.com/article/00003081-201612000-00003

394. HUNN J, RODRIGUEZ GC. Ovarian Cancer. Clinical Obstetrics and Gynecology. 2012 Mar;55(1):3–23.

395. Ali AT. Reproductive Factors and the Risk of Endometrial Cancer. International Journal of Gynecologic Cancer. 2014 Mar;24(3):384–93.

396. Collaborative Group on Hormonal Factors in Breast Cancer. Menarche, menopause, and Breast Cancer risk: Individual Participant meta-analysis, Including 118 964 Women with Breast Cancer from 117 Epidemiological Studies. The Lancet Oncology. 2012 Nov;13(11):1141–51.

397. Mikkelsen AP, Egerup P, Ebert JFM, Kolte AM, Nielsen HS, Lidegaard Ø. Pregnancy Loss and Cancer Risk: A Nationwide Observational Study. EClinicalMedicine [Internet]. 2019 Oct 9;15(2021 Nov 12;13(22):5654):80–8. Available from: https://www.ncbi.nlm.nih.gov/pmc/articles/PMC6833468/ .

398. Kuzhan A, Adli M. The Effect of Socio-Economic-Cultural Factors on Breast Cancer. The Journal of Breast Health. 2015 Jan 9;11(1):17–21.

399. Lee K, Kruper L, Dieli-Conwright CM, Mortimer JE. The Impact of Obesity on Breast Cancer Diagnosis and Treatment. Current Oncology Reports [Internet]. 2019 Mar 27;21(5). Available from:

https://www.ncbi.nlm.nih.gov/pmc/articles/PMC6437123/ .

400. Dydjow-Bendek D, Zagożdżon P. Selected dietary factors and breast cancer risk. Przeglad Epidemiologiczny. 2019;73(3)(2019):361–8.

401. McDonald JA, Goyal A, Terry MB. Alcohol Intake and Breast Cancer Risk: Weighing the Overall Evidence. Current Breast Cancer Reports. 2013 May 19;5(3):208–21.

402. Preston DL, Kitahara CM, Freedman DM, Sigurdson AJ, Simon SL, Little MP, et al. Breast cancer risk and protracted low-to-moderate dose occupational radiation exposure in the US Radiologic Technologists Cohort, 1983–2008. British Journal of Cancer [Internet]. 2016 Oct 1;115(9):1105–12. Available from: https://www.nature.com/articles/bjc2016292 .

403. Gurunath S, Pandian Z, Anderson RA, Bhattacharya S. Defining infertility—a systematic review of prevalence studies. Human Reproduction Update. 2011 Apr 14;17(5):575–88.

404. Thonneau P, Marchand S, Tallec A, Ferial ML, Ducot B, Lansac J, et al. Incidence and main causes of infertility in a resident population (1,850,000) of three French regions (1988-1989). Human reproduction (Oxford, England) [Internet]. 1991;6(6):811–6. Available from: https://www.ncbi.nlm.nih.gov/pubmed/1757519/ .

405. Farhi J, Ben-Haroush A. Distribution of causes of infertility in patients attending primary fertility clinics in Israel. The Israel Medical Association journal: IMAJ [Internet]. 2011 Jan 1;13(1):51–4. Available from: https://pubmed.ncbi.nlm.nih.gov/21446238/ .

406. Lundberg FE, Iliadou AN, Rodriguez-Wallberg K, Gemzell-Danielsson K, Johansson ALV. The risk of breast and gynecological cancer in women with a diagnosis of infertility: a nationwide population-based study. European Journal of Epidemiology [Internet]. 2019 Jan 9;34(5):499–507. Available from: https://www.ncbi.nlm.nih.gov/pmc/articles/PMC6456460/ .

407. Van den Belt-Dusebout AW, van Leeuwen FE, Burger CW. Breast Cancer Risk After Ovarian Stimulation for In Vitro Fertilization—Reply. JAMA. 2016 Oct 25;316(16):1713.

408. Cullinane C, Gillan H, Geraghty J, Evoy D, Rothwell J, McCartan D, et al. Fertility treatment and breast-cancer incidence: meta-analysis. BJS Open [Internet]. 2022 Jan 6 [cited 2022 Aug 4];6(1). Available from: https://academic.oup.com/bjsopen/article/6/1/zrab149/6526446?login=false .

409. Lundberg FE, Johansson ALV, Rodriguez-Wallberg K, Brand JS, Czene K, Hall P, et al. Association of infertility and fertility treatment with mammographic density in a large screening-based cohort of women: a cross-sectional study. Breast cancer research: BCR [Internet]. 2016 Apr 13 [cited 2023 Feb 8];18(1):36. Available from: https://pubmed.ncbi.nlm.nih.gov/27072636/ .

410. Katz D, Paltiel O, Peretz T, Revel A, Sharon N, Maly B, et al. Beginning IVF Treatments After Age 30 Increases the Risk of Breast Cancer: Results of a Case-Control Study. The Breast Journal. 2008 Nov;14(6):517–22.

411. FARHUD DD, ZOKAEI S, KEYKHAEI M, HEDAYATI M, ZARIF YEGANEH M. In-Vitro Fertilization Impact on the Risk of Breast Cancer: A Review Article. Iranian Journal of Public Health. 2021 Mar 1;50(3).

412. Bernstein L. Epidemiology of endocrine-related risk factors for breast cancer. Journal of Mammary Gland Biology and Neoplasia. 2002;7(1):3–15.

413. Key TJ, Verkasalo PK, Banks E. Epidemiology of breast cancer. The Lancet Oncology [Internet]. 2001 Mar;2(3):133–40. Available from: https://www.sciencedirect.com/science/article/abs/pii/S1470204500002540 .

375

414. McGuire WL. Estrogen Receptors in Human Breast Cancer. Journal of Clinical Investigation [Internet]. 1973 Jan 1;52(1):73–7. Available from: https://www.ncbi.nlm.nih.gov/pmc/articles/PMC302228/.

415. Bulzomi P, Bolli A, Galluzzo P, Leone S, Acconcia F, Marino M. Naringenin and 17Î2-estradiol coadministration prevents hormone-induced human cancer cell growth. IUBMB Life. 2009;52(1):73–7.

416. Sreeja S, Santhosh Kumar TR, Lakshmi BS, Sreeja S. Pomegranate extract demonstrate a selective estrogen receptor modulator profile in human tumor cell lines and in vivo models of estrogen deprivation. The Journal of Nutritional Biochemistry. 2012 Jul;23(7):725–32.

417. Fritz MA, Holmes RT, Keenan EJ. Effect of clomiphene citrate treatment on endometrial estrogen and progesterone receptor induction in women. American Journal of Obstetrics and Gynecology [Internet]. 1991 Jul 1 [cited 2023 Feb 8];165(1):177–85. Available from: https://pubmed.ncbi.nlm.nih.gov/1906682/ .

418. Sterile F. Use of clomiphene citrate in women. Fertility and Sterility. 2006 Nov;86(5):S187–93.

419. KERIN JF, LIU JH, PHILLIPOU G, YEN SSC. Evidence for a Hypothalamic Site of Action of Clomiphene Citrate in Women*. The Journal of Clinical Endocrinology & Metabolism [Internet]. 1985 Aug [cited 2021 Nov 18];61(2):265–8.Available from: https://academic.oup.com/jcem/article-abstract/61/2/265/2674877?redirectedFrom=fulltext .

420. Homburg R. Oral agents for ovulation induction – clomiphene citrate versus aromatase inhibitors. Human Fertility. 2008 Jan;11(1):17–22.

421. Homburg R. Clomiphene citrate—end of an era? a mini-review. Human Reproduction. 2005 May 5;20(8):2043–51.

422. Adonakis G, Deshpande N, Yates RW, Fleming R (1998). Luteinizing hormone increases estradiol secretion but has no effect on progesterone concentrations in the late follicular phase of in vitro fertilization cycles in women treated with gonadotropin-releasing hormone agonist and follicle-stimulating hormone. Fertil Steril, 69(3):450-3.

423. Henderson BE, Ross RK, Judd HL, Krailo MD, Pike MC. Do regular ovulatory cycles increase breast cancer risk? Cancer 1985;56(5):1206-8.

424. Henderson BE, Ross RK, Judd HL, Krailo MD, Pike MC. Do regular ovulatory cycles increase breast cancer risk? Cancer. 1985 Sep 1;56(5):1206–8.

425. Andarieh MG, Delavar MA, Moslemi D, Ahmadi MH, Zabihi E, Esmaeilzadeh S. Infertility as a risk factor for breast cancer: Results from a hospital-based case-control study. Journal of Cancer Research and Therapeutics [Internet]. 2019 [cited 2023 Feb 8];15(5):976–80. Available from: https://pubmed.ncbi.nlm.nih.gov/31603097/ .

426. Reigstad M. Risk of breast cancer following fertility treatment—a registry based cohort study of parous women in Norway. Int J Cancer. 2015;136(5):1140–8.

427. Hanson B, Johnstone E, Dorais J, Silver B, Peterson CM, Hotaling J. Female infertility, infertility-associated diagnoses, and comorbidities: a review. Journal of Assisted Reproduction and Genetics [Internet]. 2016 Nov 5;34(2):167–77. Available from: https://link.springer.com/article/10.1007%2Fs10815-016-0836-8.

428. Oktay K, Kim JY, Barad D, Babayev SN. Association of BRCA1 Mutations With Occult Primary Ovarian Insufficiency: A Possible Explanation for the Link Between Infertility and Breast/Ovarian Cancer Risks. Journal of Clinical Oncology [Internet]. 2010 Jan 10 [cited 2022 Aug 22];28(2):240–4. Available from: https://www.ncbi.nlm.nih.gov/pmc/articles/PMC3040011/ .

429. *Ford D, Easton DF, Peto J: Estimates of the gene frequency of BRCA1 and its contribution to breast and ovarian cancer incidence. Am J Hum Genet 57:1457-1462, 1995.*

430. *Warner E, Foulkes W, Goodwin P, et al: Prevalence and penetrance of BRCA1 and BRCA2gene mutations in unselected Ashkenazi Jewish women with breast cancer. J Natl Cancer Inst 91:1241-1247, 1999.*

Chapter 20

431. *Global, Regional, and National Cancer Incidence, Mortality, Years of Life Lost, Years Lived With Disability, and Disability-Adjusted Life-Years for 29 Cancer Groups, 1990 to 2017, Christina Fitzmaurice, MD, and Christopher J. L. Murray, JAMA Oncol. 2021 January 28; 7(3): 466.*

432. *The colorectal cancer epidemic: challenges and opportunities for primary, secondary and tertiary prevention, Hermann Brenner and Chen Chen, British Journal of Cancer (2018) 119:785–792.*

433. *Consensus document for management of colorectal cancer, ICMR, 2014, https://main.icmr.nic.in/sites/default/files/guidelines/Colorectal%20Cancer_0.pdf accessed 11th October 2021.*

434. *Differences in Incidence and Mortality Trends of Colorectal Cancer Worldwide Based on Sex, Age, and Anatomic Location, Martin C. S. Wong, Junjie Huang, Veeleah Lok, Clinical Gastroenterology and Hepatology 2021;19:955–966.*

435. *Colorectal cancer development and advances in screening, Karen Simon, Clinical Interventions in Aging 2016:11 967–976.*

436. *Colorectal Cancer Screening, Jesse Samuel Moore, Tess Hannah Aulet, Surg Clin N Am, 2017, 97, 487–502.*

437. *Environmental factors, gut microbiota, and colorectal cancer prevention, Mingyang Song and Andrew T. Chan, Clin Gastroenterol Hepatol. 2019 ; 17(2): 275–289.*

438. *Prevention of colorectal cancer: How many tools do we have in our basket?, Luca Roncucci *, Francesco Mariani, Eur J Intern Med, 2015, http://dx.doi.org/10.1016/j.ejim.2015.08.019.*

439. *Colorectal Cancer and Nutrition, Kannan Thanikachalam and Gazala Khan, Nutrients 2019, 11, 164.*

440. *The Immune System in Cancer Prevention, Development and Therapy, Serge M. Candéiasa and Udo S. Gaipl, Anti-Cancer Agents in Medicinal Chemistry, 2016, 16, 101-107.*

441. *The Influence of the Gut Microbiome on Cancer, Immunity, and Cancer Immunotherapy, Vancheswaran Gopalakrishnan, Beth A. Helmink, Christine N. Spencer, Cancer Cell 2018, 33, 570-579.*

442. *Sleep and immune function, Luciana Besedovsky, Tanja Lange & Jan Born, Eur J Physiol, 2012, 463:121–137*

443. *Melatonin, sleep disturbance and cancer risk, David E. Blask, Sleep Medicine Reviews 13, 2009, 257–264*

444. *Colorectal cancer and dysplasia in inflammatory bowel disease: a review of disease epidemiology, pathophysiology, and management, Parambir S. Dulai, William J. Sandborn, and Samir Gupta, Cancer Prev Res (Phila). 2016 ; 9(12): 887–894.*

Chapter 21

445. *Landgren O., Graubard B.I., Kumar S., Kyle R.A., Katzmann J.A., Murata K., Costello R., Dispenzieri A., Caporaso N., Mailankody S., et al. Prevalence of myeloma precursor state monoclonal gammopathy of undetermined*

significance in 12372 individuals 10-49 years old: A population-based study from the National Health and Nutrition Examination Survey. Blood Cancer J. 2017;7:e618. doi: 10.1038/bcj.2017.97.

446.   Vernocchi A., Longhi E., Lippi G., Gelsumini S. Increased Monoclonal Components: Prevalence in an Italian Population of 44 474 Outpatients Detected by Capillary Electrophoresis. J. Med. Biochem. 2016;35:50–54. doi: 10.1515/jomb-2015-0007.

447.   Kyle R.A., San-Miguel J.F., Mateos M.V., Rajkumar S.V. Monoclonal gammopathy of undetermined significance and smouldering multiple myeloma. Hematology/oncology Clin. N. Am. 2014;28:775–790.

448.   Baker A., Braggio E., Jacobus S., Jung S., Larson D., Therneau T., Dispenzieri A., Van Wier S.A., Ahmann G., Levy J., et al. Uncovering the biology of multiple myeloma among African Americans: A comprehensive genomics approach. Blood. 2013;121:3147–3152. doi: 10.1182/blood-2012-07-443606.

449.   Guikema J.E., Hovenga S., Vellenga E., Conradie J.J., Abdulahad W.H., Bekkema R., Smit J.W., Zhan F., Shaughnessy J., Jr., Bos N.A. CD27 is heterogeneously expressed in multiple myeloma: Low CD27 expression in patients with high-risk disease. Br. J. Haematol. 2003;121:36–43. doi: 10.1046/j.1365-2141.2003.04260.x.

450.   Hofmann J.N., Mailankody S., Korde N., Wang Y., Tageja N., Costello R., Zingone A., Hultcrantz M., Pollak M.N., Purdue M.P., et al. Circulating Adiponectin Levels Differ Between Patients with Multiple Myeloma and its Precursor Disease. Obesity. 2017;25:1317–1320. doi: 10.1002/oby.21894.

451.   Chang S.H., Luo S., O'Brian K.K., Thomas T.S., Colditz G.A., Carlsson N.P., Carson K.R. Association between metformin use and progression of monoclonal gammopathy of undetermined significance to multiple myeloma in US veterans with diabetes mellitus: A population-based retrospective cohort study. Lancet Haematol. 2015;2:e30–e36.

452.   Ravenborg N., Udd K., Berenson A., Costa F., Berenson J.R. Vitamin D levels are frequently below normal in multiple myeloma patients and are infrequently assessed by their treating physicians. Blood. 2014;124:5769.

453.   Lipe B., Kambhampati S., Veldhuizen P.V., Yacoub A., Aljitawi O., Mikhael J. Correlation between markers of bone metabolism and vitamin D levels in patients with monoclonal gammopathy of undetermined significance (MGUS) Blood Cancer J. 2017;7:646. doi: 10.1038/s41408-017-0015-x.

454. Knutson K.L. Does inadequate sleep play a role in vulnerability to obesity? Am. J. Hum. Biol. 2012;24:361–371. doi: 10.1002/ajhb.22219.

455. Gu F., Xiao Q., Chu L.W., Yu K., Matthews C.E., Hsing A.W., Caporaso N.E. Sleep duration and cancer in the NIH-AARP diet and health study cohort. PLoS ONE. 2016;11:e0161561. doi: 10.1371/journal.pone.0161561.

456. Lewis WD, Lilly S, Jones KL. Lymphoma: Diagnosis and Treatment. Am Fam Physician. 2020 Jan 1;101(1):34-41. PMID: 31894937.

457. Swerdlow SH, Campo E, Pileri SA, et al. The 2016 revision of the World Health Organization classification of lymphoid neoplasms. Blood. 2016;127(20):2375-2390. doi:10.1182/blood-2016-01-643569.

458. India Fact Sheets - International Agency for Research on Cancer [Internet]. India. The Global Cancer Observatory; 2021 [cited 2022Jun22]. Available from: https://gco.iarc.fr/today/data/factsheets/populations/356-india-fact-sheets.pdf

459. Qiu F, Liang CL, Liu H, et al. Impacts of cigarette smoking on immune responsiveness: Up and down or upside down?. Oncotarget. 2017;8(1):268-284. doi:10.18632/oncotarget.13613.

460. Tramacere I, Pelucchi C, Bonifazi M, Bagnardi V, Rota M, Bellocco R, Scotti L, Islami F, Corrao G, Boffetta P, La Vecchia C, Negri E. Alcohol drinking and non-Hodgkin lymphoma risk: a systematic review and a meta-analysis. Ann Oncol. 2012 Nov;23(11):2791-2798. doi: 10.1093/annonc/mds013. Epub 2012 Feb 22. PMID: 22357444.

461. Dai S, Mo Y, Wang Y, et al. Chronic Stress Promotes Cancer Development. Front Oncol. 2020;10:1492. Published 2020 Aug 19. doi:10.3389/fonc.2020.01492.

462. Larsson SC, Wolk A. Obesity and risk of non-Hodgkin's lymphoma: a meta-analysis. Int J Cancer. 2007 Oct 1;121(7):1564-70. doi: 10.1002/ijc.22762. PMID: 17443495.

463. Mao Y, Hu J, Ugnat AM, White K. Non-Hodgkin's lymphoma and occupational exposure to chemicals in Canada. Canadian Cancer Registries Epidemiology Research Group. Ann Oncol. 2000;11 Suppl 1:69-73. PMID: 10707783.

464. Nakamura S, Yao T, Aoyagi K, Iida M, Fujishima M, Tsuneyoshi M. Helicobacter pylori and primary gastric lymphoma. A histopathologic and immunohistochemical analysis of 237 patients. Cancer. 1997 Jan 1;79(1):3-11. PMID: 8988720.

465. Li M, Gan Y, Fan C, Yuan H, Zhang X, Shen Y, Wang Q, Meng Z, Xu D, Tu H. Hepatitis B virus and risk of non-Hodgkin lymphoma: An updated meta-analysis of 58 studies. J Viral Hepat. 2018 Aug;25(8):894-903. doi: 10.1111/jvh.12892. Epub 2018 Apr 2. PMID: 29532605.

466. Carbone A, Gloghini A. HHV-8-associated lymphoma: state-of-the-art review. Acta Haematol. 2007;117(3):129-31. doi: 10.1159/000097459. Epub 2006 Nov 29. PMID: 17135725.

467. Mahieux R, Gessain A. HTLV-1 and associated adult T-cell leukemia/lymphoma. Rev Clin Exp Hematol. 2003 Dec;7(4):336-61. PMID: 15129647.

468. Grogg KL, Miller RF, Dogan A. HIV infection and lymphoma. J Clin Pathol. 2007;60(12):1365-1372. doi:10.1136/jcp.2007.051953.

469. Heise W. GI-lymphomas in immunosuppressed patients (organ transplantation; HIV). Best Pract Res Clin Gastroenterol. 2010 Feb;24(1):57-69. doi: 10.1016/j.bpg.2010.01.001. PMID: 20206109.

470. Dracham CB, Shankar A, Madan R. Radiation induced secondary malignancies: a review article. Radiat Oncol J. 2018;36(2):85-94. doi:10.3857/roj.2018.00290.

471. Cerhan JR, Slager SL. Familial predisposition and genetic risk factors for lymphoma. Blood. 2015;126(20):2265-2273. doi:10.1182/blood-2015-04-537498.

472. Khanmohammadi S, Shabani M, Tabary M, Rayzan E, Rezaei N. Lymphoma in the setting of autoimmune diseases: A review of association and mechanisms. Crit Rev Oncol Hematol. 2020 Jun;150:102945. doi: 10.1016/j.critrevonc.2020.102945. Epub 2020 Apr 22. PMID: 32353704.

473. Tucker MA, Coleman CN, Cox RS, Varghese A, Rosenberg SA. Risk of second cancer after treatment for Hodgkin's disease. New England Journal of Medicine. 1988 Jan 14;318(2):76-81.

474. Sarkozy C, Salles G, Falandry C. The biology of aging and lymphoma: a complex interplay. Current Oncology Reports. 2015 Jul;17(7):1-0.

Chapter 22

475. Kramer IRH, Lucas RB, Pindborg JJ et al (1978) Definition of leukoplakia and related lesions: an aid to studies

on oral precancer. Oral Surg Oral Med Oral Pathol 46:518–539.

476. World Health Organization (1973) Report from a meeting of investigation on histological definition of precancerous lesions. CAN/731, Geneva.

477. Axell T, Pindborg JJ, Smith CJ et al (1996) Oral white lesions with special reference to precancerous and tobacco-related lesions. J Oral Pathol Med 25:49–54.

478. Pindborg JJ, Reichart PA, Smith CJ et al (1997) World Health Organization: Histological typing of cancer and precancer of the oral mucosa, 2nd edn. Springer, Berlin.

479. Squamous cell carcinoma. Epidemiologic patterns in Connecticut from 1935 to 1985. Cancer 1990;66:1288-1296.

480. Llewellyn CD, Johnson NW,Warnakulasuriya KA. Risk factors for squamous cell carcinoma of the oral cavity in young people—a comprehensive literature review. Oral Oncol 2001;37:401- 418.

481. Schantz SP,Yu GP. Head and neck cancer incidence trends in young Americans, 1973-1997, with a special analysis for tongue cancer. Arch Otolaryngol Head Neck Surg 2002;128:268- 274.

482. Warnakulasuriya S, Johnson NW, van der Wall I (2007) Nomenclature and classification of potentially malignant disorders of the oral mucosa. J Oral Pathol Med 36:575–580.

483. Silverman S Jr. Epidemiology. In: Silverman S Jr ed. Oral Cancer. 4th ed. Hamilton, Ontario, Canada: BC Decker Inc;1998;1-6.

484. Chen JK, Katz RV, Krutchkoff DJ. Intraoral squamous cell carcinoma. Epidemiologic patterns in Connecticut from 1935 to 1985. Cancer 1990;66:1288-1296.

485. Ries LAG, Hankey BF, Miller BA, et al. Cancer Statistics Review 1973-1988. National Cancer Institute, NIH Publication No. 91-2789, 1991.

486. Banoczy J, Sugar L (1972) Longitudinal studies in oral leukoplakias. J Oral Pathol 1:265–272.

487. Gupta PC, Mehta FS, Daftary DR et al (1980) Incidence rates of oral cancer and natural history of oral precancerous lesions in a 10years follow-up study of Indian villagers. Community Dent Oral Epidemiol 8:287–333.

488. Baric JM, Alman JE, Feldman RS et al (1982) Influence of cigarette, pipe, and cigar smoking, removable partial dentures, and age on oral leukoplakia. Oral Surg Oral Med Oral Pathol 54:424–429.

489. Mehta FS, Pindborg JJ, Gupta PC et al (1969) Epidemiologic and histologic study of oral cancer and leukoplakia among 50,915 villagers in India. Cancer (Phila) 24:832–849.

490. Gupta PC (1989) Leukoplakia and incidence of oral cancer. J Oral Pathol Med 18:17.

491. Roed-Petersen B, Renstrup G (1969) A topographical classification of oral mucosa suitable for electronic data processing its application to 560 leukoplakias. Acta Odont Scand 27:681–695.

492. Fitzpatrick SG, Hirsch SA, Gordon SC. The malignant transformation of oral lichen planus and oral lichenoid lesions: a systematic review. J Am Dent Assoc 2014;145:45- 56.

493. Amagasa T, Yamashiro M, Ishikawa H (2006) Oral leukoplakia related to malignant transformation. Oral Sci Int 3:45–55.

494. Suter VG, Morger R, Altermatt HJ et al. [Oral erythroplakia and erythroleukoplakia: red and red-white dysplastic lesions of the oral mucosa--part 1: epidemiology, etiology, histopathology and differential diagnosis]. Schweiz Monatsschr Zahnmed. 2008;118(5):390-7.

495. Tadakamadla J, Kumar S, Lalloo R et al. Impact of oral potentially malignant disorders on quality of life. J Oral Pathol Med. 2018 Jan;47(1):60-65.

496. Feijoo JF, Bugallo J, Limeres J, Peñarrocha D, Peñarrocha M, Diz P. Inherited epidermolysis bullosa: an update and suggested dental care considerations. J Am Dent Assoc. 2011 Sep;142(9):1017-25.

497. Bongiorno M, Rivard S, Hammer D, Kentosh J. Malignant transformation of oral leukoplakia in a patient with dyskeratosis congenita. Oral Surg Oral Med Oral Pathol Oral Radiol. 2017 Oct;124(4):e239-e242.

498. De Oliveira Ribeiro A, da Silva LC, Martins-Filho PR. Prevalence of and risk factors for actinic cheilitis in Brazilian fishermen and women. Int J Dermatol. 2014 53(11):1370-6.

499. Yen AM, Chen SC, Chang SH et al (2008) The effect of betel quid and cigarette on multistate progression of oral pre-malignancy. J Oral Pathol Med 37(7):417–422.

Chapter 23

500. Wright NA, Poulsom R, Stamp G, et al. Trefoil peptide gene expression in gastrointestinal epithelial cells in inflammatory bowel disease. Gastroenterology. 1993;104(1):12–20.

501. Jemal A, Bray F, Center MM, Ferlay J, Ward E, Forman D. Global cancer statistics. CA Cancer J Clin. 2011;61(2):69–90.

502. Stock M, Otto F. Gene deregulation in gastric cancer. Gene. 2005;360(1):1–19.

503. Parkin DM, Bray F, Ferlay J, Pisani P. Global cancer statistics 2002. CA Cancer J Clin. 2005;55(2):74–108.

504. Buckland G, Travier N1, Huerta JM, et al. Healthy lifestyle index and risk of gastric adenocarcinoma in the EPIC cohort study. Int J Cancer. 2015;137(3):598–606.

505. Lin SH, Li YH, Leung K, Huang CY, Wang XR. Salt processed food and gastric cancer in a Chinese population. Asian Pac J Cancer Prev. 2014;15(13):5293–5298.

506. Massarrat S, Stolte M. Development of gastric cancer and its prevention. Arch Iran Med. 2014;17(7):514–520.

507. World Cancer Research Fund/American Institute for Cancer Research. Continuous Update Project Expert Report Diet, Nutrition, Physical Activity and Stomach Cancer. Available online: https://www.wcrf.org/dietandcancer/stomach-cancer/.

508. McLean, R.M. Measuring Population Sodium Intake: A Review of Methods. Nutrients 2014, 6, 4651–4662.

509. Fox, J.G.; A Dangler, C.; Taylor, N.S.; King, A.; Koh, T.J.; Wang, T.C. High-salt diet induces gastric epithelial hyperplasia and parietal cell loss, and enhances Helicobacter pylori colonization in C57BL/6 mice. Cancer Res. 1999, 59, 4823–4828.

510. Iyengar, N.M.; Gucalp, A.; Dannenberg, A.J.; Hudis, C.A. Obesity and Cancer Mechanisms: Tumor Microenvironment and Inflammation. J. Clin. Oncol. Off. J. Am. Soc. Clin. Oncol. 2016, 34, 4270–4276.

511. Boffetta, P.; Hashibe, M. Alcohol and cancer. Lancet Oncol. 2006, 7, 149–156.

512. *International Agency for Research on Cancer. Personal Habits and Indoor Combustions. In IARC Monographs on the Evaluation of Carcinogenic Risks to Humans; International Agency for Research on Cancer: Lyon, France, 2012; Volume 100E.*

513. *Wang, Q.; Chen, Y.; Wang, X.; Gong, G.; Li, G.; Li, C. Consumption of fruit, but not vegetables, may reduce risk of gastric cancer: Results from a meta-analysis of cohort studies. Eur. J. Cancer 2014, 50, 1498–1509. [CrossRef] [PubMed].*

514. *Gonzalez, C.A.; Lujan-Barroso, L.; Bueno-de-Mesquita, H.B.A.; Jenab, M.; Duell, E.J.; Agudo, A.; Riboli, E. Fruit and vegetable intake and the risk of gastric adenocarcinoma: A reanalysis of the European Pro-spective Investigation into Cancer and Nutrition (EPIC-EURGAST) study after a longer follow-up. Int. J. Cancer 2012, 131, 2910–2919. [CrossRef] [PubMed].*

515. *Duell, E.J.; Lujan-Barroso, L.; Llivina, C.; Muñoz, X.; Jenab, M.; Boutron-Ruault, M.-C.; Clavel-Chapelon, F.; Racine, A.; Boeing, H.; Buijsse, B.; et al. Vitamin C transporter gene (SLC23A1 and SLC23A2) polymorphisms, plasma vitamin C levels, and gastric cancer risk in the EPIC cohort. Genes Nutr. 2013, 8, 549–560.*

516. *Sheikh M, Poustchi H, Pourshams A, et al. Household fuel use and the risk of gastrointestinal cancers: The Golestan Cohort Study. Environ Health Perspect 2020; 128:67002.*

517. *Coleman NC, Burnett RT, Higbee JD, et al. Cancer mortality risk, fine particulate air pollution, and smoking in a large, representative cohort of US adults. Cancer Causes Control 2020; 31:767–776.*

518. *Yu H, Xu N, Li ZK, Xia H, Ren HT, Li N, Wei JB, Bao HZ. Association of ABO Blood Groups and Risk of Gastric Cancer. Scand J Surg. 2020 Dec;109(4):309-313. doi:10.1177/1457496919863886.*

519. *IARC Working Group on the Evaluation of Carcinogenic Risks to Humans (2012). Biological Agents. Volume 100 B. A Review of Human Carcinogens. IARC Monogr. Eval. Carcinog. Risks. Hum. 100, 1–441.*

520. *Fox, J. G., and Wang, T. C. (2001). Helicobacter pylori - not a good bug after all. N. Engl. J. Med. 345, 829–832. doi: 10.1056/NEJM200109133451111.*

521. *Ansari, S., and Yamaoka, Y. (2019). Helicobacter pylori virulence factors exploiting gastric colonization and its pathogenicity. Toxins 11:E677. doi: 10.3390/toxins11110677.*

522. *Li, Q., Liu, J., Gong, Y., and Yuan, Y. (2016). Serum VacA antibody is associated with risks of peptic ulcer and gastric cancer: a meta-analysis. Microb. Pathog. 99, 220–228. doi:10.1016/j.micpath.2016.08.030.*

523. *Raju, D., Hussey, S., Ang, M., Terebiznik, M. R., Sibony, M., Galindo-Mata, E., et al. (2012). Vacuolating cytotoxin and variants in Atg16L1 that disrupt autophagy promote Helicobacter pylori infection in humans. Gastroenterology 142, 1160–1171. doi: 10.1053/j.gastro.2012.01.043.*

524. *Kamboj, A. K., Cotter, T. G., and Oxentenko, A. S. (2017). Helicobacter pylori: the past, present, and future in management. Mayo Clin. Proc. 92, 599–604. doi:10.1016/j.mayocp.2016.11.017.*

525. *Grande, R., Sisto, F., Puca, V., Carradori, S., Ronci, M., Aceto, A., et al. (2020). Antimicrobial and antibiofilm activities of new synthesized silver ultrananoclusters (SUNCs) against Helicobacter pylori. Front. Microbiol. 11:1705. doi: 10.3389/fmicb.2020.01705.*

526. *Muresan IAP, Pop LL, Dumitrascu DL. Lactobacillus reuteri versus triple therapy for the eradication of Helicobacter pylori in functional dyspepsia. Med Pharm Rep. 2019;92(4):352-355. doi:10.15386/mpr-1375.*

527. *Lahner, E., Conti, L., Cicone, F., Capriello, S., Cazzato, M., and Centanni, M. (2020). Thyroenterogastric*

autoimmunity: pathophysiology and implications for patient management. Best. Pract. Res. Clin. Endocrinol. Metab. 34, 101373. doi: 10.1016/j.beem.2019.101373.

528. *Gupta S, Li D, El Serag HB, Davitkov P, Altayar O, Sultan S, Falck-Ytter Y, Mustafa RA. AGA Clinical Practice Guidelines on Management of Gastric Intestinal Metaplasia. Gastroenterology. 2020 Feb;158(3):693-702. doi: 10.1053/j.gastro.2019.12.003. Epub 2019 Dec 6.*

Chapter 24

529. *International Agency for research on Cancer. 2020 [Internet]. Available from: https://gco.iarc.fr/today.*

530. *Mathur P, Sathishkumar K, Chaturvedi M, Das P, Sudarshan KL, Santhappan S, et al. Cancer Statistics, 2020: Report from National Cancer Registry Programme, India. JCO Glob Oncol. 2020 Nov;(6):1063–75.*

531. *Bray F, Ferlay J, Soerjomataram I, Siegel RL, Torre LA, Jemal A. Global cancer statistics 2018: GLOBOCAN estimates of incidence and mortality worldwide for 36 cancers in 185 countries. CA Cancer J Clin. 2018 Nov;68(6):394–424.*

532. *Klein AP, Brune KA, Petersen GM, Goggins M, Tersmette AC, Offerhaus GJA, et al. Prospective Risk of Pancreatic Cancer in Familial Pancreatic Cancer Kindreds. Cancer Res. 2004 Apr 1;64(7):2634–8.*

533. *American cancer society [Internet]. Available from: https://www.cancer.org/cancer/pancreatic-cancer/detection-diagnosis-staging/survival-rates.html*

534. *Midha S, Chawla S, Garg PK. Modifiable and non-modifiable risk factors for pancreatic cancer: A review. Cancer Lett. 2016 Oct;381(1):269–77.*

535. *Ezzati M, Henley SJ, Lopez AD, Thun MJ. Role of smoking in global and regional cancer epidemiology: Current patterns and data needs. Int J Cancer. 2005 Oct 10;116(6):963–71.*

536. *IARC Working Group on the Evaluation of Carcinogenic Risks to Humans. Tobacco smoke and involuntary smoking. IARC Monogr Eval Carcinog Risks Hum. 2004;83:1–1438.*

537. *Anderson MA, Zolotarevsky E, Cooper KL, Sherman S, Shats O, Whitcomb DC, et al. Alcohol and tobacco lower the age of presentation in sporadic pancreatic cancer in a dose-dependent manner: a multicenter study. Am J Gastroenterol. 2012 Nov;107(11):1730–9.*

538. *Bosetti C, Lucenteforte E, Silverman DT, Petersen G, Bracci PM, Ji BT, et al. Cigarette smoking and pancreatic cancer: an analysis from the International Pancreatic Cancer Case-Control Consortium (Panc4). Ann Oncol Off J Eur Soc Med Oncol. 2012 Jul;23(7):1880–8.*

539. *Hassan MM, Bondy ML, Wolff RA, Abbruzzese JL, Vauthey JN, Pisters PW, et al. Risk factors for pancreatic cancer: case-control study. Am J Gastroenterol. 2007 Dec;102(12):2696–707.*

540. *Lynch SM, Vrieling A, Lubin JH, Kraft P, Mendelsohn JB, Hartge P, et al. Cigarette smoking and pancreatic cancer: a pooled analysis from the pancreatic cancer cohort consortium. Am J Epidemiol. 2009 Aug 15;170(4):403–13.*

541. *Raimondi S, Maisonneuve P, Lowenfels AB. Epidemiology of pancreatic cancer: an overview. Nat Rev Gastroenterol Hepatol. 2009 Dec;6(12):699–708.*

542. *Vrieling A, Bueno-de-Mesquita HB, Boshuizen HC, Michaud DS, Severinsen MT, Overvad K, et al. Cigarette smoking, environmental tobacco smoke exposure and pancreatic cancer risk in the European Prospective Investigation*

into Cancer and Nutrition. Int J Cancer. 2010 May 15;126(10):2394–403.

543. Kuzmickiene I, Everatt R, Virviciute D, Tamosiunas A, Radisauskas R, Reklaitiene R, et al. *Smoking and other risk factors for pancreatic cancer: A cohort study in men in Lithuania. Cancer Epidemiol. 2013 Apr;37(2):133–9.*

544. Mizuno S, Nakai Y, Isayama H, Kawahata S, Saito T, Takagi K, et al. *Smoking, Family History of Cancer, and Diabetes Mellitus Are Associated With the Age of Onset of Pancreatic Cancer in Japanese Patients. Pancreas. 2014 Oct;43(7):1014–7.*

545. Pelucchi C, Galeone C, Polesel J, Manzari M, Zucchetto A, Talamini R, et al. *Smoking and Body Mass Index and Survival in Pancreatic Cancer Patients. Pancreas. 2014 Jan;43(1):47–52.*

546. Rahman F, Cotterchio M, Cleary SP, Gallinger S. *Association between Alcohol Consumption and Pancreatic Cancer Risk: A Case-Control Study. Abulseoud OA, editor. PLOS ONE. 2015 Apr 9;10(4):e0124489.*

547. Genkinger JM, Kitahara CM, Bernstein L, Berrington de Gonzalez A, Brotzman M, Elena JW, et al. *Central adiposity, obesity during early adulthood, and pancreatic cancer mortality in a pooled analysis of cohort studies. Ann Oncol Off J Eur Soc Med Oncol. 2015 Nov;26(11):2257–66.*

548. Larsson SC, Wolk A. *Red and processed meat consumption and risk of pancreatic cancer: meta-analysis of prospective studies. Br J Cancer. 2012 Jan 31;106(3):603–7.*

549. Thiébaut ACM, Jiao L, Silverman DT, Cross AJ, Thompson FE, Subar AF, et al. *Dietary fatty acids and pancreatic cancer in the NIH-AARP diet and health study. J Natl Cancer Inst. 2009 Jul 15;101(14):1001–11.*

550. Rohrmann S, Linseisen J, Nöthlings U, Overvad K, Egeberg R, Tjønneland A, et al. *Meat and fish consumption and risk of pancreatic cancer: results from the European Prospective Investigation into Cancer and Nutrition. Int J Cancer. 2013 Feb 1;132(3):617–24.*

551. Beaney AJ, Banim PJR, Luben R, Lentjes MAH, Khaw KT, Hart AR. *Higher Meat Intake Is Positively Associated With Higher Risk of Developing Pancreatic Cancer in an Age-Dependent Manner and Are Modified by Plasma Antioxidants: A Prospective Cohort Study (EPIC-Norfolk) Using Data From Food Diaries. Pancreas. 2017 May;46(5):672–8.*

552. Mancuso TF, el-Attar AA. *Cohort study of workers exposed to betanaphthylamine and benzidine. J Occup Med Off Publ Ind Med Assoc. 1967 Jun;9(6):277–85.*

553. Antwi SO, Eckert EC, Sabaque CV, Leof ER, Hawthorne KM, Bamlet WR, et al. *Exposure to environmental chemicals and heavy metals, and risk of pancreatic cancer. Cancer Causes Control CCC. 2015 Nov;26(11):1583–91.*

554. Hartwig A, Krüger I, Beyersmann D. *Mechanisms in nickel genotoxicity: the significance of interactions with DNA repair. Toxicol Lett. 1994 Jun;72(1–3):353–8.*

555. Lee YW, Klein CB, Kargacin B, Salnikow K, Kitahara J, Doujat K, et al. *Carcinogenic nickel silences gene expression by chromatin condensation and DNA methylation: a new model for epigenetic carcinogens. Mol Cell Biol. 1995 May;15(5):2547–57.*

556. Kasprzak KS. *The role of oxidative damage in metal carcinogenicity. Chem Res Toxicol. 1991 Nov;4(6):604–15.*

557. Ahamed M, Akhtar MJ, Siddiqui MA, Ahmad J, Musarrat J, Al-Khedhairy AA, et al. *Oxidative stress mediated apoptosis induced by nickel ferrite nanoparticles in cultured A549 cells. Toxicology. 2011 May;283(2–3):101–8.*

558. Bertin G, Averbeck D. Cadmium: cellular effects, modifications of biomolecules, modulation of DNA repair and genotoxic consequences (a review). Biochimie. 2006 Nov;88(11):1549–59.

559. Waalkes MP, Cherian MG, Ward JM, Goyer RA. Immunohistochemical Evidence of High Concentrations of Metallothionein in Pancreatic Hepatocytes Induced by Cadmium in Rats. Toxicol Pathol. 1992 May;20(3–1):323–6.

560. Candéias S, Pons B, Viau M, Caillat S, Sauvaigo S. Direct inhibition of excision/synthesis DNA repair activities by cadmium: Analysis on dedicated biochips. Mutat Res Mol Mech Mutagen. 2010 Dec 10;694(1–2):53–9.

561. Maisonneuve P, Amar S, Lowenfels AB. Periodontal disease, edentulism, and pancreatic cancer: a meta-analysis. Ann Oncol Off J Eur Soc Med Oncol. 2017 May 1;28(5):985–95.

562. Bosetti C, Bertuccio P, Negri E, La Vecchia C, Zeegers MP, Boffetta P. Pancreatic cancer: Overview of descriptive epidemiology. Mol Carcinog. 2012 Jan;51(1):3–13.

563. Siegel RL, Miller KD, Jemal A. Cancer statistics, 2018: Cancer Statistics, 2018. CA Cancer J Clin. 2018 Jan;68(1):7–30.

564. Arnold LD, Patel AV, Yan Y, Jacobs EJ, Thun MJ, Calle EE, et al. Are Racial Disparities in Pancreatic Cancer Explained by Smoking and Overweight/Obesity? Cancer Epidemiol Biomarkers Prev. 2009 Sep 1;18(9):2397–405.

565. Pernick NL, Sarkar FH, Philip PA, Arlauskas P, Shields AF, Vaitkevicius VK, et al. Clinicopathologic Analysis of Pancreatic Adenocarcinoma in African Americans and Caucasians: Pancreas. 2003 Jan;26(1):28–32.

566. Chari ST, Leibson CL, Rabe KG, Ransom J, de Andrade M, Petersen GM. Probability of pancreatic cancer following diabetes: a population-based study. Gastroenterology. 2005 Aug;129(2):504–11.

567. Raghavan SR, Ballehaninna UK, Chamberlain RS. The impact of perioperative blood glucose levels on pancreatic cancer prognosis and surgical outcomes: an evidence-based review. Pancreas. 2013 Nov;42(8):1210–7.

568. Rosa JA, Van Linda BM, Abourizk NN. New-onset diabetes mellitus as a harbinger of pancreatic carcinoma. A case report and literature review. J Clin Gastroenterol. 1989 Apr;11(2):211–5.

569. Permert J, Ihse I, Jorfeldt L, von Schenck H, Arnquist HJ, Larsson J. Improved glucose metabolism after subtotal pancreatectomy for pancreatic cancer. Br J Surg. 2005 Dec 6;80(8):1047–50.

570. Bosetti C, Rosato V, Li D, Silverman D, Petersen GM, Bracci PM, et al. Diabetes, antidiabetic medications, and pancreatic cancer risk: an analysis from the International Pancreatic Cancer Case-Control Consortium. Ann Oncol. 2014 Oct;25(10):2065–72.

571. Hruban RH, Canto MI, Goggins M, Schulick R, Klein AP. Update on familial pancreatic cancer. Adv Surg. 2010;44:293–311.

572. Humphris JL, Johns AL, Simpson SH, Cowley MJ, Pajic M, Chang DK, et al. Clinical and pathologic features of familial pancreatic cancer. Cancer. 2014 Dec 1;120(23):3669–75.

573. Lynch HT, Smyrk T, Kern SE, Hruban RH, Lightdale CJ, Lemon SJ, et al. Familial pancreatic cancer: a review. Semin Oncol. 1996 Apr;23(2):251–75.

574. Catts ZAK, Baig MK, Milewski B, Keywan C, Guarino M, Petrelli N. Statewide Retrospective Review of Familial Pancreatic Cancer in Delaware, and Frequency of Genetic Mutations in Pancreatic Cancer Kindreds. Ann Surg Oncol. 2016 May;23(5):1729–35.

575. Wang L, Brune KA, Visvanathan K, Laheru D, Herman J, Wolfgang C, et al. Elevated Cancer Mortality in the Relatives of Patients with Pancreatic Cancer. Cancer Epidemiol Biomarkers Prev. 2009 Nov;18(11):2829–34.

576. Couch FJ, Johnson MR, Rabe KG, Brune K, de Andrade M, Goggins M, et al. The Prevalence of BRCA2 Mutations in Familial Pancreatic Cancer. Cancer Epidemiol Biomarkers Prev. 2007 Feb 1;16(2):342–6.

577. Risch HA, Yu H, Lu L, Kidd MS. ABO Blood Group, Helicobacter pylori Seropositivity, and Risk of Pancreatic Cancer: A Case-Control Study. JNCI J Natl Cancer Inst. 2010 Apr 7;102(7):502–5.

578. Chen XZ, Schöttker B, Castro FA, Chen H, Zhang Y, Holleczek B, et al. Association of helicobacter pylori infection and chronic atrophic gastritis with risk of colonic, pancreatic and gastric cancer: A ten-year follow-up of the ESTHER cohort study. Oncotarget. 2016 Mar 29;7(13):17182–93.

579. Rahbari NN, Bork U, Hinz U, Leo A, Kirchberg J, Koch M, et al. ABO blood group and prognosis in patients with pancreatic cancer. BMC Cancer. 2012 Dec;12(1):319.

580. Lowenfels A, Maisonneuve P, Whitcomb D. RISK FACTORS FOR CANCER IN HEREDITARY PANCREATITIS. Med Clin North Am. 2000 May 1;84(3):565–73.

581. Howes N, Lerch MM, Greenhalf W, Stocken DD, Ellis I, Simon P, et al. Clinical and genetic characteristics of hereditary pancreatitis in Europe. Clin Gastroenterol Hepatol. 2004 Mar;2(3):252–61.

582. Parkin DM, Boyd L, Walker LC. 16. The fraction of cancer attributable to lifestyle and environmental factors in the UK in 2010: Summary and conclusions. Br J Cancer. 2011 Dec;105(S2):S77–81.

583. Bao Y, Hu FB, Giovannucci EL, Wolpin BM, Stampfer MJ, Willett WC, et al. Nut consumption and risk of pancreatic cancer in women. Br J Cancer. 2013 Nov;109(11):2911–6.

584. Paluszkiewicz P, Smolińska K, Dębińska I, Turski WA. Main dietary compounds and pancreatic cancer risk. The quantitative analysis of case–control and cohort studies. Cancer Epidemiol. 2012 Feb;36(1):60–7.

Chapter 25

585. https://www.cancer.org/cancer/ovarian-cancer/about/key-statistics.html

586. Siegel RL, Miller KD and Jemal A: Cancer statistics. Cancer J Clin. 2019; 69:7–34.

587. Burger CW, Kenemans P. Post-menopausal hormone replacement therapy and cancer of the female genital tract and breast. Curr Opin Obstet Gynecol. 1998;10(1):41-45.

588. Danforth KN, Im TM, Whitlock EP. Addendum to Screening for Ovarian Cancer: Evidence Update for the US Preventive Services Task Force Reaffirmation Recommendation Statement. AHRQ Publication No. 12-05165-EF4. Rockville, MD: Agency for Healthcare Research and Quality; April 2012

589. Matz M, Coleman MP, Carreira H, et al. Worldwide comparison of ovarian cancer survival: Histological group and stage at diagnosis (CONCORD-2) [published correction appears in Gynecol Oncol. 2017 Dec;147(3):725]. Gynecol Oncol. 2017;144(2):396-404.

590. Wright JD, Chen L, Tergas AI, et al. Trends in relative survival for ovarian cancer from 1975 to 2011. Obstet Gynecol. 2015;125(6):1345-1352.

591. Kurnit, Katherine C. MD, MPH; Fleming, Gini F. MD; Lengyel, Ernst MD, PhD Updates and New Options in Advanced Epithelial Ovarian Cancer Treatment, Obstetrics & Gynecology: January 2021 - Volume 137 - Issue 1 - p 108-121

592. Patni R. Screening for Ovarian Cancer: An Update. J Midlife Health. 2019;10(1):3-5.

593. Devouassoux-Shisheboran M, Genestie C. Pathobiology of ovarian carcinomas. Chin J Cancer. 2015;34(1):50-55.

594. Kurman RJ, Carcangiu ML, Herrington CS, et al. WHO classification of tumors of female reproductive organs. Lyon: IARC Press; 2014.

595. Koshiyama M, Matsumura N, Konishi I. Recent concepts of ovarian carcinogenesis: type I and type II. Biomed Res Int. 2014; 2014:934261. doi:10.1155/2014/934261.

596. Babaier A, Ghatage P. Mucinous Cancer of the Ovary: Overview and Current Status. Diagnostics (Basel). 2020;10(1):52.

597. Khunamornpong S, Suprasert P, Chiangmai WN, Siriaunkgul S. Metastatic tumors to the ovaries: a study of 170 cases in northern Thailand. Int J Gynecol Cancer. 2006;16 Suppl 1:132-138.

598. Obata K, Morland SJ, Watson RH, et al. Frequent PTEN/MMAC mutations in endometrioid but not serous or mucinous epithelial ovarian tumors. Cancer Res. 1998;58(10):2095-2097.

599. Sato N, Tsunoda H, Nishida M, et al. Loss of heterozygosity on 10q23.3 and mutation of the tumor suppressor gene PTEN in benign endometrial cyst of the ovary: possible sequence progression from benign endometrial cyst to endometrioid carcinoma and clear cell carcinoma of the ovary. Cancer Res. 2000;60(24):7052-7056.

600. Lee Y, Miron A, Drapkin R, et al. A candidate precursor to serous carcinoma that originates in the distal fallopian tube [published correction appears in J Pathol. 2007 Sep;213(1):116] J Pathol. 2007;211(1):26-35.

601. Folkins AK, Jarboe EA, Saleemuddin A, et al. A candidate precursor to pelvic serous cancer (p53 signature) and its prevalence in ovaries and fallopian tubes from women with BRCA mutations. Gynecol Oncol. 2008;109(2):168-173.

602. Diep CH, Daniel AR, Mauro LJ, Knutson TP, Lange CA. Progesterone action in breast, uterine, and ovarian cancers. J Mol Endocrinol. 2015;54(2): R31-R53.

603. Lukanova A, Kaaks R. Endogenous hormones and ovarian cancer: epidemiology and current hypotheses. Cancer Epidemiol Biomarkers Prev. 2005;14(1):98-107.

604. Newhouse ML, Pearson RM, Fullerton JM, Boesen EA, Shannon HS. A case-control study of carcinoma of the ovary. Br J Prev Soc Med. 1977;31(3):148-153. doi:10.1136/jech.31.3.148.

605. Casagrande JT, Louie EW, Pike MC, Roy S, Ross RK, Henderson BE. "Incessant ovulation" and ovarian cancer. Lancet. 1979;2(8135):170-173. doi:10.1016/s0140-6736(79)91435-1.

606. Hankinson SE, Colditz GA, Hunter DJ, Spencer TL, Rosner B, Stampfer MJ. A quantitative assessment of oral contraceptive use and risk of ovarian cancer. Obstet Gynecol. 1992;80(4):708-714.

607. Beral V, Doll R, Hermon C, Peto R, Reeves G. Ovarian cancer and oral contraceptives: collaborative reanalysis of data from 45 epidemiological studies including 23,257 women with ovarian cancer and 87,303 controls. Lancet. 2008;371(9609):303-314.

608. Anderson GL, Judd HL, Kaunitz AM, et al. Effects of estrogen plus progestin on gynecologic cancers and associated diagnostic procedures: the Women's Health Initiative randomized trial. JAMA.2003;290(13):17391748.

609. Beral V; Million Women Study Collaborators, Bull D, Green J, Reeves G. Ovarian cancer and hormone replacement therapy in the Million Women Study. Lancet. 2007;369(9574):1703-1710.

610. Pearce CL, Chung K, Pike MC, Wu AH. Increased ovarian cancer risk associated with menopausal estrogen therapy is reduced by adding a progestin. Cancer. 2009;115(3):531-539.

611. Cottreau CM, Ness RB, Modugno F, Allen GO, Goodman MT. Endometriosis and its treatment with danazol or lupron in relation to ovarian cancer. Clin Cancer Res. 2003;9(14):5142-5144.

612. Olsen CM, Green AC, Nagle CM, et al. Epithelial ovarian cancer: testing the 'androgens hypothesis'. Endocr Relat Cancer. 2008;15(4):1061-1068.

613. Langdon SP, Herrington CS, Hollis RL, Gourley C. Estrogen Signaling and Its Potential as a Target for Therapy in Ovarian Cancer. Cancers (Basel). 2020;12(6):1647.

614. Park SH, Cheung LW, Wong AS, Leung PC. Estrogen regulates Snail and Slug in the down-regulation of E-cadherin and induces metastatic potential of ovarian cancer cells through estrogen receptor alpha. Mol Endocrinol. 2008;22(9):2085-2098.

615. Kuiper GG, Enmark E, Pelto-Huikko M, Nilsson S, Gustafsson JA. Cloning of a novel receptor expressed in rat prostate and ovary. Proc Natl Acad Sci U S A. 1996;93(12):5925-5930.

616. Byers M, Kuiper GG, Gustafsson JA, Park-Sarge OK. Estrogen receptor-beta mRNA expression in rat ovary: down-regulation by gonadotropins. Mol Endocrinol. 1997;11(2):172-182.

617. Brandenberger AW, Tee MK, Jaffe RB. Estrogen receptor alpha (ER-alpha) and beta (ER-beta) mRNAs in normal ovary, ovarian serous cystadenocarcinoma and ovarian cancer cell lines: down-regulation of ER-beta in neoplastic tissues. J Clin Endocrinol Metab. 1998;83(3):1025-1028.

618. Hillier SG, Anderson RA, Williams AR, Tetsuka M. Expression of oestrogen receptor alpha and beta in cultured human ovarian surface epithelial cells. Mol Hum Reprod. 1998;4(8):811-815.

619. Lau KM, Mok SC, Ho SM. Expression of human estrogen receptor-alpha and -beta, progesterone receptor, and androgen receptor mRNA in normal and malignant ovarian epithelial cells. Proc Natl Acad Sci U S A. 1999;96(10):5722-5727.

620. Bardin A, Hoffmann P, Boulle N, et al. Involvement of estrogen receptor beta in ovarian carcinogenesis [retracted in: Lazennec G. Cancer Res. 2005 Jun 15;65(12):5480]. Cancer Res. 2004;64(16):5861-5869.

621. Lazennec G. Estrogen receptor beta, a possible tumor suppressor involved in ovarian carcinogenesis. Cancer Lett. 2006;231(2):151-157

622. Chan KK, Wei N, Liu SS, Xiao-Yun L, Cheung AN, Ngan HY. Estrogen receptor subtypes in ovarian cancer: a clinical correlation. Obstet Gynecol. 2008;111(1):144-151.

623. Geisler HE. The use of high dose megestrol acetate in the treatment of ovarian adenocarcinoma. Semin Oncol. 1985;12(1 Suppl 1):20-22.

624. Suzuki F, Akahira J, Miura I, et al. Loss of estrogen receptor beta isoform expression and its correlation with aberrant DNA methylation of the 5'-untranslated region in human epithelial ovarian carcinoma. Cancer Sci. 2008;99(12):2365-2372.

625. Yap OW, Bhat G, Liu L, Tollefsbol TO. Epigenetic modifications of the Estrogen receptor beta gene in epithelial ovarian cancer cells. Anticancer Res. 2009;29(1):139-144.

626. Rao BR, Slotman BJ. Endocrine factors in common epithelial ovarian cancer. Endocr Rev. 1991;12(1):14-26. doi:10.1210/edrv-12-1-14

627. Bossard C, Busson M, Vindrieux D, et al. Potential role of estrogen receptor beta as a tumor suppressor of epithelial ovarian cancer [published correction appears in PLoS One. 2013;8(5). doi:10.1371/annotation/480acc26-456b-4e06-8cb6-2834bd6f5553]. PLoS One. 2012;7(9):e44787.

628. Pujol P, Rey JM, Nirde P, et al. Differential expression of estrogen receptor-alpha and -beta messenger RNAs as a potential marker of ovarian carcinogenesis. Cancer Res. 1998;58(23):5367-5373.

629. Chan KK, Leung TH, Chan DW, et al. Targeting estrogen receptor subtypes (ERa and ERβ) with selective ER modulators in ovarian cancer. J Endocrinol. 2014;221(2):325-336.

630. Langdon SP, Gabra H, Bartlett JM, et al. Functionality of the progesterone receptor in ovarian cancer and its regulation by estrogen. Clin Cancer Res. 1998;4(9):2245-2251.

631. Lau KM, Mok SC, Ho SM. Expression of human estrogen receptor-alpha and -beta, progesterone receptor, and androgen receptor mRNA in normal and malignant ovarian epithelial cells. Proc Natl Acad Sci U S A. 1999;96(10):5722-5727.

632. Akahira J, Suzuki T, Ito K, et al. Differential expression of progesterone receptor isoforms A and B in the normal ovary, and in benign, borderline, and malignant ovarian tumors. Jpn J Cancer Res. 2002;93(7):807-815.

633. Gabra H, Watson JE, Taylor KJ, et al. Definition and refinement of a region of loss of heterozygosity at 11q23.3-q24.3 in epithelial ovarian cancer associated with poor prognosis. Cancer Res. 1996;56(5):950-954.

634. Edmondson RJ, Monaghan JM. The epidemiology of ovarian cancer. Int J Gynecol Cancer. 2001;11(6):423-429

635. Reid BM, Permuth JB, Sellers TA. Epidemiology of ovarian cancer: a review. Cancer Biol Med. 2017;14(1):9-32.

636. Mendelson CR. Minireview: fetal-maternal hormonal signaling in pregnancy and labor. Mol Endocrinol. 2009;23(7):947-954.

637. Akahira J, Inoue T, Suzuki T, et al. Progesterone receptor isoforms A and B in human epithelial ovarian carcinoma: immunohistochemical and RT-PCR studies. Br J Cancer. 2000;83(11):1488-1494.

638. Akahira J, Suzuki T, Ito K, et al. Differential expression of progesterone receptor isoforms A and B in the normal ovary, and in benign, borderline, and malignant ovarian tumors. Jpn J Cancer Res. 2002;93(7):807-815.

639. Lenhard M, Tereza L, Heublein S, et al. Steroid hormone receptor expression in ovarian cancer: progesterone receptor B as prognostic marker for patient survival. BMC Cancer. 2012; 12:553.

640. Hempling RE, Piver MS, Eltabbakh GH, Recio FO. Progesterone receptor status is a significant prognostic variable of progression-free survival in advanced epithelial ovarian cancer. Am J Clin Oncol. 1998;21(5):447-451.

641. Münstedt K, Steen J, Knauf AG, Buch T, von Georgi R, Franke FE. Steroid hormone receptors and long-term survival in invasive ovarian cancer. Cancer. 2000;89(8):1783-1791.

642. Lindgren P, Bäckström T, Mählck CG, Ridderheim M, Cajander S. Steroid receptors and hormones in relation to cell proliferation and apoptosis in poorly differentiated epithelial ovarian tumors. Int J Oncol. 2001;19(1):31-38.

643. Lee P, Rosen DG, Zhu C, Silva EG, Liu J. Expression of progesterone receptor is a favourable prognostic marker in ovarian cancer. Gynecol Oncol. 2005;96(3):671-677.

644. Høgdall EV, Christensen L, Høgdall CK, et al. Prognostic value of estrogen receptor and progesterone receptor tumor expression in Danish ovarian cancer patients: from the 'MALOVA' ovarian cancer study. Oncol Rep. 2007;18(5):1051-1059.

645. *Sinn BV, Darb-Esfahani S, Wirtz RM, et al. Evaluation of a hormone receptor-positive ovarian carcinoma subtype with a favourable prognosis by determination of progesterone receptor and oestrogen receptor 1 mRNA expression in formalin-fixed paraffin-embedded tissue. Histopathology. 2011;59(5):918-927.*

646. *Chodankar R, Kwang S, Sangiorgi F, et al. Cell-nonautonomous induction of ovarian and uterine serous cystadenomas in mice lacking a functional Brca1 in ovarian granulosa cells. Curr Biol. 2005;15(6):561-565.*

647. *Hong H, Yen HY, Brockmeyer A, et al. Changes in the mouse estrus cycle in response to BRCA1 inactivation suggest a potential link between risk factors for familial and sporadic ovarian cancer. Cancer Res. 2010;70(1):221-228.*

648. *Yen HY, Gabet Y, Liu Y, et al. Alterations in Brca1 expression in mouse ovarian granulosa cells have short-term and long-term consequences on estrogen-responsive organs. Lab Invest. 2012;92(6):802-811.*

649. *Widschwendter M, Rosenthal AN, Philpott S, et al. The sex hormone system in carriers of BRCA1/2 mutations: a case-control study. Lancet Oncol. 2013;14(12):1226-1232*

650. *Bu SZ, Yin DL, Ren XH, et al. Progesterone induces apoptosis and up-regulation of p53 expression in human ovarian carcinoma cell lines. Cancer. 1997;79(10):1944-1950.*

651. *Keith Bechtel M, Bonavida B. Inhibitory effects of 17beta-estradiol and progesterone on ovarian carcinoma cell proliferation: a potential role for inducible nitric oxide synthase. Gynecol Oncol. 2001;82(1):127-138.*

652. *Syed V, Ho SM. Progesterone-induced apoptosis in immortalized normal and malignant human ovarian surface epithelial cells involves enhanced expression of FasL. Oncogene. 2003;22(44):6883-6890.*

653. *Faivre EJ, Daniel AR, Hillard CJ, Lange CA. Progesterone receptor rapid signaling mediates serine 345 phosphorylation and tethering to specificity protein 1 transcription factors. Mol Endocrinol. 2008;22(4):823-837.*

654. *Pierson-Mullany LK, Lange CA. Phosphorylation of progesterone receptor serine 400 mediates ligand-independent transcriptional activity in response to activation of cyclin-dependent protein kinase 2. Mol Cell Biol. 2004;24(24):10542-10557.*

655. *Hagan CR, Regan TM, Dressing GE, Lange CA. ck2-dependent phosphorylation of progesterone receptors (PR) on Ser81 regulates PR-B isoform-specific target gene expression in breast cancer cells. Mol Cell Biol. 2011;31(12):2439-2452.*

656. *Modugno F, Laskey R, Smith AL, Andersen CL, Haluska P, Oesterreich S. Hormone response in ovarian cancer: time to reconsider as a clinical target? Endocr Relat Cancer. 2012;19(6):R255-R279.*

657. *Sieh W, Köbel M, Longacre TA, et al. Hormone-receptor expression and ovarian cancer survival: an Ovarian Tumor Tissue Analysis consortium study. Lancet Oncol. 2013;14(9):853-862.*

658. *Kim O, Park EY, Kwon SY, et al. Targeting progesterone signaling prevents metastatic ovarian cancer. Proc Natl Acad Sci U S A. 2020;117(50):31993-32004.*

659. *Paleari L, DeCensi A. Endocrine therapy in ovarian cancer: where do we stand? Curr Opin Obstet Gynecol. 2018;30(1):17-22.*

660. *Miyamoto H, Messing EM, Chang C. Androgen deprivation therapy for prostate cancer: current status and future prospects. Prostate. 2004;61(4):332-353.*

661. *Mizushima T, Tirador KA, Miyamoto H. Androgen receptor activation: a prospective therapeutic target for bladder cancer? Expert Opin Ther Targets. 2017;21(3):249-257.*

662. Shi P, Zhang Y, Tong X, Yang Y, Shao Z. Dihydrotestosterone induces p27 degradation via direct binding with SKP2 in ovarian and breast cancer. Int J Mol Med. 2011;28(1):109-114.

663. Gogoi R, Kudla M, Gil O, Fishman D. The activity of medroxyprogesterone acetate, an androgenic ligand, in ovarian cancer cell invasion. Reprod Sci. 2008;15(8):846-852.

664. Ligr M, Patwa RR, Daniels G, et al. Expression and function of androgen receptor coactivator p44/Mep50/WDR77 in ovarian cancer [published correction appears in PLoS One. 2011;6(10) 26250.

665. Cuzick J, Bulstrode JC, Stratton I, Thomas BS, Bulbrook RD, Hayward JL. A prospective study of urinary androgen levels and ovarian cancer. Int J Cancer. 1983;32(6):723-726.

666. Lukanova A, Kaaks R. Endogenous hormones and ovarian cancer: epidemiology and current hypotheses. Cancer Epidemiol Biomarkers Prev. 2005;14(1):98-107.

667. von Wolff M, Stute P, Eisenhut M, Marti U, Bitterlich N, Bersinger NA. Serum and follicular fluid testosterone concentrations do not correlate, questioning the impact of androgen supplementation on the follicular endocrine milieu. Reprod Biomed Online. 2017;35(5):616-623.

668. Mizushima T, Miyamoto H. The Role of Androgen Receptor Signaling in Ovarian Cancer. Cells. 2019;8(2):176.

669. Chamberlain NL, Driver ED, Miesfeld RL. The length and location of CAG trinucleotide repeats in the androgen receptor N-terminal domain affect transactivation function. Nucleic Acids Res. 1994;22(15):3181-3186. doi:10.1093/nar/22.15.3181.

670. Tut TG, Ghadessy FJ, Trifiro MA, Pinsky L, Yong EL. Long polyglutamine tracts in the androgen receptor are associated with reduced trans-activation, impaired sperm production, and male infertility. J Clin Endocrinol Metab. 1997;82(11):3777-3782. doi:10.1210/jcem.82.11.4385.

671. Li AJ, Scoles DR, Armstrong KU, Karlan BY. Androgen receptor cytosine-adenine-guanine repeat polymorphisms modulate EGFR signaling in epithelial ovarian carcinomas. Gynecol Oncol. 2008;109(2):220-225.

672. Li AJ, Baldwin RL, Karlan BY. Short androgen receptor allele length is a poor prognostic factor in epithelial ovarian carcinoma. Clin Cancer Res. 2003;9(10 Pt 1):3667-3673.

673. Tan J, Song C, Wang D, et al. Expression of hormone receptors predicts survival and platinum sensitivity of high-grade serous ovarian cancer. Biosci Rep. 2021;41(5): BSR20210478.

674. Badgwell D, Bast RC Jr. Early detection of ovarian cancer. Dis Markers. 2007;23(5-6):397-410.

675. Troisi R, Bjørge T, Gissler M, et al. The role of pregnancy, perinatal factors, and hormones in maternal cancer risk: a review of the evidence. J Intern Med. 2018;283(5):430-445.

676. Babic A, Sasamoto N, Rosner BA et al. Association Between Breastfeeding and Ovarian Cancer Risk. JAMA Oncol. 2020 Jun 1;6(6): e200421.

677. Gaitskell K, Green J, Pirie K, Reeves G, Beral V; Million Women Study Collaborators. Tubal ligation and ovarian cancer risk in a large cohort: Substantial variation by histological type. Int J Cancer. 2016;138(5):1076-1084.

Chapter 26

678. Cervix uteri - global cancer observatory. (2020). https://gco.iarc.fr/today/data/factsheets/cancers/23-Cervix-uteri-fact-sheet.pdf

679. Cohen, P. A., Jhingran, A., Oaknin, A., & Denny, L. (2019). Cervical cancer. The Lancet, 393(10167), 169–182. https://doi.org/10.1016/s0140-6736(18)32470-x

680. Basu, P., Mittal, S., Bhadra Vale, D., & Chami Kharaji, Y. (2018). Secondary Prevention of Cervical Cancer. Best Practice & Research Clinical Obstetrics & Gynaecology, 47, 73–85. https://doi.org/10.1016/j.bpobgyn.2017.08.012.

681. Kaarthigeyan, K. (2012). Cervical cancer in India and HPV vaccination. Indian Journal of Medical and Paediatric Oncology, 33(01), 7–12. https://doi.org/10.4103/0971-5851.96961

682. Cervical cancer prevention (PDQ®)–patient version. National Cancer Institute. (2021) https://www.cancer.gov/types/cervical/patient/cervical-prevention-pdq

683. Cervical cancer risk factors: Risk factors for cervical cancer. American Cancer Society. (2020).https://www.cancer.org/cancer/cervical-cancer/causes-risks-prevention/risk-factors.html

684. Goodman, H., & Stump-Sutliff, K. (2022). Cervical cancer: Risk factors. Cervical Cancer: Risk Factors - Health Encyclopedia - University of Rochester Medical Center. https://www.urmc.rochester.edu/encyclopedia/content.aspx?ContentTypeID=34&ContentID=17227-1

685. Mishra, G. A., Pimple, S. A., & Shastri, S. S. (2016). Prevention of cervix cancer in India. Oncology, 91(Suppl. 1), 1–7. https://doi.org/10.1159/000447575

686. Aggarwal, P. (2014). Cervical cancer: Can it be prevented? World Journal of Clinical Oncology, 5(4), 775. https://doi.org/10.5306/wjco.v5.i4.775

687. World Health Organization. (2022). Cervical cancer. World Health Organization. https://www.who.int/news-room/fact-sheets/detail/cervical-cancer#:~:text=Key%20facts,%2Dincome%20countries%20(1).

688. Cervical cancer screening (PDQ®)–patient version. National Cancer Institute. (2022). https://www.cancer.gov/types/cervical/patient/cervical-screening-pdq

Chapter 27

(Am J Respir Crit Care Med Vol. 190, P7-P8, 2014, ATS Patient Education Series © 2020 American Thoracic Society)

(WattenbergLW.Chemopreventionofcancer.CancerRes1985;45(1):1–8)

Chapter 28

689. Varmus H. The new era in cancer research. Science. 2006 May 26;312(5777):1162–5.

690. Sonnenschein C, Soto AM. THEORIES of CARCINOGENESIS: An Emerging Perspective. Semin Cancer Biol. 2008 Oct;18(5):372–7.

691. Soto AM, Sonnenschein C. Regulation of cell proliferation: the negative control perspective. Ann N Y Acad Sci. 1991;628:412–8.

692. The Society of Cells – Cancer and control of cell proliferation. C. Sonnenschein and A. M. Soto. Bios Scientific,

Oxford, 1999. No. of pages: 154. Price: £18.95. ISBN: 1 85996 276 9 (US Publisher: Springer-Verlag, New York. Price: US $34.95. ISBN 0 387 91583 4.). J Pathol. 2000;190(4):518–9.

693. Moro L, Arbini AA, Marra E, Greco M. Mitochondrial DNA depletion reduces PARP-1 levels and promotes progression of the neoplastic phenotype in prostate carcinoma. Cell Oncol Off J Int Soc Cell Oncol. 2008;30(4):307–22.

694. Hoye AT, Davoren JE, Wipf P, Fink MP, Kagan VE. Targeting mitochondria. Acc Chem Res. 2008 Jan;41(1):87–97.

695. Cancer statistics, 2017 - Siegel - 2017 - CA: A Cancer Journal for Clinicians - Wiley Online Library [Internet]. [cited 2021 Sep 29]. Available from: https://acsjournals.onlinelibrary.wiley.com/doi/full/10.3322/caac.21387

696. Cumberbatch MG, Rota M, Catto JWF, Vecchia CL. The Role of Tobacco Smoke in Bladder and Kidney Carcinogenesis: A Comparison of Exposures and Meta-analysis of Incidence and Mortality Risks. Eur Urol. 2016 Sep 1;70(3):458–66.

697. Weikert S, Boeing H, Pischon T, Weikert C, Olsen A, Tjonneland A, et al. Blood Pressure and Risk of Renal Cell Carcinoma in the European Prospective Investigation into Cancer and Nutrition. Am J Epidemiol. 2008 Feb 15;167(4):438–46.

698. Capitanio U, Bensalah K, Bex A, Boorjian SA, Bray F, Coleman J, et al. Epidemiology of Renal Cell Carcinoma. Eur Urol. 2019 Jan;75(1):74–84.

699. Ito R, Narita S, Huang M, Nara T, Numakura K, Takayama K, et al. The impact of obesity and adiponectin signaling in patients with renal cell carcinoma: A potential mechanism for the "obesity paradox." PLOS ONE. 2017 Feb 8;12(2):e0171615.

700. Ljungberg B, Campbell SC, Cho HY, Jacqmin D, Lee JE, Weikert S, et al. The Epidemiology of Renal Cell Carcinoma. Eur Urol. 2011 Oct 1;60(4):615–21.

701. Port FK, Ragheb NE, Schwartz AG, Hawthorne VM. Neoplasms in dialysis patients: a population-based study. Am J Kidney Dis Off J Natl Kidney Found. 1989 Aug;14(2):119–23.

702. Al-Bayati O, Hasan A, Pruthi D, Kaushik D, Liss MA. Systematic review of modifiable risk factors for kidney cancer. Urol Oncol. 2019 Jun;37(6):359–71.

703. Shuch B, Vourganti S, Ricketts CJ, Middleton L, Peterson J, Merino MJ, et al. Defining Early-Onset Kidney Cancer: Implications for Germline and Somatic Mutation Testing and Clinical Management. J Clin Oncol. 2014 Feb 10;32(5):431–7.

704. Islami F, Stoklosa M, Drope J, Jemal A. Global and Regional Patterns of Tobacco Smoking and Tobacco Control Policies. Eur Urol Focus. 2015 Aug;1(1):3–16.

705. Burger M, Catto JWF, Dalbagni G, Grossman HB, Herr H, Karakiewicz P, et al. Epidemiology and risk factors of urothelial bladder cancer. Eur Urol. 2013 Feb;63(2):234–41.

706. Steinmaus C, Ferreccio C, Acevedo J, Yuan Y, Liaw J, Durán V, et al. Increased lung and bladder cancer incidence in adults after in utero and early-life arsenic exposure. Cancer Epidemiol Biomark Prev Publ Am Assoc Cancer Res Cosponsored Am Soc Prev Oncol. 2014 Aug;23(8):1529–38.

707. Tuccori M, Filion KB, Yin H, Yu OH, Platt RW, Azoulay L. Pioglitazone use and risk of bladder cancer: population based cohort study. BMJ. 2016 Mar 30;352:i1541.

708. Faurschou M, Mellemkjaer L, Voss A, Keller KK, Hansen IT, Baslund B. Prolonged risk of specific malignancies following cyclophosphamide therapy among patients with granulomatosis with polyangiitis. Rheumatol Oxf Engl. 2015 Aug;54(8):1345–50.

709. Vermeulen SH, Hanum N, Grotenhuis AJ, Castaño-Vinyals G, van der Heijden AG, Aben KK, et al. Recurrent urinary tract infection and risk of bladder cancer in the Nijmegen bladder cancer study. Br J Cancer. 2015 Feb 3;112(3):594–600.

710. Ho C-H, Sung K-C, Lim S-W, Liao C-H, Liang F-W, Wang J-J, et al. Chronic Indwelling Urinary Catheter Increase the Risk of Bladder Cancer, Even in Patients Without Spinal Cord Injury. Medicine (Baltimore). 2015 Oct 30;94(43):e1736.

711. Teleka S, Häggström C, Nagel G, Bjørge T, Manjer J, Ulmer H, et al. Risk of bladder cancer by disease severity in relation to metabolic factors and smoking: A prospective pooled cohort study of 800,000 men and women. Int J Cancer. 2018 Dec 15;143(12):3071–82.

712. Rouprêt M, Yates DR, Comperat E, Cussenot O. Upper urinary tract urothelial cell carcinomas and other urological malignancies involved in the hereditary nonpolyposis colorectal cancer (lynch syndrome) tumor spectrum. Eur Urol. 2008 Dec;54(6):1226–36.

713. Jelaković B, Karanović S, Vuković-Lela I, Miller F, Edwards KL, Nikolić J, et al. Aristolactam-DNA adducts are a biomarker of environmental exposure to aristolochic acid. Kidney Int. 2012 Mar;81(6):559–67.

714. Nortier JL, Martinez MC, Schmeiser HH, Arlt VM, Bieler CA, Petein M, et al. Urothelial carcinoma associated with the use of a Chinese herb (Aristolochia fangchi). N Engl J Med. 2000 Jun 8;342(23):1686–92.

715. Steffens J, Nagel R. Tumours of the renal pelvis and ureter. Observations in 170 patients. Br J Urol. 1988 Apr;61(4):277–83.

716. Kiciński M, Vangronsveld J, Nawrot TS. An epidemiological reappraisal of the familial aggregation of prostate cancer: a meta-analysis. PloS One. 2011;6(10):e27130.

717. Nyberg T, Frost D, Barrowdale D, Evans DG, Bancroft E, Adlard J, et al. Prostate Cancer Risks for Male BRCA1 and BRCA2 Mutation Carriers: A Prospective Cohort Study. Eur Urol. 2020 Jan;77(1):24–35.

718. Tang B, Han C-T, Gan H-L, Zhang G-M, Zhang C-Z, Yang W-Y, et al. Smoking increased the risk of prostate cancer with grade group ≥ 4 and intraductal carcinoma in a prospective biopsy cohort. The Prostate. 2017 Jun;77(9):984–9.

719. Perez-Cornago A, Appleby PN, Pischon T, Tsilidis KK, Tjønneland A, Olsen A, et al. Tall height and obesity are associated with an increased risk of aggressive prostate cancer: results from the EPIC cohort study. BMC Med. 2017 Jul 13;15(1):115.

720. Rao D, Yu H, Bai Y, Zheng X, Xie L. Does night-shift work increase the risk of prostate cancer? a systematic review and meta-analysis. OncoTargets Ther. 2015 Oct 5;8:2817–26.

721. Ju-Kun S, Yuan D-B, Rao H-F, Chen T-F, Luan B-S, Xu X-M, et al. Association Between Cd Exposure and Risk of Prostate Cancer: A PRISMA-Compliant Systematic Review and Meta-Analysis. Medicine (Baltimore). 2016 Feb;95(6):e2708.

722. Multigner L, Ndong JR, Giusti A, Romana M, Delacroix-Maillard H, Cordier S, et al. Chlordecone exposure and risk of prostate cancer. J Clin Oncol Off J Am Soc Clin Oncol. 2010 Jul 20;28(21):3457–62.

723. Risk factors for the onset of prostatic cancer: age, location, and behavioral correlates - PubMed [Internet]. [cited 2022

Jan 23]. Available from: https://pubmed.ncbi.nlm.nih.gov/22291478/

724. Stevenson SM, Lowrance WT. Epidemiology and Diagnosis of Testis Cancer. Urol Clin North Am. 2015 Aug;42(3):269–75.

725. Emmanuel A, Nettleton J, Watkin N, Berney DM. The molecular pathogenesis of penile carcinoma-current developments and understanding. Virchows Arch Int J Pathol. 2019 Oct;475(4):397–405.

726. Leto M das GP, Santos Júnior GFD, Porro AM, Tomimori J. Human papillomavirus infection: etiopathogenesis, molecular biology and clinical manifestations. An Bras Dermatol. 2011 Apr;86(2):306–17.

727. Spiess PE, Dhillon J, Baumgarten AS, Johnstone PA, Giuliano AR. Pathophysiological basis of human papillomavirus in penile cancer: Key to prevention and delivery of more effective therapies. CA Cancer J Clin. 2016 Nov 12;66(6):481–95.

728. Larke NL, Thomas SL, dos Santos Silva I, Weiss HA. Male circumcision and penile cancer: a systematic review and meta-analysis. Cancer Causes Control CCC. 2011 Aug;22(8):1097–110.

729. Clouston D, Hall A, Lawrentschuk N. Penile lichen sclerosus (balanitis xerotica obliterans). BJU Int. 2011 Nov;108 Suppl 2:14–9.

730. Barnes KT, McDowell BD, Button A, Smith BJ, Lynch CF, Gupta A. Obesity is associated with increased risk of invasive penile cancer. BMC Urol. 2016 Jul 13;16(1):42.

731. Harish K, Ravi R. The role of tobacco in penile carcinoma. Br J Urol. 1995 Mar;75(3):375–7.

732. Vieira CB, Feitoza L, Pinho J, Teixeira-Júnior A, Lages J, Calixto J, et al. Profile of patients with penile cancer in the region with the highest worldwide incidence. Sci Rep. 2020 Feb 19;10(1):2965.

733. Stern RS, Bagheri S, Nichols K, PUVA Follow Up Study. The persistent risk of genital tumors among men treated with psoralen plus ultraviolet A (PUVA) for psoriasis. J Am Acad Dermatol. 2002 Jul;47(1):33–9.

734. Definition of premalignant - NCI Dictionary of Cancer Terms - National Cancer Institute [Internet]. 2011 [cited 2021 Dec 31]. Available from: https://www.cancer.gov/publications/dictionaries/cancer-terms/def/premalignant

735. Khani F, Robinson BD. Precursor Lesions of Urologic Malignancies. Arch Pathol Amp Lab Med. 2017 Dec 1;141(12):1615–1615.

736. Schoots IG, Zaccai K, Hunink MG, Verhagen PCMS. Bosniak Classification for Complex Renal Cysts Reevaluated: A Systematic Review. J Urol. 2017 Jul;198(1):12–21.

737. H M, PA H, TM U, VE R. WHO Classification of Tumours of the Urinary System and Male Genital Organs [Internet]. [cited 2022 Jan 23]. Available from: https://publications.iarc.fr/Book-And-Report-Series/Who-Classification-Of-Tumours/WHO-Classification-Of-Tumours-Of-The-Urinary-System-And-Male-Genital-Organs-2016.

738. Hodges KB, Lopez-Beltran A, Davidson DD, Montironi R, Cheng L. Urothelial dysplasia and other flat lesions of the urinary bladder: clinicopathologic and molecular features. Hum Pathol. 2010 Feb;41(2):155–62.

739. Cheng L, Cheville JC, Neumann RM, Bostwick DG. Natural history of urothelial dysplasia of the bladder. Am J Surg Pathol. 1999 Apr;23(4):443–7.

740. Epstein JI, Herawi M. Prostate needle biopsies containing prostatic intraepithelial neoplasia or atypical foci suspicious for carcinoma: implications for patient care. J Urol. 2006 Mar;175(3 Pt 1):820–34.

741. *Borboroglu PG, Comer SW, Riffenburgh RH, Amling CL. Extensive repeat transrectal ultrasound guided prostate biopsy in patients with previous benign sextant biopsies. J Urol. 2000 Jan;163(1):158–62.*

742. *Tosoian JJ, Alam R, Ball MW, Carter HB, Epstein JI. Managing high-grade prostatic intraepithelial neoplasia (HGPIN) and atypical glands on prostate biopsy. Nat Rev Urol. 2018 Jan;15(1):55–66.*

743. *Porter WM, Francis N, Hawkins D, Dinneen M, Bunker CB. Penile intraepithelial neoplasia: clinical spectrum and treatment of 35 cases. Br J Dermatol. 2002 Dec;147(6):1159–65.*

744. *Bleeker MCG, Heideman D a. M, Snijders PJF, Horenblas S, Dillner J, Meijer CJLM. Penile cancer: epidemiology, pathogenesis and prevention. World J Urol. 2009 Apr;27(2):141–50.*

745. *Buechner SA. Common skin disorders of the penis. BJU Int. 2002 Sep;90(5):498–506.*

746. *Kim B, Garcia F, Touma N, Moussa M, Izawa JI. A rare case of penile cancer in situ metastasizing to lymph nodes. Can Urol Assoc J. 2007 Nov;1(4):404–7.*

747. *Diet, nutrition, physical activity and kidney cancer. 2015;46.*

748. *Behrens G, Leitzmann MF. The association between physical activity and renal cancer: systematic review and meta-analysis. Br J Cancer. 2013 Mar 5;108(4):798–811.*

749. *Shivappa N, Steck SE, Hurley TG, Hussey JR, Hébert JR. Designing and developing a literature-derived, population-based dietary inflammatory index. Public Health Nutr. 2014 Aug;17(8):1689–96.*

750. *Dietary Inflammatory Index and Renal Cell Carcinoma Risk in an Italian Case–Control Study: Nutrition and Cancer: Vol 69, No 6 [Internet]. [cited 2022 Jan 26]. Available from: https://www.tandfonline.com/doi/full/10.1080/01635581.2017.1339815*

751. *Does beer, wine or liquor consumption correlate with the risk of renal cell carcinoma? A dose-response meta-analysis of prospective cohort studies - PubMed [Internet]. [cited 2022 Jan 26]. Available from: https://pubmed.ncbi.nlm.nih.gov/25965820/*

752. *Antwi SO, Eckel-Passow JE, Diehl ND, Serie DJ, Custer KM, Arnold ML, et al. Coffee consumption and risk of renal cell carcinoma. Cancer Causes Control CCC. 2017 Aug;28(8):857–66.*

753. *Zhang S, Jia Z, Yan Z, Yang J. Consumption of fruits and vegetables and risk of renal cell carcinoma: a meta-analysis of observational studies. Oncotarget. 2017 Apr 25;8(17):27892–903.*

754. *Usher-Smith J, Simmons RK, Rossi SH, Stewart GD. Current evidence on screening for renal cancer. Nat Rev Urol. 2020 Nov;17(11):637–42.*

755. *Farivar-Mohseni H, Perlmutter AE, Wilson S, Shingleton WB, Bigler SA, Fowler JE. Renal cell carcinoma and end stage renal disease. J Urol. 2006 Jun;175(6):2018–20; discussion 2021.*

756. *Hurst FP, Jindal RM, Graham LJ, Falta EM, Elster EA, Stackhouse GB, et al. Incidence, predictors, costs, and outcome of renal cell carcinoma after kidney transplantation: USRDS experience. Transplantation. 2010 Oct 27;90(8):898–904.*

757. *Beisland C, Guðbrandsdottir G, Reisæter LAR, Bostad L, Hjelle KM. A prospective risk-stratified follow-up programme for radically treated renal cell carcinoma patients: evaluation after eight years of clinical use. World J Urol. 2016 Aug;34(8):1087–99.*

758. Stewart-Merrill SB, Thompson RH, Boorjian SA, Psutka SP, Lohse CM, Cheville JC, et al. Oncologic Surveillance After Surgical Resection for Renal Cell Carcinoma: A Novel Risk-Based Approach. J Clin Oncol Off J Am Soc Clin Oncol. 2015 Dec 10;33(35):4151–7.

759. Massari F, Di Nunno V, Mollica V, Graham J, Gatto L, Heng D. Adjuvant Tyrosine Kinase Inhibitors in Treatment of Renal Cell Carcinoma: A Meta-Analysis of Available Clinical Trials. Clin Genitourin Cancer. 2019 Apr;17(2):e339–44.

760. Li Y, Tindle HA, Hendryx MS, Xun P, He K, Liang X, et al. Smoking Cessation and the Risk of Bladder Cancer among Post-menopausal Women. Cancer Prev Res Phila Pa. 2019 May;12(5):305–14.

761. Al-Zalabani AH, Stewart KFJ, Wesselius A, Schols AMWJ, Zeegers MP. Modifiable risk factors for the prevention of bladder cancer: a systematic review of meta-analyses. Eur J Epidemiol. 2016;31(9):811–51.

762. Khochikar MV. Rationale for an early detection program for bladder cancer. Indian J Urol IJU J Urol Soc India. 2011;27(2):218–25.

763. Pradere B, Lotan Y, Roupret M. Lynch syndrome in upper tract urothelial carcinoma: significance, screening, and surveillance. Curr Opin Urol. 2017 Jan;27(1):48–55.

764. Lippman SM, Klein EA, Goodman PJ, Lucia MS, Thompson IM, Ford LG, et al. Effect of selenium and vitamin E on risk of prostate cancer and other cancers: the Selenium and Vitamin E Cancer Prevention Trial (SELECT). JAMA. 2009 Jan 7;301(1):39–51.

765. Thompson IM, Goodman PJ, Tangen CM, Lucia MS, Miller GJ, Ford LG, et al. The influence of finasteride on the development of prostate cancer. N Engl J Med. 2003 Jul 17;349(3):215–24.

766. Effect of Dutasteride on the Risk of Prostate Cancer | NEJM [Internet]. [cited 2022 Jan 28]. Available from: https://www.nejm.org/doi/full/10.1056/nejmoa0908127

767. Theoret MR, Ning Y-M, Zhang JJ, Justice R, Keegan P, Pazdur R. The risks and benefits of 5α-reductase inhibitors for prostate-cancer prevention. N Engl J Med. 2011 Jul 14;365(2):97–9.

768. Andriole GL, Crawford ED, Grubb RL, Buys SS, Chia D, Church TR, et al. Prostate cancer screening in the randomized Prostate, Lung, Colorectal, and Ovarian Cancer Screening Trial: mortality results after 13 years of follow-up. J Natl Cancer Inst. 2012 Jan 18;104(2):125–32.

769. Schröder FH, Hugosson J, Roobol MJ, Tammela TLJ, Zappa M, Nelen V, et al. Screening and prostate cancer mortality: results of the European Randomised Study of Screening for Prostate Cancer (ERSPC) at 13 years of follow-up. Lancet Lond Engl. 2014 Dec 6;384(9959):2027–35.

770. Moyer VA, U.S. Preventive Services Task Force. Screening for prostate cancer: U.S. Preventive Services Task Force recommendation statement. Ann Intern Med. 2012 Jul 17;157(2):120–34.

771. de Koning HJ, Gulati R, Moss SM, Hugosson J, Pinsky PF, Berg CD, et al. The efficacy of prostate-specific antigen screening: Impact of key components in the ERSPC and PLCO trials. Cancer. 2018 Mar 15;124(6):1197–206.

772. Eeles R, Goh C, Castro E, Bancroft E, Guy M, Al Olama AA, et al. The genetic epidemiology of prostate cancer and its clinical implications. Nat Rev Urol. 2014 Jan;11(1):18–31.

773. Wood HM, Elder JS. Cryptorchidism and testicular cancer: separating fact from fiction. J Urol. 2009 Feb;181(2):452–61.

774. Thornton CP. Best Practice in Teaching Male Adolescents and Young Men to Perform Testicular Self-Examinations: A Review. J Pediatr Health Care Off Publ Natl Assoc Pediatr Nurse Assoc Pract. 2016. Dec;30(6):518–27.

775. Ilic D, Misso ML. Screening for testicular cancer. Cochrane Database Syst Rev. 2011 Feb 16;(2):CD007853.

776. Balawender K, Orkisz S, Wisz P. Testicular microlithiasis: what urologists should know. A review of the current literature. Cent Eur J Urol. 2018;71(3):310–4.

777. Thomas A, Necchi A, Muneer A, Tobias-Machado M, Tran ATH, Van Rompuy A-S, et al. Penile cancer. Nat Rev Dis Primer. 2021 Feb 11;7(1):1–24.

778. Obara W, Kanehira M, Katagiri T, Kato R, Kato Y, Takata R. Present status and future perspective of peptide-based vaccine therapy for urological cancer. Cancer Sci. 2018 Mar;109(3):550–9.

ABOUT THE EDITORIAL TEAM

Dr. Nanda Rajaneesh

Dr. Nanda Rajaneesh is a GI Laparoscopic, breast, bariatric surgeon, and surgical oncologist with over 20 years of experience. She is the Founder and Chairman of the Society for Prevention of Cancer (SPOC). This non-profit organization works to raise awareness about cancer and promote early detection and prevention. She holds a Fellowship in GI and Minimally Invasive Surgery. Dr. Nanda Rajaneesh is a leading expert in breast cancer surgery. She is also a passionate advocate for breast cancer awareness and prevention. She was the founding member of the team at Nova that pioneered the concept of short-stay surgeries. She has given numerous lectures and talks on the subject and has published several papers on breast cancer. She is the author of two books, "Life with Fibromyalgia" (which is based on her own story) and "Risk factors in breast cancer." She recently completed a surgical leadership program at Harvard.

Dr. M Vijayakumar

Dr. M Vijaykumar is a senior surgical oncologist with over 40 years of experience. He is Professor of Surgical Oncology in Zulekha Yenepoya Institute of Oncology (Yenepoya Medical College Hospital) and the Vice Chancellor of Yenepoya (Deemed to be University), Mangalore, India. He is the former director of the KIDWAI Cancer Institute. He is a Fellow of the Royal College of Physicians & Surgeons, Glasgow, the International College of Surgeons, and the American College of Surgeons. He has published over 60 papers in peer-reviewed journals and contributed to numerous chapters and textbooks. Recently, he co-edited "Yenepoya Student Series Vol -I, Oral Cancer." He is an accomplished teacher and surgeon. His areas of interest include cancer surgery, cancer prevention, and cancer awareness.

Dr. Rohan Thomas Mathew

Dr. Rohan Thomas Mathew is an Oral and Maxillofacial Surgeon with over seven years of experience in head and neck oncology. He has extensive experience in diagnosing, treating, and rehabilitating patients with oral cancer and salivary gland tumors. Dr. Rohan is a passionate advocate for early cancer detection and prevention. He is also a co-editor of the book "Yenepoya Student Series Vol -I, Oral Cancer." He is presently working in Zulekha Yenepoya Institute of Oncology (Yenepoya Medical College Hospital), Mangalore.

Dr. Rohan is the Co-founder and Director of Emys Bionics Pvt. Ltd., a healthcare start-up that develops affordable patient-specific implants and post-treatment rehabilitation for cancer patients.

Made in the USA
Columbia, SC
20 March 2025

55429591R00255